T0220359

Case Reports in Cardiology

From the earliest days of medicine to the present, case reports have been a critical aspect of clinical education and knowledge development. In this comprehensive volume, Dr. William C. Roberts, a renowned expert in the field, explores the rich history and ongoing importance of case reports in cardiology.

Through engaging and insightful analysis, the book demonstrates how case reports have provided physicians with crucial insights into rare diseases, complex conditions, and ground-breaking treatments. Drawing on a vast range of sources, from seminal manuscripts to cutting-edge journals, it offers a unique perspective on the role of case reports in medical education and practice of congenital heart diseases and associated cardiac complications. It underscores how case reports can be used to enhance diagnostic accuracy, identify new treatment options, and promote innovation in the field. In addition, the book provides valuable insights into the process of writing and publishing case reports, including tips for young physicians looking to break into the field.

The book will be an indispensable guide to the history, practice, and ongoing significance of case reports for medical students, physicians, and researchers alike.

KEY FEATURES

- Provides a rich repository of diverse case reports in cardiology published by the editor and his colleagues over 61 years

- Features 52 clinical case studies related to Congenital Heart Disease, useful for medical students and practicing cardiologists

- It is a valuable resource for young physicians seeking to establish a foothold in medical research and academics

Case Reports in Cardiology Series

Series Editor

William C. Roberts, MD

Baylor Heart and Vascular Institute, Baylor University Medical Center, Dallas

Case Reports in Cardiology: Congenital Heart Disease
Edited by Dr. William C. Roberts, MD

Case Reports in Cardiology: Valvular Heart Disease
Edited by Dr. William C. Roberts, MD

Case Reports in Cardiology: Coronary Heart Disease and Hyperlipidemia
Edited by Dr. William C. Roberts, MD

Case Reports in Cardiology: Cardiomyopathy
Edited by Dr. William C. Roberts, MD

Case Reports in Cardiology: Cardiac Neoplasm
Edited by Dr. William C. Roberts, MD

Case Reports in Cardiology: Cardiovascular Diseases with a Focus on Aorta
Edited by Dr. William C. Roberts, MD

For more information on this series, please visit https://www.routledge.com/Case-Reports-in-Cardiology/book-series/CRIC

Case Reports in Cardiology
Congenital Heart Disease

Edited by
William C. Roberts, MD

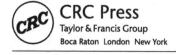

CRC Press
Taylor & Francis Group
Boca Raton London New York

CRC Press is an imprint of the
Taylor & Francis Group, an **informa** business

Designed cover image: Shutterstock

First edition published 2024
by CRC Press
2385 NW Executive Center Drive, Suite 320, Boca Raton FL 33431

and by CRC Press
4 Park Square, Milton Park, Abingdon, Oxon, OX14 4RN

CRC Press is an imprint of Taylor & Francis Group, LLC

ISBN: 978-1-032-52946-2 (hbk)
ISBN: 978-1-032-52945-5 (pbk)
ISBN: 978-1-003-40934-2 (ebk)

DOI: 10.1201/9781003409342

Typeset in Palatino LT Std
by Apex CoVantage, LLC

William Clifford Roberts, MD [1932–2023]
A Remembrance

As a cardiac surgical associate at the NIH in Bethesda for 2 years, I attended my father's Monday conference regularly. There was a case of a healed traumatic aortic rupture. The fellow discovered that the patient was in a motor vehicle accident "several years before death." To this fellow, WCR said, "Write this case up and have it on my desk by Friday." He added, "It takes about as long to write a brief report as it does to write up the chart. Know the case precisely before going to the library to search the literature." He told the fellow to put the aorta in his pocket to remind him what it looked like. "This is a single task, a single mission." What to search for in the library? "Are there any cases of healed traumatic aneurysm of the descending thoracic aorta." In 30 years, WCR had seen only 1 other, who died 7 days later, not 7 years. This was 1989, of course, before the ubiquitous use of CT scans.

The material for his case reports was this weekly conference in cardiovascular pathology over 6 decades. During these conferences, WCR would personally examine each surgical and autopsy cardiovascular specimen that was submitted—a heart or valve or aorta—and a chart would be created for each patient. He would typically examine each specimen as "an unknown." To him it was a provocative way to conduct the conference. He urged his students and residents and fellows to "remember one thing about each case." To him that was >600 "new things" a year. He believed that studying the case at hand was better than general reading.

In a personal review of his own publications, William Clifford Roberts, MD (WCR) listed 269 case reports out of a total of 1784 publications over a 60-year period, 1961–2022. This sheer number of case reports by one physician in cardiovascular disease is perhaps a record in the field.

As an editor in chief of 2 medical journals, he carefully considered the value of case reports:

> Usually, case reports have only 1 point, and information not pertinent to that point is unnecessary. Indeed, unnecessary words and nonessential details actually prevent clear focus on the patient. Thus, these "Brief Reports" must be brief—no more than 2 or 3 double-spaced typed pages with few references. Reports only 1 page long will be favored over those 3 pages long. Pertinent illustrations may be the dominant element in conveying the message . . . Brief Reports require clear thinking. Each word must count.

In nearly every case report of WCR, there is an illustration or photograph. WCR preferred "drawings not words." He would say, "There is nothing more important than absolutely perfect photographs." In his first 20 years at NIH, he spent every Tuesday and Thursday morning from 9am to noon with a photographer. He believed the subject should occupy "85% of the frame."

WCR graduated from Southern Methodist University (1954) and Emory University School of Medicine (1958), then had 6 years of residency training. For the next 60 years (1964–2023), he focused exclusively on cardiovascular pathology. The first 30 years were spent at NIH in Bethesda and the second 30 years at Baylor University Medical Center in Dallas. He held his weekly conference past 90 years of age.

My younger brother, John David Roberts, observed that WCR was "an intense scholar, but also a loving person. He had both qualities. He was loved for the person, not the accomplishments. One would never know he was a physician in daily interactions. He was satisfied to be unknown. Though in the Public Health Service for 30 years, he never wore the Navy uniform, even when it was recommended at NIH. As a father he required respect, which included "Yes Sir" and "No Sir." Manners were important to him, especially at the table for the evening meal, where each of his children was asked to express what he or she learned that day."

He will be remembered by his family not only for his contribution to the field of medicine, but for his hungry intellect, his indominable work ethic, his high standards, and his loyalty to loved ones.

Charles Stewart Roberts, MD
October 1, 2023

Contents

*Note: Cases are numbered based on their number in WCR's CV.

CONTENTS

Preface

When these case reports (numbering 272) were sent to the publisher my intention was that all would be published in one or two volumes. The publisher, however, convinced me that the collection of case reports would be too large if they were all published together, and that decision resulted into dividing the collection into six smaller books arranged by subject. I find case reports useful and often they are the first publication of many authors. William Osler published many case reports in the later decades of the 19th century. Today, the JACC has a journal devoted solely to case reports. The doctor-patient relationship is one on one. Most journals today publish case reports, but their name is usually disguised as something else.

William C. Roberts, MD

About the Editor

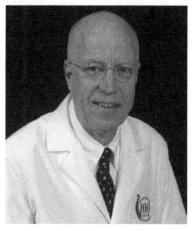 **William C. Roberts, MD,** was born in Atlanta, Georgia, on September 11, 1932. He graduated from Southern Methodist University (1954) and Emory University School of Medicine (1958). He did his training in internal medicine at the Boston City Hospital and at The Johns Hopkins Hospital. He had a 1-year fellowship in cardiology at the National Heart, Lung and Blood Institute. He did his training in anatomic pathology at the National Institutes of Health (1959–1962). From July 1964 to March 1993, he was Chief of Pathology at the National Heart, Lung, and Blood Institute, National Institutes of Health, Bethesda, Maryland. He has written 1784 articles. Additionally, he has edited 31 books and lectured in more than 2200 cities around the world.

From December 1992 through December 2018, Dr. Roberts was program director of the Williamsburg Conference on Heart Disease held every December in Williamsburg, Virginia. The American College of Cardiology Foundation sponsored this conference for 30 years. Since March 1993, Dr. Roberts had been the executive director of the Baylor Heart and Vascular Institute at Baylor University Medical Center in Dallas, Texas. He served as the editor in chief of the *Baylor University Medical Center Proceedings* from 1994 to 2022 (29 years) and the editor in chief of *The American Journal of Cardiology* from June 1982 until July 2022 (40 years).

He received many honors, including the 1978 Gifted Teacher Award from The American College of Cardiology; the 1983 College Medalist Award of the American College of Chest Physicians; the Public Health Service Commendation Medal in 1979; the 1984 Richard and Hilda Rosenthal Foundation Award from the Council of Cardiology of the American Heart Association; an honorary Doctor of Science degree from Far Eastern University, Manila, Philippines in 1995; the designation of *Master* from The American College of Cardiology in 2004; the Lifetime Achievement Award of The American College of Cardiology in 2016; and the Lifetime Achievement Award for D's CEO's Excellence in Healthcare Awards in 2021.

Sadly, Dr. William C. Roberts passed away in June 2023 at the age of 90, just as this book series went into production.

Introduction

Case reports have had a long history. Many diseases have been reported initially as a case report. The first publication of many authors, including the present author, was a case report. William Osler's curriculum vitae (CV) is loaded with individual case studies on a variety of conditions. Paul Dudley White's CV, particularly his early publications, is loaded with individual case reports. Indeed, he indicated that he tried to write a case report on a variety of cardiovascular conditions to familiarize himself quickly with them.

The physician-patient relationship is a one-on-one encounter. Although randomized clinical trials are favored today, often it is difficult to fit a single patient into these types of studies due to the heterogeneous nature of the populations. Some patients or circumstances cannot be described except in the case-report format. An example might be case #342 included in volume 6, which described a man who was shot; the bullet coursed through the right atrium and then through the right ventricular outflow tract, preventing flow to the left side of the heart. Autopsy disclosed the left atrial appendage to have protruded through the mitral orifice, suggesting that the left ventricle had a negative pressure during ventricular diastole, something confirmed physiologically in a subsequent publication. We recently received a manuscript describing a young boy who was thrown from his vehicle and landed on a rattlesnake who bit him on his leg that was the site of a compound fracture suffered during the accident. The case-report format is the only mechanism to report such events.

Many disease entities have been described initially as case reports: Ochronosis by Rudolph Virchow (1821–1920), sickle-cell anemia by James B. Herrick (1861–1954), and the Pickwickian syndrome (obesity-hyperventilation syndrome) by Charles Sydney Burwell (1893–1967) are just a few examples. Multiple first operations were described initially in the case report format, as well as the first effective anesthetic drug.

Another benefit of case reports is that they provide the opportunity for young physicians to break into the medical publishing arena. They can be used to describe a new facet of a disease or provide a fuller description of an entity described previously. New journals often begin by publishing case reports. (See the early issues of the *Mayo Clinic Proceedings* or the *Cleveland Clinic Medical Quarterly* or the *Baylor University Medical Center Proceedings*.)

Some authors, editors, and readers minimize the usefulness of case reports to medical education. We recently received a case report from an important and established investigator who indicated that he was really not in favor of publishing case reports but that his was "special" and deserved rapid acceptance and publication. This type of comment is fairly frequent.

In more modern times, several collections of case reports have been published. *The New England Journal of Medicine* calls them "Images in Clinical Medicine" or "Case Records of the Massachusetts General Hospital"; *The Lancet* calls them "Clinical Picture"; *Circulation* calls them "Cardiovascular Images" or "Cases and Traces" or "ECG Challenge"; *JAMA Cardiology* calls them "JAMA Cardiology Clinical Challenge"; and *The American Journal of Medicine* calls them "Diagnostic Dilemma" or "Images in Dermatology" or "Images in Radiology" or "ECG Image of the Month," to name a few examples. *The Journal of the American College of Cardiology* has an entire journal devoted to case reports (*JACC Case Reports*).

The present collection of case reports, of course, is not the first. An early collection of case studies was by Ambroise Pare called *Oeuvres* in 1628 (in French) and compiled and edited by Wallace B. Hamby and titled *The Case Reports and Autopsy Records of Ambroise Pare* (in English) in 1960. These short descriptions of patients are fascinating and enjoyable reading. Richard C. Cabot, who started the clinicopathologic conferences at the Massachusetts General Hospital, published *Case Teaching in Medicine—A Series of Graduated Exercises in the Differential Diagnosis, Prognosis and Treatment of Actual Cases of Disease* in 1906. Cabot described 78 patients, most of whom went to autopsy and some to surgery. The collection included patients with a variety of conditions. Cabot's 1906 book led to "The Case History Series": *Case Histories in Pediatrics* by John Lovett Morse; *Surgical Problems* by James G. Mumford in 1911 (100 cases); and *Case Histories in Neurology* by E. W. Taylor in 1911.

In more modern times, several collections of case reports have been published. The most popular are under the general heading of *Clinicopathologic Conferences of The Massachusetts General Hospital:* the collection of cases, published individual books, are variously titled *Selected Medical Cases; Surgical; Bone and Joint; Neurologic;* and *Cardiac.* The latter by Benjamin Castleman and Roman W. De Sanctis presents 50 cases of various cardiovascular diseases studied both clinically and at necropsy. (The gross photos of the hearts cannot be recommended.)

Finally, case reports are fun reading (particularly Ambroise Pare's *Selections*). They are a "break" from the data-heavy multicenter placebo-controlled trials and metaanalyses.

When these 272 case reports were sent to the publisher, my intention was that all would be published in one or two volumes. The publisher, however, convinced me that the collection of case reports would be too large if they were all published together, and that decision resulted into dividing the collection into six smaller books arranged by subject:

1. Congenital Heart Disease
2. Valvular Heart Disease
3. Coronary Heart Disease and Hyperlipidemia
4. Cardiomyopathy
5. Cardiac Neoplasm
6. Cardiovascular Diseases with a Focus on Aorta

The case reports were written by me and colleagues over a 61-year period (1961 to 2022). All 272 describe a single patient with a cardiovascular disease, nearly all of whom were studied both clinically and morphologically, i.e., at autopsy or after cardiac transplantation or after another cardiovascular operation. Thus, the collection is unique. Each report is numbered as it appears in my CV, which includes as of August 15, 2022, a total of 1784 publications (Table 1). Some were book chapters, published interviews of prominent physicians, or published symposia in which I participated, but most (952) were patient-centered studies.

William C. Roberts, MD
May 5, 2022

Disclaimer:

All case reports are reprinted exactly as first published.

Table 1: Number and types of articles published by William C. Roberts, MD, 1961–2022

Article type		N
1. Patient-centered studies		952
a. Single patient	269	
b. Multipatient	666	
c. Nonpatient	17	
2. From-the-editor columns		342
a. AJC (1982–2022)	234	
b. BUMC (1994–2021)	108	
3. Other editorials, mini reviews, forewords, historical pieces (all journals)		67
4. Chapters in books		143
5. Interviews		197
a. AJC	77	
b. BUMC	96	
c. Visiting professors	24	
6. Published symposia ("AJC editor's roundtable")		43
7. AJC in month (25 years earlier) (May 1983–August 1988)		40
Total		**1784**

AJC indicates American Journal of Cardiology;
BUMC, Baylor University Medical Center Proceedings.
Note: Additional publications were added after this table was compiled, including additional case studies, with a new total of 272.

Case 1 Differential Diagnosis of Mitral Regurgitation in Childhood

Clinical Pathological Conference at the National Institutes of Health*

Moderator: Eugene Braunwald, MD, Discussants: Richard S. Ross, MD, F.A.C.P.
Baltimore, Maryland

Andrew G. Morrow, MD, and William C. Roberts, MD
Bethesda, Maryland

DR. EUGENE BRAUNWALD: The patient whose records form the basis of this conference taught a good deal to those of us who were involved in his care, and for this reason his case was selected for this presentation.

He was a 13-year-old colored male who was the product of a normal full term pregnancy and delivery and who weighed over six pounds at birth. His growth and development were retarded, walking occurring at 18 months and talking after the age of two years. His mother felt that he had always been small and sickly compared with his siblings.

He was not examined by a physician until the age of six years when he was hospitalized because of fever and tachypnea. Physical examination revealed a pulse of 108, and blood pressure of 120/75 mm. Hg. The lungs were clear. A grade IV, high pitched, systolic murmur was heard at the apex; there was a protodiastolic sound at the apex and a questionable presystolic murmur at the apex. Chest x-rays revealed cardiomegaly with a cardiothoracic ratio of 0.61. The left ventricle was considered to be greatly enlarged and there was slight fullness in the area of the pulmonary conus. The electrocardiogram was said to show prolongation of the PR interval when age and rate were considered. Acute rheumatic fever was diagnosed and, following discharge from the hospital, the patient was placed on oral penicillin. Examination eight months later showed a regular rhythm, a systolic thrill and loud systolic murmur at the apex, and a questionable presystolic murmur at the apex. The electrocardiogram showed a PR interval of 0.19 sec. and a heart rate of 110/min.

He convalesced slowly but was not able to resume normal activity. He was hospitalized near his home four times because of fever, with abdominal pain on one occasion, and symptoms of left and right sided heart failure on three occasions. His C-reactive protein and antistreptolysin titer were always unremarkable. Cardiac examination always revealed systolic and diastolic murmurs, and during the latter two hospitalizations he was in atrial fibrillation which converted to sinus rhythm upon administration of quinidine. The electrocardiograms showed left atrial and ventricular enlargement with a first degree heart block.

* Received for publication March 17, 1961.

This is an edited transcription of a clinical pathological conference at the Clinical Center, Bethesda, Md., by the National Heart Institute, National Institutes of Health, Public Health Service, Department of Health, Education, and Welfare.

Requests for reprints should be addressed to Eugene Braunwald, M.D., Chief, Cardiology Branch, National Heart Institute, Bethesda, Md.

DOI: 10.1201/9781003409342-1

He was referred to the National Heart Institute because of persistent dyspnea and orthopnea. On physical examination the patient was a small, poorly developed, undernourished boy who appeared to be chronically ill. Blood pressure was 110/87 mm. Hg and the pulse rate was 100/min. and grossly irregular. The neck veins were dilated and pulsated vigorously when he was in the sitting position. There was a prominent precordial bulge, a striking left ventricular lift, and a modest right ventricular lift. The second heart sound was palpable along the left sternal border. On auscultation this sound was split with a loud pulmonic component. The phonocardiogram showed that P_2 remained split even after the Valsalva maneuver. A grade 3/6 pansystolic murmur was best heard at the apex but was well transmitted to the axilla and over the entire precordium. A grade 3/6 mid-diastolic, rumbling murmur and an early diastolic sound were heard at the apex. The liver edge was palpable five fingerbreadths below the costal margin. The complete blood count, sedimentation rate, serology, urinalysis, CRP, ASO, blood electrolytes, and "liver chemistries" were unremarkable. The electrocardiogram is reproduced in Figure 1 and the chest roentgenograms in Figures 2 and 3.

Our discussant today is Dr. Richard S. Ross, Associate Professor of Medicine and Radiology at the Johns Hopkins University School of Medicine. Dr. Ross had only the above protocol on hand for the preparation of his initial discussion.

DR. RICHARD S. ROSS: The electrocardiogram shows left axis deviation and atrial fibrillation. There is no R wave in Lead V_1. Deep S waves are present over the right precordium. The R wave is 24 mm. in Lead V_6, and small Q waves are present over the left precordium. The sagging of the ST segments and inversion of T waves in Lead V_6 are characteristic of left ventricular hypertrophy or, in older terminology, "left ventricular strain." On the roentgenograms the heart is huge and there appears to be enlargement of all chambers. There is fullness in the region of the pulmonary artery and there is a double density which I believe represents the left atrium. I think the little prominence on the right border of the heart is also part of a giant left atrium. In the lateral and right oblique views, there is posterior deviation of the esophagus, which makes me feel that this individual had a greatly enlarged left atrium. In the right oblique projection, the left atrium bulges out behind the esophagus. The left oblique film shows the left ventricle to be enlarged and it is seen to project posteriorly well beyond the spine. In summary, the x-rays show enlargement

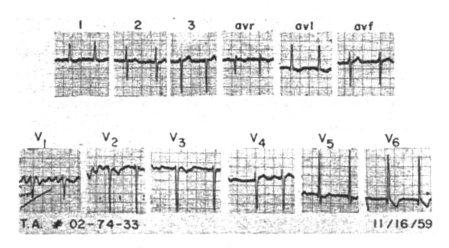

Figure 1 Electrocardiogram of patient T. A.

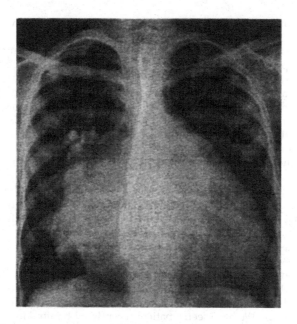

Figure 2 Chest roentgenogram of patient T.A.

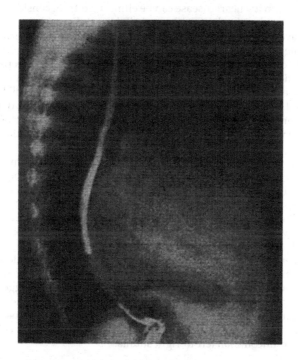

Figure 3 Lateral roentgenogram of patient T. A.

of the left atrium and left ventricle and slight fullness of the right ventricular out-flow tract.

There was an excellent history of retarded growth and development which can be used to support the contention that the disease was congenital. The febrile illness may or may not be significant, but it could have been either rheumatic fever or bacterial endocarditis. The most prominent physical sign was a loud apical pansystolic murmur which was noted by several observers. It was heard maximally at the apex, but also at other places on the precordium. Throughout the history there was evidence of both right and left ventricular failure. The patient was dyspneic and tachypneic, but he also had a large liver and distended neck veins.

Occasionally, the heart may be enlarged, or may function abnormally from extracardiac causes, and this possibility must always be considered first. In this case we can say, from the size of the heart and other findings, that this individual had primary heart disease. The intensity of the murmur and the coexisting thrill makes me feel certain that this patient had either valvular disease, a septal defect, or obstruction to the outflow tract in one or the other of the cardiac chambers. A murmur of this intensity, associated with a thrill, is not heard in the absence of one of these recognized causes of turbulence within the heart.

We next come to the question of whether this be congenital or acquired heart disease. The early appearance of the murmur and the retarded growth and development indicate that it was congenital heart disease. It is possible to have rheumatic fever at an early age. We have seen a patient recently with mitral insufficiency who had unequivocal chronic rheumatic valvular disease at the age of six years, but this is not the usual situation. There were no associated manifestations of rheumatic fever in the case under discussion today and the laboratory studies for detecting active rheumatic fever were negative. In difficult clinical situations such as this, the C-reactive protein and antistreptolysin titer are most useful when they are negative. At this point, rheumatic heart disease can be eliminated from consideration, and the patient can be considered to have had congenital heart disease.

We then have to reconsider the two general categories of diseases in which murmurs of this intensity are heard—septal defects and valvular diseases. On the x-rays the lung fields did not appear to be abnormally vascular. The electrocardiogram showed no evidence of right ventricular hypertrophy or right axis deviation, and I was unable to explain the giant atrium on the basis of any of the well known septal abnormalities. I considered ventricular septal defect, atrial septal defect, a shunt from the left ventricle to the right atrium, and a patent ductus arteriosus. I did not give specific consideration to right-to-left shunts because no mention was made of cyanosis.

The ostium primum defects and the varieties of persistent common atrioventricular canal receive special attention because these defects are frequently associated with mitral valve abnormalities. The electrocardiogram in the ostium primum defects always shows some evidence of right ventricular hypertrophy, and this was lacking in today's patient. Furthermore, the left atrium is never enlarged to this degree. These two facts allowed me to eliminate ostium primum defects from this initial discussion.

The left ventriculo-right atrial communications were considered with Dr. Braunwald's article as the reference.[1] The electrocardiogram in his patients showed right ventricular hypertrophy, combined hypertrophy, or ". . . a suggestion of left." Thus, left axis deviation and left ventricular hypertrophy were inconsistent with ventriculo-atrial shunt. Left atrial enlargement would not be expected in these patients and it was not present in the reported patients. At this point I eliminated all the common and uncommon left-to-right shunts.

The category of valvular and obstructive lesions must be considered next. Because of the massive dilatation of the left atrium and the left ventricle, attention was directed to the left side of the heart. Valvular aortic stenosis seemed an unlikely cause of this murmur. Subvalvular aortic stenosis could produce a murmur in this location. We have seen a few cases of a subvalvular obstruction in which the murmur was maximal at the apex or near the apex; in one case, there was a thrill at the apex in association with the murmur.

In favor of the diagnosis of subvalvular aortic stenosis, we might list the signs of left ventricular hypertrophy on the electrocardiogram and the large left ventricle on the x-ray. The left atrium may be enlarged in aortic stenosis but I have never seen a left atrium attain the size which our patient's did in the presence of aortic stenosis alone. Therefore, against the diagnosis of aortic stenosis would be this tremendous enlargement of the left atrium and the description of the murmur as pansystolic. This is unusual even for the murmurs in subaortic stenosis which are usually confined to the early part of systole. Obstruction to left ventricular outflow did not offer an adequate explanation for all the important findings and therefore was excluded.

Mitral insufficiency, the other cause of murmurs of this type, offered the best explanation for the enlarged left atrium. The left atrium may reach this size in mitral stenosis, but the more common cause of giant atrium is mitral insufficiency. The signs of left ventricular hypertrophy on physical examination, the enlarged left ventricle on x-ray, and the electrocardiographic findings were perfectly compatible with this diagnosis. The murmur was much more compatible with mitral insufficiency than it was with aortic stenosis.

I had some reservations about the electrocardiogram because, though left axis deviation and left ventricular hypertrophy occur in mitral insufficiency, the axis is usually not much to the left of 0°. Furthermore, this particular type of ST segment is uncommon in mitral insufficiency. There were minor objections and I concluded that congenital mitral insufficiency was the best diagnosis.

This led to a consideration of the various anatomic lesions which result in mitral regurgitation (Table 1).

The literature contains descriptions of valves with fused, fixed cusps, valves with a cleft leaflet in association with the ostium primum defect and without this lesion, perforated valve leaflets, valves with a double orifice, and cusps with anomalous insertion of the chordae tendineae in such a way as to hold the valve open. This latter lesion may be associated with corrected transposition of the great vessels. Corrected transposition of the great vessels is associated with another interesting mitral valve lesion, referred to as Ebstein's malformation of the left AV valve, in which the left AV valve, which looks like the normal tricuspid valve, is displaced

Table 1: Congenital mitral insufficiency

1. Fused fixed valve.
2. Cleft mitral leaflet.
3. Perforated mitral leaflet.
4. Double orifice of the mitral valve.
5. Anomalous insertion of chordae tendineae.
6. Corrected transposition of great vessels.
   a. Anomalous insertion of chordae tendineae.
   b. Ebstein's malformation, left.
7. Fibroelastosis of left ventricle.

downward into the left ventricle and may be incompetent. Finally, fibroelastosis of the left ventricle may cause mitral regurgitation by sticking the leaflets to the wall of the ventricle and holding the valve open.

Without much difficulty, we can dispose of diagnoses 6 and 7 in Table 1. The mitral lesions associated with the corrected transpositions can be excluded by the electrocardiogram which, in our patient, has definite Q waves in Leads V_5 and V_6. This electrocardiographic pattern is almost never seen with corrected transposition.[2] There were several other points against corrected transpositions. First, when mitral insufficiency occurs in this malformation, it is usually not this severe and clinically dominant, and it is not associated with a giant left atrium. Second, there was no evidence of any of the defects commonly associated with corrected transposition, such as ventricular septal defect and pulmonary stenosis. Fibroelastosis is unlikely because patients with this disease usually die earlier and murmurs are usually not a prominent feature. Murmurs of such intensity are not heard in this disease, and the left atrium, though enlarged, is never this big.

At this point I was left with an isolated congenital mitral insufficiency, which was probably anatomically one of the first five diagnoses in Table 1. In this malformation, the left atrium may be large, there is an early history of failure, growth is retarded, and the electrocardiogram shows left ventricular hypertrophy. There is no certain way of differentiating between the first five types of congenital mitral insufficiency. In Dr. H. B. Taussig's book[3] there is a drawing of a heart exhibiting a kind of mitral insufficiency in which the mitral valve is replaced by a perforated diaphragm. The clinical course in this patient was similar to that of the subject of today's conference. There was auricular fibrillation, a huge left atrium, and an enlarged left ventricle. I thought the patient under discussion today would have a similar mitral valve.

Therefore, in summary, on the basis of the protocol, x-rays, and electrocardiogram before I received the catheterization data, my diagnosis was congenital mitral insufficiency due to a fused fixed perforated diaphragm in place of the mitral valve.

DR. EUGENE BRAUNWALD: A right heart catheterization was carried out and the pressure in the right atrium was markedly elevated with V wave peaks of 17 mm. Hg and a mean pressure of 13 mm. Hg. The catheter crossed an atrial communication into the left atrium where the pressure pulse was found to have V wave peaks of 27 mm. Hg and the mean pressure in the left atrium was 15 mm. Hg, only slightly but distinctly higher than the mean pressure in the right atrium. The contours of the two pressure pulses were also quite different. The systolic pressure in the right ventricle was elevated to 55 mm. Hg; the end-diastolic pressure was 15 mm. Hg; the femoral arterial oxygen saturation was normal.

The krypton[85] inhalation test[4] for the characterization of left-to-right shunts indicated a value of 46% in the right atrium. The upper limit of normal is 15%, and the value observed in our patient represents a left-to-right shunt entering the right atrium. The value of 34% in the right ventricle confirmed the fact that a left-to-right shunt existed.

Indicator dilution curves were obtained. Injection of indocyanine dye into the left atrium and sampling from the femoral artery resulted in a curve which indicated the presence of a left-to-right shunt. Injection of dye into the inferior vena cava showed no evidence of a right-to-left shunt, but showed a broad diffuse curve which was compatible with congestive heart failure and/or a left-to-right shunt. The levels of pressure in the various cardiac chambers and the results of the krypton[85] test and of the dye dilution curves were then sent to Dr. Ross *after* he had prepared the foregoing discussion. However, we did not indicate how the left atrium was entered.

DR. RICHARD S. ROSS: I should have asked a question when I first got the catheterization data because I have just realized for the first time that the catheter entered the left atrium. I had assumed that the transseptal technic[5] had been employed, and I am distressed to learn that the left atrium was entered without puncture of the septum.

The catheterization report adds four important facts to the list of clinical evidence we have already considered:

1. Evidence of a left-to-right shunt into the right atrium.
2. Right ventricular systolic hypertension.
3. No right-to-left shunt.
4. Tall V waves in the left atrium.

The next step is to consider the clinical diagnosis of congenital mitral insufficiency in the light of the catheterization data. Certainly, the tall V waves support this diagnosis and the right ventricular hypertension was consistent with it. The evidence of the left-to-right shunt into the right atrium was difficult to reconcile with the large left atrium. It is difficult to see how the left atrium could have reached this size if there were an atrial septal defect, as the atrial septal defect would tend to decompress the left atrium. It is well recognized that in Lutembacher's syndrome, in which the hemodynamic situation is similar, though the mitral valve is involved in a different way, the left atrium is not huge.

We have seen three patients who have mitral insufficiency and an ostium secundum defect. These people by and large have not been severely ill, and the left atrium has not been as big as we would have expected it to be on the basis of the mitral valvular disease alone. They have not had signs of gross left ventricular hypertrophy on electrocardiogram or on x-ray. The systolic murmurs were far less impressive than the one heard in this patient.

A similar set of cases has been reported by Bashour and Simmons.[6] None of their cases of mitral insufficiency and ostium secundum atrial septal defects had a left atrium as large as did our patient. Of course, it could be said that in this particular case there was more than the usual amount of mitral insufficiency and a very small atrial defect, and that this accounted for the unusual clinical picture.

Before settling on this diagnosis, I thought I should consider some other possibilities, so I began to consider the possible sources of a left-to-right shunt of oxygenated blood into the right atrium. The various possibilities are:

1. Aorta to right atrium.
2. Left ventricle to right ventricle—tricuspid insufficiency to right atrium.
3. Left ventricle to right atrium.
4. Left atrium to right atrium.

The simple atrial defect can be excluded because of the size of the left atrium. The aorta to right atrium shunt can be excluded on the basis of physical findings; patients with this communication almost always have a continuous murmur, are usually sicker, and the disease runs a more rapid course. The possibility of the ventricular septal defect with a regurgitant tricuspid valve seemed real, but on the basis of the electrocardiogram, it was excluded. If the right side of the heart were overloaded by a ventricular septal defect and tricuspid insufficiency, there would certainly be evidence of right hypertrophy in the electrocardiogram. The absence of right hypertrophy on the electrocardiogram was also the major objection to the diagnosis of ostium primum defect. The objections were the same as those raised in the earlier discussion.

The diagnosis selected will have to provide an explanation for the following findings:

1. Oxygenated blood to right atrium.
2. Incompetent mitral valve.

3. Huge left atrium (intact atrial septum).
4. Left ventricular hypertrophy.

The large left atrium excluded the existence of a significant atrial septal defect and yet we had evidence of oxygenated blood entering the right atrium. The left ventricular hypertrophy that we saw in the EKG suggested that there might be a cause of ventricular overloading other than the mitral insufficiency.

In a search for other causes of left ventricular hypertrophy, I considered various kinds of aortic stenosis and found an illustration in Dr. Taussig's book[3] which shows an infundibular aortic stenosis with anomalous insertion of the chordae of the mitral valve. This insertion caused the aortic leaflet of the mitral valve to be pulled away from the mural leaflet. The patient died, presumably due to a combination of mitral insufficiency and an infundibular aortic stenosis. This malformation would have explained all the findings in today's case except for the shunt. From this case, I was led to a case reported by Dr. Charlotte Ferencz in 1957 which had all of the features necessary to explain the findings in the case today.

In conclusion, I believe the patient under discussion today had the malformation described by Ferencz. The x-ray findings in this malformation are almost identical with those presented today. The left atrium is equally prominent and gives the same configuration to the right heart border in the PA projection (Figure 4). The other projections show the massive dilatation of the left atrium and the enlarged left ventricle. The electrocardiogram is also similar to that of today's patient. The tall R waves over the left precordium are accompanied by similar ST segment changes.

The anatomy of the heart in Ferencz' patient can be seen in Figure 5. The chordae from the aortic leaflet of the mitral valve were attached to the ventricular septum and the mitral valve was rendered incompetent. These same anomalous chordae formed a network in the outflow tract of the left ventricle and interfered with left ventricular emptying. There was a communication between the left ventricle and the right atrium which would explain very nicely the left-to-right shunt with an

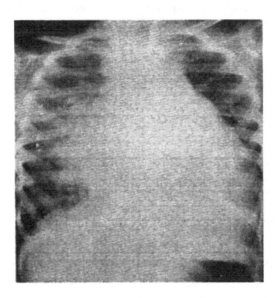

Figure 4 Chest roentgenogram of patient described by Ferencz.[7] (Reproduced by permission of Bull. Johns Hopkins Hosp. 100: 209, 1957.)

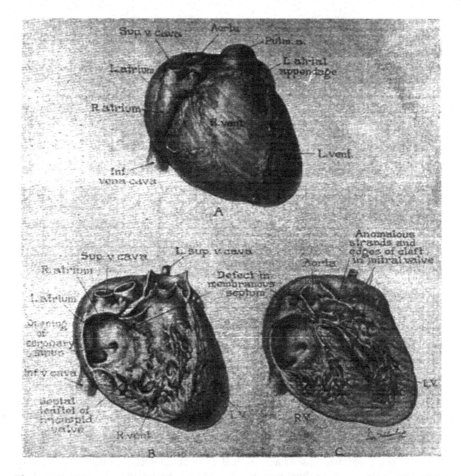

Figure 5 Drawing of the heart in the case described by Ferencz. (Reproduced by permission of Bull. Johns Hopkins Hosp. **100**: 209, 1957.)

intact atrial septum. Before hearing Dr. Braunwald's discussion of the catheterization I had assumed that the atrial septum was intact, and I still feel it hard to explain the large left atrium in any other way.

The diagram in Figure 6 shows how the heart in Ferencz' patient would function. If this isn't the right diagnosis, I'm quite sure that it would give an identical clinical picture. The chordae from the mitral valve are shown extending across the outflow tract of the left ventricle. There is a communication between the left ventricle and the right atrium. There is a huge left atrium, which of course has many hemodynamic factors operating to make it so large: first, there is an intact septum; second, the mitral valve is incompetent; third, there is left ventricular outflow obstruction so that the pressure in the left ventricle is very high; and fourth, there is a left-to-right shunt so that the return of blood to the left atrium from the lung would be increased.

Therefore, in conclusion, I think the correct diagnosis is left ventriculo-right atrial communication, with mitral insufficiency due to anomalous insertion of the chordae tendineae, and obstruction of left ventricular outflow due to the chordae tendineae extending across the left ventricular outflow tract.

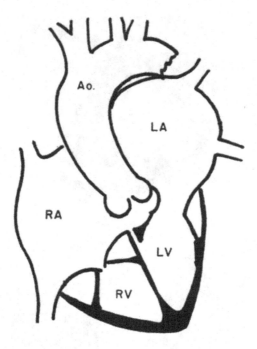

Figure 6 Diagrammatic representation of the lesion in the case described by Ferencz.

DR. EUGENE BRAUNWALD: Thank you very much for this most instructive discussion, Dr. Ross. In passing the catheter from the right atrium to the left, we didn't assume that it had passed across an atrial septal defect because the left atrium was so large and because there was a distinct pressure difference between the two atria. The possibility was considered that the catheter had been passed across a patent foramen ovale. Dr. Morrow operated upon this patient and I will ask him to describe the operative findings and the clinical course.

DR. ANDREW G. MORROW: I'm glad that we did not have to deal with the type of anomaly reported by Ferencz and which you discussed, Dr. Ross. Before the operation we were not certain of the exact diagnosis, but it seemed clear that mitral regurgitation was the dominant lesion and the one which should receive first consideration. For this reason we made a bilateral anterior thoracotomy so that we might approach any chamber of the heart and would also have optimal exposure of the left atrium.

The entire heart, as you might imagine, was enormous, and the left atrium was particularly prominent. It bulged out behind the right atrium and venae cavae, extending several centimeters beyond the border of the right chambers of the heart. The right atrium was also strikingly enlarged, and there was a faint systolic thrill over it. Over the exposed posterior portion of the left atrium, however, there was an intense systolic thrill.

The digital intracardiac exploration, through the right atrial appendage, was revealing. In the region of the foramen ovale I could feel no interatrial communication but low in the right atrium, immediately above the tricuspid annulus, was a tiny defect which would not admit my finger. Most strikingly, one could feel an intense systolic jet of blood impinging on the interatrial septum from the left side. There was also evidence of a moderate jet of tricuspid regurgitation.

When the cannulations and other preparations for bypass had been completed, I introduced my finger into the left atrium. I could reach the mitral valve only with some difficulty because of the size of the atrium but could easily feel an intense regurgitant jet of blood coming through it. By palpation the jet did not seem to be localized to a commissure but more to the central portion of the valve. We then went on bypass and opened the left atrium from the right side. When the blood had been evacuated we could see a small interatrial communication which lay immediately above the atrioventricular ring. This was less than a centimeter in diameter. Coming through the opening from the right side was dark blood, the coronary return.

Inspection of the mitral valve revealed that the posterior or mural leaflet was somewhat thickened but was essentially normal. In the anterior or aortic leaflet of the mitral valve, however, there was a complete cleft which extended from the common endocardial cushion through the length of the valve to its free margin. The cleft was of the type typically seen in the partial form of persistent atrioventricular canal. We closed the interatrial septal defect from the left side with a few sutures and then approximated the valve cleft with a series of reinforced interrupted mattress sutures. After it had been repaired the valve seemed to be competent.

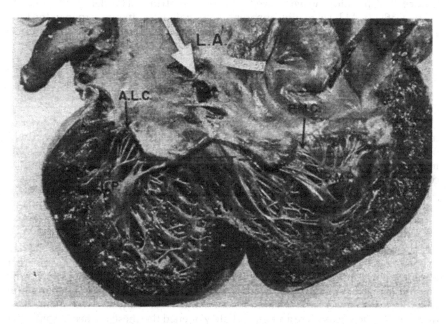

Figure 7 The left atrium (L.A.), mitral valve, and left ventricle (L.V.) are opened. The left atrium is markedly dilated and the left ventricle is hypertrophied and dilated. The sutures closing the ostium primum defect (white arrow) have been removed. The defect is located at the apex of the cleft in the anterior mitral leaflet. The chordae tendineae extending to the anterolateral (A.L.P.) and posteromedial (P.M.P.) papillary muscles are normal. The anterolateral (A.L.C.) and posteromedial (P.M.C.) commissures are designated for orientation purposes.

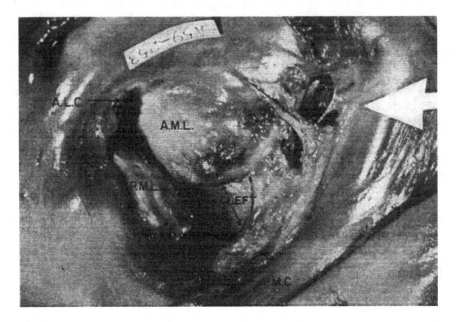

Figure 8 The mitral valve viewed from the left atrium. The cleft in the anterior mitral leaflet (A.M.L.) is readily apparent. The small defect (white arrow) in the lowest portion of the atrial septum is located at the apex of the cleft. The posterior mitral leaflet (P.M.L.) is unremarkable. The posteromedial (P.M.C.) and the anterolateral (A.L.C.) commissures are evident.

The left atriotomy was then closed and we opened the right atrium in order to inspect the tricuspid valve. There was obvious tricuspid regurgitation, but we could find no discrete lesion that seemed amenable to repair. There was no distinct cleft in any of the leaflets. The regurgitation through the tricuspid valve seemed to be coming from the commissure between the septal and posterior leaflets and it was felt that it might be corrected by an annuloplasty. This was performed with three or four mattress sutures placed through the annulus at the commissure described.

We then came off bypass and the child maintained his circulation well. There was still enlargement of the left atrium and it was quite tense, but we could not feel systolic thrill in the left atrium after the repair. The child did well during the day of operation and that night. On one occasion his blood pressure fell for no apparent reason, but it responded immediately to a single small dose of metaraminol. On the day following the operation, he was sitting up in bed. The nurse was having him cough to evacuate secretions. He did cough, and vigorously, and that moment he died. The resident was there and immediately opened the chest; the heart was found to be in arrest and could not be resuscitated.

DR. EUGENE BRAUNWALD: The pathologic findings will now be presented and discussed by Dr. Roberts.

DR. WILLIAM C. ROBERTS: The complete cleavage or cleft in the anterior or aortic leaflet of the mitral valve produced a wide-open canal between the left atrium and the left ventricle (Figures 7, 8). The mitral regurgitation led to extreme dilatation of the left atrium and to moderate hypertrophy and dilatation of the left ventricle. A small defect, measuring only 1 cm. in its largest diameter, was present in the lower portion of the atrial septum—a so-called ostium primum type atrial septal defect. In addition, the tricuspid valve was abnormal. Although there was no cleavage of its septal leaflet, the most superior portion of the septal leaflet was absent, and the remaining portion of this leaflet was shortened. These abnormalities prevented complete closure of the tricuspid valve during ventricular systole, and tricuspid regurgitation resulted. Other cardiovascular findings included anomalous chordae tendineae from the anterior leaflet of the mitral valve, a quadricuspid pulmonic valve, and moderate hypoplasia of the right coronary artery. The lungs were collapsed bilaterally; the liver and spleen showed marked changes of chronic passive congestion.

The normal mitral valve consists of two leaflets, the anterior, which is the larger and which is continuous with the aortic valve, and the posterior. Normally chordae tendineae from the margins of each of the two leaflets insert only into the two papillary muscles of the left ventricle. In the patient under discussion the anterior mitral leaflet was divided by the cleft into two halves, which may be designated "anterior" and "posterior." Chordae tendineae not only inserted into the two papillary muscles of the left ventricle, but chordae from the "anterior" portion of the anterior mitral leaflet also inserted into the crest of the muscular ventricular septum immediately beneath the aortic valve (Figure 9). These thickened and fused anomalous chordae, which have no counterpart in the normal heart, are always present when there is a cleft anterior mitral leaflet. They are important because, as emphasized by Edwards,[8] if they are not divided at the time the cleft is repaired, some mitral insufficiency will invariably remain. Caution must be exerted by the surgeon, however, when cutting these accessory chordae in order not to lacerate an aortic valve cusp or perforate the membranous ventricular septum. In addition, as already stressed by Dr. Ross, these anomalous chordae may interfere with the outflow of blood from the left ventricle and thus produce a form of subaortic stenosis.

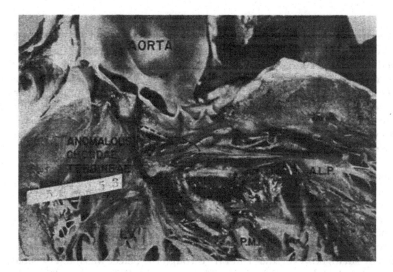

Figure 9 The left ventricle (L.V.), aortic valve, and aorta are opened. The anomalous chordae tendineae, enclosed by the broken lines, extend from the anterior portion of the cleft anterior mitral leaflet to the crest of the ventricular septum immediately beneath the aortic valve cusps. The anterolateral (A.L.P.) and posteromedial (P.M.P.) papillary muscles are labeled.

PERSISTENT COMMON ATRIOVENTRICULAR CANAL

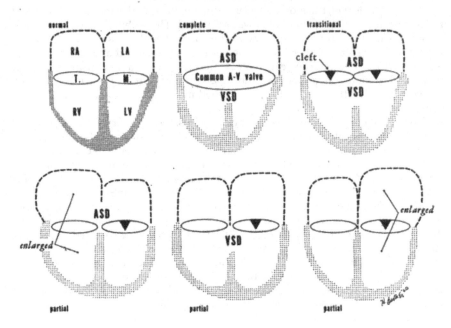

Figure 10 Diagrammatic representation of various forms of persistent common AV canal. RA, right atrium, LA, left atrium, RV, right ventricle, LV, left ventricle; T, tricuspid valve ring; M, mitral valve ring; ASD, atrial septal defect; VSD, ventricular septal defect

A cleft anterior mitral valve and an ostium primum defect, both of which were present in this patient, are two of the components of the complex anomaly variously termed persistent common atrioventricular canal, atrioventricularis communis, and endocardial cushion defect. Persistent common atrioventricular canal has been divided by Wakai and Edwards[9, 10] into three forms: complete, transitional or intermediate, and partial (Figure 10). In the complete form there is only one valve common to both sides of the heart; an atrial septal defect of the ostium primum type and a high ventricular septal defect are also present. In the transitional form (Figure 10, upper right diagram) the common valve meets in the midline, forming two atrioventricular valves. A cleft is present in the septal leaflet of the tricuspid valve as well as in the anterior leaflet of the mitral valve. The partial forms (Figure 10, lower diagrams) are characterized by the presence of a cleft in the anterior mitral valve and by the absence of a cleft in the tricuspid valve, although portions of the latter may be shortened or absent.

The patient under discussion had a cleft mitral valve and an atrial septal defect (Figure 10, lower left diagram). Since the atrial septal defect in this patient was extremely small, however, the "run-off" through the defect was likewise small, and consequently (as illustrated in Figure 10, lower right diagram) left atrial dilatation and left ventricular hypertrophy occurred, rather than right atrial and right ventricular enlargement.

In the 109 specimens with congenital malformations of the heart and great vessels in the pathologic collection of the Clinical Center, there are 12 instances of persistent common AV canal (Table 2). The subject of this conference is case 12. The age range of these 12 patients is nine months to 54 years. The partial form of AV canal was the most common. The complete type, the most frequent in most series, was absent. The anterior mitral valve was cleft in all but two patients. In contrast, the septal tricuspid valve was cleft in only one patient and normal in only two. In eight, there was either partial or total absence of the septal leaflet. When the ventricular septal defects were present, they were quite small, except in two patients. The two patients with the large ventricular septal defects had no ostium primum type atrial septal defect, but did have cleft anterior mitral valves. It is not necessary for an ostium primum type atrial septal defect to be present in order that the diagnosis of persistent common atrioventricular canal be made. The one anatomic feature noted in all patients listed in Table 2 is the presence of anomalous chordae tendineae from the mitral valve to the ventricular septum (Figure 9). I therefore consider anomalous chordae tendineae to be a hallmark of the complex anomaly of persistent common atrioventricular canal. Thus, the patient described by Ferencz[7] and discussed by Dr. Ross may perhaps be considered to have had an unusual form of the persistent common atrioventricular canal.

A patent foramen ovale was present in eight of the 12 patients whom we have examined. In three of these eight cases the valve guarding the foramen was incompetent. Of special note is the presence of right ventricular hypertrophy in all patients in this series, except case 12, the patient under discussion, who had isolated left ventricular hypertrophy.

DR. EUGENE BRAUNWALD: The unusual anatomic features presented by this patient and discussed by Drs. Roberts and Morrow were responsible for the clinical and hemodynamic findings which are unusual for patients with the partial form of persistent AV canal. The majority of these patients have a large atrial septal defect and a mild or moderate degree of mitral regurgitation. Clinically, although they present with a loud pansystolic apical murmur they usually have only mild left atrial and left ventricular enlargement. In general the lung fields are plethoric on roentgenograms of the chest and these patients have all of the other clinical features associated with a large left-to-right shunt and increased pulmonary blood flow. The electrocardiograms usually show more marked left axis deviation of the terminal forces than our patient did. In addition, there is evidence of "right ventricular diastolic overload," i.e., an RSR' configuration in right precordial leads. The absence of this feature in our patient may reasonably be attributed to the small left-to-right shunt and the only slightly augmented right ventricular output (Figure 1). The prolonged PR interval, which our patient exhibited on several EKGs prior to the development of atrial fibrillation, could have been a clue to the diagnosis since this finding is common in patients with AV canal.

The clinical findings in this patient, and in one other patient with identical anatomic findings, were those of massive mitral regurgitation; there was a prominent apical holosystolic murmur which was transmitted well into the axilla and over the precordium. Prominent left ventricular lifts were palpable. The roentgenographic findings were of left atrial enlargement rather than of increased pulmonary blood flow. Since the atrial septal defect was very small it could not adequately decompress the left atrium, and a pressure gradient between these two chambers was present throughout the cardiac cycle, particularly during ventricular systole when a large V wave was present in the left atrial pressure pulse; the latter was related to massive mitral regurgitation and is not usually present in patients with mitral regurgitation and a large atrial septal defect.

I shall now ask Dr. Morrow to discuss some of the surgical considerations in persistent AV canal.

Table 2: A summary of the anatomic features in 12 patients with persistent common atrioventricular canal studied at the clinical center

Case	Age Sex, Race	Type	Mitral Valve* (Ant. leaf.)	Tricuspid Valve (Septal leaf.)	VSD	Ostium Primum Defect	Patent Foramen Ovale	Cardiomegaly	Associated Anomalies
1. A54–66	9 mo. N F	Partial	Cleft	Absent (partial)	+ (minute)	+	+	RVH	0
2. A56–111	17 mo. W M	Partial	Short	Absent (partial)	+ (minute)	+	+	RVH	0
3. A57–117	26 W F	Partial	Cleft	Normal	0	+	+ (valv. incomp.)	RVH	0
4. A57–184	14 W F	Partial	Cleft	Absent (partial)	0	+	+ (valv. incomp.)	RVH	0
5. A57–195	42 N M	Partial	Cleft	Absent (partial)	0	+	0	RVH	0
6. A57–226	2 W F	Trans.	Cleft	Cleft	+ (small)	+	+	RVH LVH	Mongolism
7. A59–12	23 W M	Partial	Cleft	Absent	+ (minute)	+	+ (valv. incomp.)	RVH	Rt. PV→RA† LSCV→CS‡
8. A59–207	54 W F	Partial	Cleft (partial)	Absent	0	+	+	RVH	CS→LA§
9. A60–41	13 W F	Partial	Cleft (partial)	Normal	+ (large)	0	+	RVH	0
10. A60–84	13 W F	Partial	No cleft	Anomalous * chordae	+ (large)	0	0	RVH LVH	LSVC→CS‡ Bicuspid pul. valve
11. A60–276	31 W F	Partial	Cleft	Absent (partial)	0	+ (small)	0	RVH LVH	0
12. A59–253	14 N M	Partial	Cleft	Absent (partial)	0	+ (small)	0	LVH	0

All patients had anomalous chordae tendineae from the mitral valve to the ventricular septum.

† Rt. PV→RA: The right pulmonary veins drained only into the right atrium.

‡ LSCV→CS: A left superior vena cava drained into the coronary sinus.

§ CS→LA: The coronary sinus drained only into the left atrium. The right atrial ostium of the coronary sinus was atretic.

* Double orifice, tricuspid valve.

DR. ANDREW G. MORROW: From the standpoint of making a decision as to whether a given child or adult with a variety of AV canal should be operated upon, I think that one important consideration is whether the lesion is the complete, the transitional, or the partial form of the anomaly. In other words, if one has to deal only with a cleft anterior leaflet of the mitral valve and to close an inter-atrial communication, a completely corrective operation can be carried out with an acceptable risk. In a child or a young adult who presents with these findings and no other contraindications we now recommend that operation be undertaken electively, regardless of the presence or absence of symptoms. Our feeling about operation is somewhat less optimistic when the complete form of AV canal is present and there is an associated large interventricular communication. The bundle of His lies immediately under the endocardium, on top of the ventricular septum, and the difficulty in repairing a complete persistent canal is to close the interventricular communication without producing complete heart block. This complication has unfortunately occurred in a large percentage of such patients who were operated upon.

In a patient such as the one described today, i.e., one who presents with the primary problem of mitral regurgitation but in whom a shunt into the right atrium is also present, another problem presents itself. First, it is difficult, I think, to be certain before operation that the patient does not have a small atrial septal defect of the ostium secundum type and a mitral valve which is not congenitally cleft but which has been damaged in another fashion, as by rheumatic fever. The importance of this differential diagnosis is that, in general, a cleft mitral valve can be repaired without undue difficulty and a competent valve can be established. On the other hand, the problem of the treatment of rheumatic mitral regurgitation, at this time in our unenlightenment, remains an extremely difficult one.

I feel that one of the reasons this child died may have been the fact that Edwards, at the time of the operation, had not yet published his article about the abnormal chordae tendineae which are present in AV canal.[8] He points out, on morphologic grounds, that if one does not divide these abnormal chordae, although the anterior leaflet is reconstituted, the chordae may restrict the motion of the valve and hold it down in the left ventricle during ventricular systole. Thus even though the leaflet itself appears competent there still may be significant mitral regurgitation. At the time of the operation we were unaware of the existence or the importance of these structures. Perhaps if we had done a more effective repair the child might have survived.

DR. EUGENE BRAUNWALD: It is technically simpler to close the atrial septal defect than it is to restore complete competency to the mitral valve in patients with the lesion which our patient presented. If this occurs the patient can actually be made worse by operation, since the atrial defect does serve as a type of escape valve for the distended left atrium. In the other patient with this malformation whom we have encountered, the pulmonary artery pressure prior to operation was 22/8 mm. Hg. Following operation, the defect remained closed but mitral regurgitation persisted, the pulmonary artery pressure rose to 54/20 mm. Hg, and the patient required a second operation.

Dr. Ross, do you have any further comments?

DR. RICHARD S. ROSS: Do you think that the anomalous chordae produced left ventricular outflow obstruction in this case? If they did, and if the mitral valve were repaired but the left ventricular outflow obstruction were allowed to remain, a satisfactory result could not be anticipated.

DR. EUGENE BRAUNWALD: At the time of the left ventricular catheterization there was no gradient between the left ventricle and the aorta; therefore there is little hemodynamic evidence that the chordae interfered with left ventricular ejection.

DR. RICHARD S. ROSS: I see. I think I erred in making the categorical assumption that the atrial septum might be intact to explain the giant left atrium. In general this is true, but, as has been pointed out, the atrial size is more a function of the ratio of the magnitude of mitral regurgitation to the size of the atrial septal defect. If there is a lot of mitral regurgitation and a small atrial septal defect, there can be a large left atrium.

QUESTION: How can one differentiate preoperatively the lesion which this patient presented from that described by Dr. Ferencz?

DR. EUGENE BRAUNWALD: Since we have not encountered the latter anomaly I can only speculate: (1) A selective left ventricular angiocardiogram or preferably a selective cine-angiogram with left ventricular injection would show immediate opacification of both atria, while this type of study in our patient would show left atrial opacification prior to right atrial opacification. The value of selective left ventricular angiocardiography in the differential diagnosis of the various forms of persistent common AV canal and of related anomalies has recently been discussed elsewhere in detail.[11] (2) The anomalous chordae in Ferencz' patient presumably resulted in a pressure gradient between the left ventricle and the aorta. This did not occur in our patient. (3) A cardiac catheter could be passed from the right to the left atrium in our patient, but this would not be possible in Ferencz' patient, who had an intact interatrial septum.

QUESTION: What was the cause of the diastolic rumbling murmur at the apex? There was no evidence of mitral stenosis at autopsy.

DR. EUGENE BRAUNWALD: In patients with pure mitral regurgitation of large degree a diastolic rumbling murmur is frequently audible at the apex. This is related to the flow of abnormally large volumes of blood from the left atrium to the left ventricle during diastole.

SUMMARIO IN INTERLINGUA

Le patiente esseva un puero de 13 annos de etate in qui—al etate de sex annos, durante le curso de un maladia febril—un forte murmure systolic apical e cardiomegalia habeva essite constatate. In le curso del sequente annos, ille esseva hospitalisate repetitemente a causa de congestive disfallimento cardiac. Le examine physic monstrava pulsante venas in le collo, un allargate hepate, e un forte e findite secunde sono cardiac in le area pulmonal. Forte murmures systolic e diastolic esseva audibile al apice. Le electrocardiogramma revelava fibrillation atrial e deviation axial al sinistra. Le catheterismo cardiac monstrava hypertension systolic dexteroventricular, un micre derivation sinistro-dextere que entrava in le atrio dextere, alte undas V in le pulso de pression sinistro-atrial, e un distincte gradiente de pression inter le duo atrios. Le diagnose differential inter iste lesion e regurgitation mitral in le pueritia es discutite in detalio.

Al operation il esseva trovate que le patiente habeva un micre defecto atrioseptal del typo de atrio prime e un complete scission in le lobo anterior del valvula mitral. Le duo lesiones esseva reparate, sed le patiente moriva le die post le operation:

Es discutite le aspectos anatomic, pathologic, e clinic de persistente canal atrioventricular.

BIBLIOGRAPHY

1. Braunwald, E., Morrow, A. G.: Left ventriculo-right atrial communication. *Amer. J. Med.* **28**: 913–920, 1960.

2. Anderson, R. C., Lillehei, C. W., Lester, R. G.: Corrected transposition of the great vessels of the heart. A review of 17 cases. *Pediatrics* **20**: 626–646, 1957.

3. Taussig, H. B.: Congenital malformations of the heart. Rev. Ed. Harvard University Press, Cambridge, MA, 1960.

4. Sanders, R. J., Morrow, A. G.: The identification and quantification of left-to-right circulatory shunts: a new diagnostic method utilizing the inhalation of a radioactive gas, Kr[85]. *Amer. J. Med.* **26**: 508–516, 1959.

5. Ross, J., Jr., Braunwald, E., Morrow, A. G.: Left heart catheterization by the transseptal route. A description of the technic and its applications. *Circulation* **22**: 927–934, 1960.

6. Bashour, F. A., Simmons, D. H.: Atrial septal defect with mitral valvulitis: clinical and catheterization diagnosis. *Ann. Intern. Med.* **48**: 1194–1204, 1958.

7. Ferencz, C.: Atrioventricular defect of the membranous septum. Left ventricular-right atrial communication with malformed mitral valve simulating aortic stenosis. Report of a case. *Bull. Johns Hopkins Hosp.* **100**: 209–222, 1957.

8. Edwards, J. E.: The problem of mitral insufficiency caused by accessory chordae tendineae in persistent common atrioventricular canal. *Proc. Mayo Clin.* **35**: 299–305, 1960.

9. Wakai, C. S., Edwards, J. E.: Developmental and pathologic considerations in persistent common atrioventricular canal. *Proc. Mayo Clin.* **31**: 487–500, 1956.

10. Wakai, C. S., Edwards, J. E.: Pathologic study of persistent common atrioventricular canal. *Amer. Heart J.* **56**: 779–794, 1958.

11. Braunwald, E., Morrow, A. G., Cooper, T.: Left ventricular angiocardiography in the diagnosis of persistent atrioventricular canal and related anomalies. *Amer. J. Cardiol.* **4**: 802–808, 1959.

Case 3 Increased Bronchial Collateral Circulation in a Patient with Transposition of the Great Vessels and Pulmonary Hypertension*

Roland Folse, MD, William C. Roberts, MD, and William P. Cornell, MD
Bethesda, Maryland

IT IS WELL established that patients with cyanotic congenital heart disease characterized by diminished pulmonary blood flow have increased collateral circulation to the lungs through enlarged bronchial arteries. The incidence, stimuli for development and structural arrangement of these collateral vessels are not well understood.

Large bronchial vessels are commonly found in patients with stenotic lesions in the right side of the heart or the pulmonary artery producing an intracardiac right to left shunt such as is seen in tetralogy of Fallot, pulmonic stenosis with atrial septal defect or tricuspid atresia. In these patients the pulmonary artery pressure and blood flow are diminished. Intravascular thromboses in the pulmonary vascular bed, presumably secondary to capillary stasis and polycythemia, may further diminish the pulmonary blood flow and thus further the need for bronchial collaterals.[1] Likewise, in patients with complete absence or atresia of the pulmonary arteries, communications arising directly from the aorta persist from fetal life and are essential not only for the nourishment of the pulmonary structures but also for supplying the lungs with desaturated blood in order to provide for exchange of gases.[2]

Bronchial collaterals may also develop in acyanotic patients. For example, the congenital absence of one main pulmonary artery is associated with enlarged bronchial arteries to that lung.[3] In other diseases, additional mechanisms may lead to increased collateral circulation to the lungs. Patients without heart disease, such as those with pulmonary infarction, bronchiectasis, tuberculosis, emphysema or lung tumors, may have increased bronchial blood flow to the diseased portions of the lungs.

It has not been generally appreciated that patients with cyanotic congenital heart disease and pulmonary hypertension may also have extensive collateral circulation to the lungs. This communication describes an infant with complete transposition of the great vessels, a ventricular septal defect and pulmonary hypertension, who also had markedly increased pulmonary collateral blood flow.

CLINICAL SUMMARY

T. N., a fourteen month old male infant, had been cyanotic since birth. His early growth and development were somewhat retarded and he had frequent respiratory infections but no episodes of severe cyanosis or squatting. He was described as being an active child with some limitation due to fatigability. There was no history of heart failure.

* From the Clinic of Surgery, National Heart Institute and Department of Pathologic Anatomy, the Clinical Center, National Institutes of Health, Bethesda, Maryland.

DOI: 10.1201/9781003409342-2

On examination the patient was moderately cyanotic at rest and had evidence of clubbing of the digits. He was somewhat small for his age, his weight being in the tenth percentile on the anthropometric chart. The heart was enlarged to both the right and left sides of the sternum. There was a lift over the lower left sternal area, but no thrill was palpable. The second sound at the base was slightly accentuated and was thought to be single. There was a soft, grade 1–6 early systolic murmur heard along the lower left sternal border. The hematocrit was 75 per cent and the hemoglobin 21.5 gm. per 100 ml. The electrocardiogram demonstrated right atrial enlargement, right axis deviation and right ventricular hypertrophy (Figure 1). Cardiac fluoroscopy revealed enlargement of both ventricles with narrowing of the base of the heart. The horizontal course of tortuous vessels in the hilar regions suggested the presence of prominent bronchial arteries.

At catheterization the pulmonary artery was not entered. The systemic arterial oxygen saturation was 43 per cent under general anesthesia. *A selective right ventricular angiocardiogram* (Figure 2) was performed which demonstrated that the aorta arose from the anatomic right ventricle. The left ventricle and pulmonary artery were not opacified in the early films. Large bronchial arteries were seen to arise from the descending aorta and appeared to be equally distributed to all parts of both lungs. The right main pulmonary artery visualized well in the later films, suggesting that it was filled by communications with the bronchial arteries. Because of the lack of prominent pulmonary vascularity on the roentgenogram of the chest and the presence of extremely prominent collateral vessels, it was believed that the patient

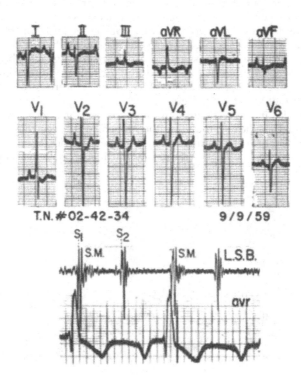

Figure 1 Electrocardiogram and phonocardiogram. S.M. = systolic murmur; L.S.B. = left sternal border.

had complete transposition of the great vessels with associated pulmonic stenosis and would, therefore, benefit from a subclavian-pulmonary artery anastomosis.

At operation the pulmonary artery, which was approximately the same size as the aorta, was observed to arise from the left ventricle and in a position directly posterior to the aorta. Pressures measured simultaneously in the pulmonary artery and aorta were equal. A large number of dilated bronchial arteries and veins were present in the hili of the lungs, in the interlobar fissures and along the subpleural surface of the lungs. Because of the high pressure in the pulmonary artery, an anastomosis was not performed. Postoperatively, the patient became progressively more cyanotic, and his condition gradually deteriorated until he died eighteen hours after operation.

PATHOLOGIC FINDINGS

Necropsy confirmed the operative finding of complete transposition of the great vessels. The aorta arose exclusively from the right ventricle (Figure 3) and the pulmonary trunk from the left ventricle. The ascending aorta lay directly anterior to the pulmonary trunk. Both ventricles were hypertrophied; the left measured 0.1 cm. and the right, 0.9 cm. in greatest thickness. A ventricular septal defect was present immediately inferior to the supraventricularis muscle (Figure 3). Both atria were dilated, the right more than the left. The atrial appendages were normally situated. A valvular-competent foramen ovale was present. The venae cavae entered the right atrium, and the pulmonary veins entered the left atrium in a normal manner. The atrioventricular valves were normally developed. The pulmonic valve lay posteriorly and joined the anterior mitral leaflet in a manner similar to the connections between the mitral and aortic valves in a normal heart. The cusps of the pulmonic and aortic valves were delicate and pliable and there was no evidence of stenosis. Three large bronchial arteries arose directly from the descending thoracic aorta (Figure 4) and coursed along the posterior aspect of the lower trachea and main bronchi before entering the hili of the lungs (Figure 5). No atherosclerotic changes were present in the pulmonary artery or aorta. The ostia of the coronary arteries arose from the two posterior sinuses of Valsalva (Figure 3).

Microscopically, in the sections from the hili of the lungs many dilated, thick-walled bronchial arteries surrounding the bronchi were seen (Figure 6A). Also, there was proliferation of the intima of some bronchial arteries (Figure 6B), a finding which has not received attention in the past. Many dilated bronchial veins were seen

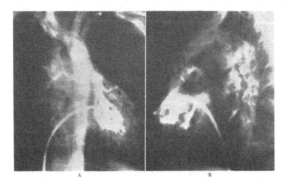

Figure 2 Selective right ventricular angiocardiogram demonstrating complete transposition of the great vessels and large bronchial arteries arising from the descending thoracic aorta. *A*, posteroanterior view: *B*. lateral view.

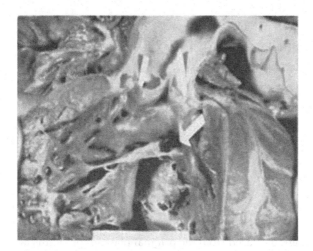

Figure 3 The right ventricle, aortic valve and aorta are opened. The aorta lies anteriorly and arises exclusively from the right ventricle. The coronary arteries arise from the aorta (narrow white pointers). A ventricular septal defect (thick white arrow) is located immediately inferior to the supraventricular muscle. Note the large size of the coronary arteries.

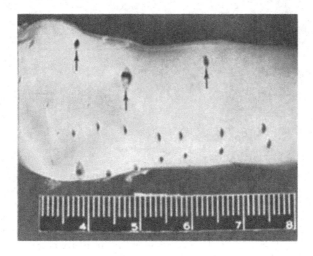

Figure 4 Descending thoracic aorta demonstrating the markedly dilated ostia (arrows) of the bronchial arteries.

in the subpleural areas of the lungs, particularly the hilar regions. Sections from the main pulmonary arteries showed the elastic fibers arranged in an orderly fashion similar to those found in a fetal pulmonary artery (Figure 7). This picture is noted in the lungs of patients in whom pulmonary hypertension has been present from birth and in whom the normal transition to the adult type of pulmonary artery has not taken place.[4] The elastic and muscular pulmonary arteries were dilated, and the latter showed medial hypertrophy and occasional intimal thickening. The lumina of the pulmonary arterioles were narrowed by intimal proliferation (Figure 8).

23

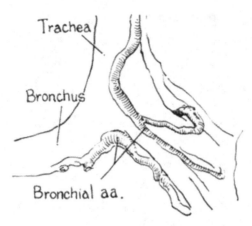

Figure 5 Diagram (traced from the original photograph of this area) illustrating the large bronchial arteries coursing along the posterior aspect of the lower trachea and main bronchi before entering the hili of the lungs.

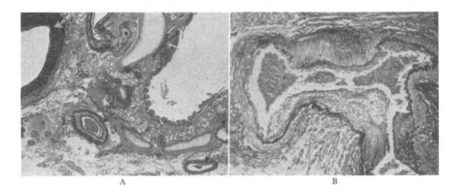

Figure 6 *A*, photomicrograph of lung in hilar region demonstrating thick-walled, dilated bronchial arteries (black arrows) surrounding a bronchus. There is intimal thickening in addition to medial hypertrophy of the bronchial artery in the uppermost portion of the figure. A large elastic pulmonary artery (white arrow) of the fetal type is present in the left upper corner of the figure. (Elastic van Giesson stain, original magnification × 17.) *B*, close-up view of the large bronchial artery appearing in A. Note the marked intimal proliferation and medial hypertrophy. (Elastic van Giesson stain, original magnification × 120.)

COMMENTS

It was demonstrated early in experiments on dogs by Mathes and associates[5] that bronchial collateral circulation to the lungs will develop following obstruction of the pulmonary artery. Liebow et al.[6] have traced the pathway of development of collateral vessels from the bronchial artery to the pulmonary artery to the pulmonary capillaries, with drainage directly into the pulmonary veins or into the azygos system by way of the bronchial veins.

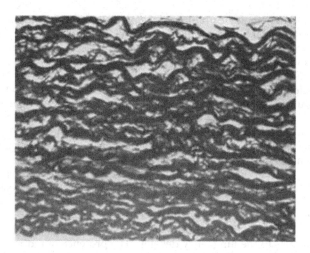

Figure 7 Photomicrograph of main pulmonary artery demonstrating the aorta-like fetal configuration of the elastic lamellae. (Elastic van Giesson stain, original magnification × 450.)

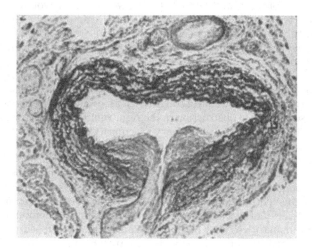

Figure 8 Photomicrograph of pulmonary artery demonstrating marked intimal proliferation and narrowing at the junction of an arteriolar branch. (Elastic van Giesson stain, original magnification × 155.)

There are few documented reports in the literature of augmentation of the bronchial circulation in association with transposition of the great vessels. The combination of complete transposition of the great vessels with pulmonary hypertension and enlarged bronchial arteries in particular, has not been well described previously. The case of transposition of the great vessels which Cockle[7] described in 1863 had enlarged bronchial vessels and probably a normal or increased pulmonary artery pressure, since there was no stenosis of the pulmonic valve and the pulmonary artery was larger than the aorta. Also, no obstruction of the pulmonary valve was noted in pathologic findings of the patient with complete transposition in whom Cudkowicz et al.[8] demonstrated extensive bronchial collateral circulation by injection technics. The pulmonary arteries were dilated and communicated freely with the vasa vasorum supplied by the bronchial arteries.

Bronchopulmonary arterial communications may be found in patients with single ventricle and pulmonary hypertension as in the case reported by Heath,[9] in which bronchial collaterals were prominent in the adventitia of large arteries, surrounding the bronchi and along the visceral pleura. In a similar case illustrated by Liebow,[10] proliferated bronchial arteries were demonstrated to communicate with tortuous pulmonary vessels. In the lungs of patients with Eisenmenger's complex, collateral channels in the form of angiomatoid lesions may connect the pulmonary and bronchial circulations.[11] Similar lesions have been reported in patients with patent ductus arteriosus with pulmonary hypertension[12, 13] and in those with atrial septal defect and pulmonary hypertension[14]; these vessels may divert blood to the alveolar capillaries.

It appears, therefore, that there is a wide spectrum of malformations in which collateral channels to the lungs may develop. The presence of reduced pulmonary blood flow or the absence of elevated pulmonary vascular resistance should not be suspected in a patient with cyanotic congenital heart disease merely because of the existence of enlarged bronchial vessels. Catheterization of the pulmonary artery is difficult or impossible in patients with transposition of the great vessels, single ventricle, truncus arteriosus and other complicated forms of cyanotic heart disease; therefore, the use of right- and left-sided angiocardiography would be valuable in assessing the size of the pulmonary artery, the relative amount of pulmonary blood flow and in estimating the pulmonary artery pressure.

In the patient reported herein a right ventricular angiocardiogram was performed, but because of the presence of complete transposition of the great vessels only the aorta was opacified; the pulmonary artery could not be visualized. As this case illustrates, the clinical picture associated with cyanotic heart disease and pulmonary hypertension may be confused with that associated with obstruction to pulmonary flow secondary to obstruction in the right ventricular outflow tract or at the pulmonary valve. The reduced pulmonary vascularity on the roentgenogram in this patient was suggestive of a reduced pulmonary artery pressure. The closely split second heart sound heard at the base resulted from the presence of equal pressures in the great vessels rather than from an obstruction to right ventricular outflow. The very soft systolic murmur probably indicated that only a small amount of blood passed across the ventricular septal defect, due to the equal ventricular pressures. Accordingly, it is essential that a thorough angiographic and hemodynamic evaluation of the pulmonary vascular bed precede any operative procedure designed to increase pulmonary blood flow in patients with transposition of the great vessels.

SUMMARY

The clinical, diagnostic and pathologic findings in a fourteen month old infant with complete transposition of the great vessels, ventricular septal defect and pulmonary hypertension with increased bronchial collateral circulation are presented. It is emphasized that the presence of increased bronchial collateral blood flow is not necessarily associated with decreased pulmonary blood flow due to obstruction to right ventricular outflow, but may also be associated with pulmonary hypertension and elevation of pulmonary vascular resistance. Thus, the presence of enlarged bronchial vessels should not indicate that the patient will benefit from an operation designed to increase the pulmonary blood flow. The importance of right and left ventricular angiocardiograms in the preoperative assessment of the pulmonary vascular bed is discussed.

REFERENCES

1. RICH, A. R. A hitherto unrecognized tendency to the development of widespread vascular obstruction in patients with congenital pulmonary stenosis (tetralogy of Fallot). *Bull. Johns Hopkins Hosp.*, **82**: 389, 1958.

2. TOBIN, C. E. The bronchial arteries and their connections with other vessels in the human lung. *Surg. Gynec. & Obst.*, **95**: 741, 1957.

3. TABAKIN, B. S., HANSON, J. S., ADHIKARI, P. K. and MILLER, D. B. Physiologic studies in congenital absence of the left main pulmonary artery. *Circulation*, **22**: 1107, 1960.

4. HEATH, D., DUSHANE, J. W., WOOD, E. H. and EDWARDS, J. E. The structure of the pulmonary trunk at different ages and in cases of pulmonary hypertension and pulmonary stenosis. *J. Path. Bact.*, **77**: 443, 1959.

5. MATHES, M. E., HOLMAN, E. and REICHERT, F. L. A study of the bronchial, pulmonary, and lymphatic circulations of the lung under various pathologic conditions experimentally produced. *J. Thoracic Surg.*, **1**: 339, 1932.

6. LIEBOW, A. A., HALES, M. R., HARRISON, W., BLOOMER, W. E. and LINDSKOG, G. F. The genesis and functional implications of collateral circulation to the lungs. *Yale J. Biol. & Med.*, **22**: 637, 1950.

7. COCKLE, J. Case of transposition of the great vessels of the heart. *Tr. Med.-Chir. Soc. London*, **46**: 193, 1863.

8. CUDKOWICZ, L. and ARMSTRONG, J. B. Injection of the bronchial circulation in a case of transposition. *Brit. Heart J.*, **14**: 374, 1952.

9. HEATH, D. Cor triloculare biatriatum. *Circulation*, **15**: 701, 1957.

10. LIEBOW, A. A. *Pathology of the Heart*, Chap. 15. Edited by GOULD, S. E. Springfield, IL, Charles C. Thomas, 1960.

11. BREWER, D. B. and HEATH, D. Pulmonary vascular changes in Eisenmenger's complex. *J. Path. Bact.*, **77**: 141, 1959.

12. BREWER, D. B. Fibrous occlusion and anastomosis of the pulmonary vessels in a case of pulmonary hypertension associated with patent ductus arteriosus. *J. Path. Bact.*, **70**: 299, 1955.

13. DAMMANN, J. F., JR., BERTHRONG, M. and BING, R. J. Reverse ductus: a presentation of the syndrome of patency of the ductus arteriosus with pulmonary hypertension and a shunting of blood flow from pulmonary artery to aorta. *Bull. Johns Hopkins Hosp.*, **92**: 128, 1953.

14. ROSSALL, R. E. and THOMPSON, H. Formation of new vascular channels in the lungs of a patient with secondary pulmonary hypertension. *J. Path. Bact.*, **76**: 593, 1958.

Case 12 Anomalous Origin of Both Coronary Arteries from the Pulmonary Artery*

William C. Roberts, MD†
Bethesda, Maryland

ANOMALOUS origin of either one or both coronary arteries from the pulmonary artery is rare. Less than 70 cases involving the left coronary artery have been reported. About 15 per cent of the patients lived to adulthood and had no recognizable clinical abnormalities;[1] the other 85 per cent had clinical and electrocardiographic features characteristic of this condition (Bland-White-Garland syndrome[2]) and died in infancy. Recognition of this anomaly is important because surgical treatment appears beneficial.[3, 4] Anomalous origin of the right coronary is even less common, about 20 patients having been reported. These patients characteristically have no clinical symptoms referable to the anomaly, which is usually only an incidental finding at autopsy. Origin of both coronary arteries from the pulmonary artery is exceedingly rare, only seven patients having previously been reported.[5–11] This report describes another patient who died of this anomaly.

CASE REPORT

N. M., a male Indian born of a normal pregnancy and delivery, died on his seventh day of life in the Turtle Mountain Indian Hospital, Belcourt, North Dakota. He had cyanosis and labored respirations at birth, and these symptoms progressively worsened until his death. No heart murmur was ever heard. The heart was normal in size by chest roentgenogram. He was treated with oxygen and digitalis without benefit.

Autopsy was performed at the Indian Hospital, and subsequently the heart and other tissues were submitted to the National Institutes of Health for examination. The heart (Figure 1) weighed 27 gm., and the right atrium, right ventricle and left ventricle were dilated and hypertrophied. The wall of each ventricle measured up to 0.4 cm. in thickness. The endocardium of the outflow tract of the left ventricle was mildly but uniformly opaque. The four cardiac valves were normal. The foramen ovale was closed. Both coronary arteries originated from the pulmonary artery. The ostium of the right coronary artery was located in the right posterior sinus, and the left one in the left posterior pulmonic sinus. No coronary arteries arose from the aortic valve sinuses (Figure 2); the course of distribution of the coronary arteries, which were of equal size, from there on was normal. The lungs were dark purple, virtually solid and without crepitation.

Histologically, the coronary arteries had the structure of arterial channels (Figure 3A), although they carried only venous blood. Sections through both ventricles (Figure 3B) disclosed minimal interstitial myocardial edema but no myocardial fibrosis nor inflammation. Myocardial fibers were fragmented, and cross-striations (phosphotungstic acid-hematoxylin stain) were poorly preserved. Some of the myocardial nuclei appeared enlarged, but most were normal. There was no periodic

* From the Pathologic Anatomy Department, Clinical Center, National Institutes of Health, Bethesda, Maryland.

† Present address: Department of Medicine, The Johns Hopkins Hospital, Baltimore 5, Maryland.

DOI: 10.1201/9781003409342-3

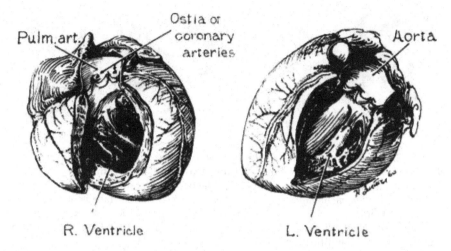

Figure 1 Drawing of heart. *Left*, the right ventricle, pulmonary valve and pulmonary trunk are opened. Both coronary arteries arise from the base of the main pulmonary artery. *Right*, the left ventricle, aortic valve and ascending aorta are opened. No coronary arterial ostia are present.

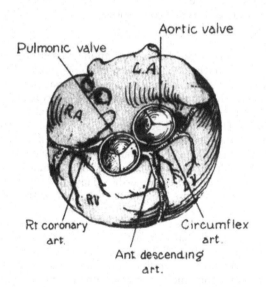

Figure 2 Sketch of heart showing both coronary arteries arising from the pulmonic valve sinuses. The left coronary artery arises from the left posterior sinus and is composed of a circumflex branch which courses anterior to the aortic valve to lie in the left atrioventricular sulcus, and an anterior descending branch which descends in the anterior interventricular sulcus. The right main coronary artery arises in the right posterior pulmonic sinus and lies in the right atrioventricular sulcus, giving off several small branches, and at the base of the posterior interventricular sulcus becomes the posterior descending coronary artery.

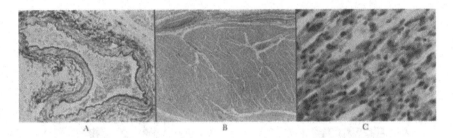

Figure 3 Histologic sections. *A, photomicrograph of the anterior descending branch of the left coronary artery* 1.5 cm. from its ostium. This vessel has the histologic features of a muscular artery. Verhoeff-Van Gieson elastic tissue stain, original magnification, ×155. *B, photomicrograph of left ventricle.* The epicardial surface is at the top of the figure. Hematoxylin and eosin stain, original magnification, ×30. *C, fat stain of left ventricular myocardium.* Cross striations are apparent. Oil red O stain on frozen section, original magnification, ×480.

acid-Schiff-positive material in the myocardium. Fat stain (Oil red O) on the frozen-sectioned myocardium was negative (Figure 3C). Cross-striations in the myocardial fibers were easily discernible in the frozen section. Section of the main pulmonary artery stained for elastic fibers (Verhoeff-Van Giesen method) disclosed a fetal, i.e., aortic-like, configuration of the elastica of this vessel. In the sections from the lungs there were extensive atelectasis and congestion.

COMMENT

Clinical Features: In contrast to the diagnosis of anomalous origin of the left coronary artery from the pulmonary artery, the antemortem diagnosis of anomalous origin of both coronary arteries from the pulmonary artery has not been reported. The probable reason is that this latter condition has not been considered clinically, and thus remains only a postmortem curiosity. However, the clinical features in both conditions are similar (Table 1) and sufficiently characteristic so that the diagnosis might be suggested before death. The newborn is cyanotic and dyspneic from birth or shortly thereafter. On the other hand, patients with only the left coronary artery originating from the pulmonary artery are normal at birth and usually remain so for one to three months when evidence of heart failure, irritability or discomfort, and respiratory infection appears. The heart in children with two anomalous coronary arteries is usually enlarged (as it is in those with anomalous left coronary artery), sometimes reaching huge proportions, as in the patient reported by Swann and Werthammer.[9] No precordial murmurs are heard unless there is an associated defect of the heart or great vessels. Frank signs of heart failure are usually apparent, and these progressively worsen. Feedings are poorly tolerated. The electrocardiogram is virtually pathognomonic in the symptomatic infant with anomalous left coronary artery,[2, 12] but no tracing has been made in reported cases of anomalous origin of both coronary arteries from the pulmonary artery. Findings of left ventricular ischemia would be expected. Breathing gradually becomes more labored, and life ends before two weeks have elapsed.

Pathologic Features: At autopsy, the ventricles, particularly the left one, are typically dilated and hypertrophied, and the endocardium of the left ventricle may be thickened. The coronary arteries, which arise from the right and left sinuses of the pulmonic valve (the anterior sinus being the noncoronary one), are normally distributed. Histologically, they may have the same morphologic features herein described;

Table 1: Anomalous origin of both coronary arteries from the pulmonary artery

Author Year	Sex	Age at Death	Condition at Birth	Weight of Heart (gm.)	Associated Cardiovascular Anomalies	Distribution of Coronary Arteries	Histologic Structure of Coronary Arteries	Histologic Structure of Myocardium	Other Findings
1. Grayzel & Tennant[5] 1934	F	9 hours	Cyanosis	19*	Atresia, tricuspid valve; VSD (2). Origin rt. PA from As.Ao; CS → LA & RA; PDA; PFO; hypoplasia, RV, PV, PA	Normal			Atelectasis, lungs. Hemorrhage, cerebellum
2. Limbourg[6] 1937	M	10 days	Cyanosis Unconsciousness	15	PDA	Normal		Fat droplets, focal, in myocardial fibers	Hemorrhage, subarachnoid, from tentorial tear Atelectasis, lungs
3. Williams, Johnson, Boulware[7] 1951	F	4 days	"Normal" Cyanosis on 2nd day, Systolic murmur	36	VSD, PS, PDA, PFO	Normal			
5. Tedeschi & Helpern[3] 1954	F	13 days	Cyanosis Dyspnea	39	PDA	Normal	Thickening of walls due to intimal fibrous proliferation & focal edema of media & adventitia	Norma	0
4. Swann & Werthammer[9] (Case 3) 1955	M	2 days	Cyanosis Dyspnea	56	PDA, PFO	Normal		Hypertrophy of myocardial fibers of both RV & LV. Fat positive vacuoles in myocardial fibers	Congestive heart failure
6. Alexander & Griffith[10] 1956	M	2 days	Cyanosis		PDA, PFO	Normal			Atelectasis, lungs
7. Schulze & Rodin[11] 1961	F	8 hours	Cyanosis	18	PDA	Normal	Vein-like	Nuclear pyknosis, loss of cross-striations, & interstitial edema with inflammatory cell infiltration	Congestive heart failure. Hyaline membrane disease, lungs
8. Present Author 1961	M	7 days	Cyanosis Dyspnea	27	0	Normal	Arterial	Normal	Atelectasis, lungs. Congestive heart failure

* Average normal heart weight for full-term newborn = 17 gms.
VSD = ventricular septal defect; PV = pulmonic valve; RV = right ventricle; CS = coronary sinus; LA = left atrium; RA = right atrium; PDA = patent ductus arteriosus; PS = pulmonic stenosis; PFO = patent foramen ovale; PA = pulmonary artery; As.Ao. = ascending aorta.

the vein-like structure reported by Schulze and Rodin[11] or the intimal fibrous proliferation observed by Tedeschi and Helpern.[8] Although there may be some focal degenerative changes of the myocardial fibers suggestive of ischemia, there is no fibrous scarring nor other evidence of myocardial infarction. Major associated congenital cardiac defects have been recorded twice. The patient reported by Grayzel and Tennant[5] had tricuspid atresia, two ventricular septal defects, anomalous drainage of the coronary sinus into the left atrium, and origin of the right pulmonary artery from the ascending aorta. An anatomic tetralogy of Fallot was present in the patient described by Williams et al.[7] The lungs are usually collapsed and congested.

Mechanism for Heart Failure: The clinical manifestations of double anomalous coronary arteries appear to be attributable to left ventricular failure. It is now well established[3, 4, 13] that when only the left coronary artery arises anomalously from the pulmonary artery, the blood contained in the aberrant vessel is fully saturated and flows away from the left ventricle in a retrograde fashion toward the pulmonary artery. When both coronary arteries arise from the pulmonary artery, however, blood in the anomalous vessels is poorly saturated and flows from the pulmonary artery toward the myocardium.

The lowered oxygen content of the blood in the anomalous coronary arteries is certainly not the cause of the left ventricular failure. Some patients with congenital cyanotic heart disease and normally arising coronary arteries have an arterial oxygen saturation below that of venous blood and live for a number of years. The heart failure appears to be the result of low perfusion pressure in the two anomalous coronary arteries. At birth, the pressures in the right ventricle and in the pulmonary trunk are at or near normal systemic levels. Within a matter of hours or days after birth, however, the pressure in the pulmonary artery falls, and consequently, in patients with both coronary arteries arising from the pulmonary artery, the coronary arterial perfusion pressure diminishes. Finally, about two weeks following birth, the perfusion pressure apparently is completely inadequate to supply the nutritional requirements of the left ventricle, and life ends.

Surgical therapy in this condition would necessarily be directed toward increasing the coronary arterial perfusion pressure. Theoretically, this could be done by either transplanting or connecting the ostia of the coronary arteries with a systemic artery, or by constricting the pulmonary trunk above the anomalous coronary arterial ostia. Obviously, neither of these procedures has been performed in a patient with double anomalous coronary arteries. However, each procedure has been carried out in patients with an aberrant left coronary artery arising from the pulmonary artery. Mustard[14] ligated the anomalous left coronary artery in his patient and anastomosed it to a systemic artery. He demonstrated that this procedure was technically feasible, but his patient died eight hours following operation. An operating dissecting microscope may be of real use in this procedure. Morrow[3] constricted the pulmonary trunk in a patient with an aberrant left coronary artery, but ventricular fibrillation occurred after completion of the supravalvular pulmonic stenosis, and the patient died.

Embryology: The embryologic basis for anomalous development of both coronary arteries from the pulmonary artery has recently been thoroughly reviewed by Schulze and Rodin.[11] Briefly, two theories, septal deviation and involution-persistence, have received considerable attention. Abrikossoff[14] suggested that either the truncus arteriosus is abnormally divided so that the two coronary anlagen are included with the pulmonary artery (Figure 4), or that a coronary bud arises anomalously from a part of the truncus destined to become the pulmonary artery. The involution-persistence theory suggested recently by Hackensellner[15] provides explanations for several anomalies of the coronary arteries which the former theories failed to do, and it appears more acceptable. He described the occurrence of

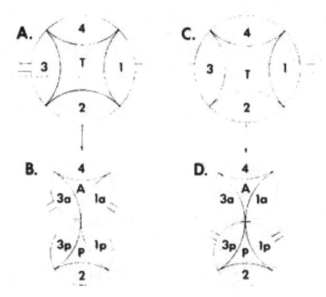

Figure 4 *Illustration to demonstrate Abrikossoff's theory of normal and abnormal development of the coronary arteries.* A and B, normal division of the truncus arteriosus by a septum (dotted line) so that two coronary anlagen are included with the aorta. C and D, abnormal division of the truncus arteriosus by a deviated septum so that the two coronary anlagen are included with the pulmonary artery. T = truncus arteriosus; A = aorta; P = pulmonary artery; 1a = left aortic valve cusp; 3a = right aortic valve cusp; 1p = left pulmonic valve cusp; 3p = right pulmonic valve cusp; 2 = anterior pulmonic valve cusp; 4 = posterior aortic valve cusp.

an anlage of a coronary artery in each of the six regions of the semilunar valves of the aorta and pulmonary trunk. Normally, permanent coronary arteries arise from anlagen in two aortic sinuses, and the anlagen in the other aortic and in all three pulmonic valvular sinuses either are not formed or are rapidly involuted (Figure 5). Thus, the combination of persistence of two normally involuted pulmonary coronary buds and involution of two normally persistent aortic coronary buds would result in anomalous origin of both coronary arteries.

SUMMARY

The clinical and pathologic features of a 7 day old infant in whom both coronary arteries arose from the pulmonary artery is presented, and information derived from the 7 previously reported patients with this anomaly is summarized. Characteristically, these infants have cyanosis and dyspnea at birth or shortly thereafter, cardiac enlargement and no heart murmur, and rapidly progress to heart failure. All reported patients with this condition have died within two weeks after birth. None of the reported patients with double anomalous coronary arteries has been diagnosed ante mortem.

ACKNOWLEDGMENTS

I wish to thank Dr. Benjamin Highman, Chief, Section of Pathology Anatomy, Laboratory of Experimental Pathology, National Institute of Arthritis and Metabolic

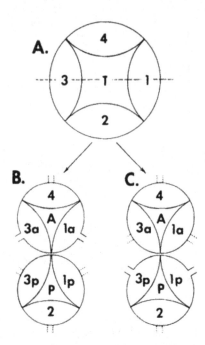

Figure 5 *Illustration to demonstrate Hackensellner's theory of normal and abnormal development of the coronary arteries.* A, normal division of the truncus arteriosus before formation of coronary anlagen. B, normal involution of all coronary anlagen (dotted lines) except the two that arise from the right and left aortic valve sinuses. C, involution of the two normally persisting aortic coronary anlagen (at 3a and 1a), with persistence of two normally involuted pulmonary coronary anlagen (at 3p and 1p). The result is anomalous origin of both coronary arteries from the pulmonary artery.

Diseases, for his kindness in referring this case and for allowing me to publish it. Also, I am grateful to Dr. Louis B. Thomas, Chief of the Surgical and Postmortem Service, National Cancer Institute, and to Dr. Ross C. MacCardle, Laboratory of Pathology, National Cancer Institute, for reviewing the manuscript.

REFERENCES

1. KEITH, J. D. The anomalous origin of the left coronary artery from the pulmonary artery. *Brit. Heart J.*, 21: 149, 1959.
2. BLAND, E. F., WHITE, P. D. and GARLAND, J. Congenital anomalies of coronary arteries. Report of an unusual case associated with cardiac hypertrophy. *Am. Heart J.*, 8: 787, 1933.
3. CASE, R. B., MORROW, A. G., STAINSBY, W. and NESTOR, J. O. Anomalous origin of the left coronary artery. The physiologic defect and suggested surgical treatment. *Circulation*, 17: 1062, 1958.
4. SABISTON, D. C., JR., NEILL, C. A. and TAUSSIG, H. B. The direction of blood flow in anomalous left coronary artery arising from the pulmonary artery. *Circulation*, 22: 591, 1960.
5. GRAYZEL, D. and TENNANT, R. Congenital atresia of tricuspid orifice and anomalous origin of coronary arteries from pulmonary artery. *Am. J. Path.*, 10: 791, 1934.

6. LIMBOURG, M. Uber den Ursprung der Kranzarterien des Herzens aus der Arteria pulmonalis. *Beitr. Path. Anat.*, 100: 191, 1937.

7. WILLIAMS, J. W., JOHNSON, W. S. and BOULWARE, J. R. A case of tetralogy of Fallot with both coronary arteries arising from the pulmonary artery. *J. Florida M. A.*, 37: 561, 1951.

8. TEDESCHI, C. G. and HELPERN, M. M. Heterotopic origin of both coronary arteries from the pulmonary artery. Review of literature and report of a case not complicated by associated defects. *Pediatrics*, 14: 53, 1954.

9. SWANN, W. C. and WERTHAMMER, S. Aberrant coronary arteries. Experiences in diagnosis with report of three cases. *Ann. Int. Med.*, 42: 873, 1955.

10. ALEXANDER, R. W. and GRIFFITH, G. C. Anomalies of the coronary arteries and their clinical significance. *Circulation*, 14: 800, 1956.

11. SCHULZE, W. B. and RODIN, A. E. Anomalous origin of both coronary arteries. Report of a case with discussion of teratogenic theories. *Arch. Path.*, 72: 36, 1961.

12. TAUSSIG, H. B. *Congenital Malformations of the Heart*, p. 324. New York, The Commonwealth Fund, 1947.

13. EDWARDS, J. E. Symposium on cardiovascular diseases. Functional pathology of congenital cardiac disease. *Pediat. Clin. North America*, 1: 13, 1954.

14. ABRIKOSSOFF, A. Aneurysma des linken Herzventrikels mit abnormer Abgangsstelle der linken Koronararterie von der Pulmonalis bei einem fünfmonatlichen Kinde. *Arch. Path. Anat.*, 203: 413, 1911.

15. HACKENSELLNER, H. A. Akzessorsiche Kranzgefässanlagen der Arteria pulmonalis under 63 menschlichen Embryonenserien mit einer grössten Länge von 12 bis 36 mm. *Ztschr. Mikroscopischanat. Forsch.*, 62: 153, 1956.

Case 15 Survival to Adulthood in a Patient with Complete Transposition of the Great Vessels*

Including a Note on the Association of Endocrine Tumors with Heart Disease

William C. Roberts, MD, Dean T. Mason, MD, and Eugene Braunwald, MD
Bethesda, Maryland

THE MAJORITY OF PATIENTS with complete transposition of the great vessels die in infancy. The subject of this paper is a man who lived for 21 years with this malformation, which was associated with several other cardiac defects. A Blalock-Taussig procedure had been performed at the age of 10 years. An adrenal cortical tumor was discovered at autopsy, and this finding provided the stimulus to review the association of endocrine tumors with heart disease.

REPORT OF PATIENT

A 21-year-old white man, a furniture maker, was admitted to the National Heart Institute on September 20, 1961. A heart murmur and cyanosis had been discovered in infancy. Growth and development had been subnormal, and fatigue, dyspnea, and squatting on exertion had been noted frequently. At the age of 10 years, a diagnosis of tetralogy of Fallot was made at another hospital following an angiogram, and a left subclavian-left pulmonary arterial anastomosis was performed. Following surgery, cardiac symptoms and cyanosis decreased, and the patient was able to finish high school and subsequently to maintain a good employment record. In September 1960, cyanosis began to increase progressively and in June 1961, the patient suddenly developed right hemiparesis and was hospitalized. Hematocrit reading at the time was 70%. It was believed that he had had a cerebral thrombosis, and he was treated with serial phlebotomies, anticoagulants, and physical therapy.

On admission to the Clinical Center, he was critically ill, and had marked generalized cyanosis and digital clubbing. Blood pressure was 120/80 mm Hg, and pulse rate was 110/min. There were slight bilateral papilledema and retinal venous congestion. The neck veins were flat, the lungs, clear, and the extremities and sacrum, free of edema. There were a prominent right ventricular lift, a loud, single, palpable, basal second sound, and a coarse grade 4/6 systolic ejection murmur in the third left intercostal space. The patient had an expressive aphasia, right facial paralysis, right spastic hemiparesis, and bilateral extensor plantar responses.

Hematocrit reading was 55%; the white blood cell count, platelets, and serum electrolytes were normal except for a sodium value of 129 mEq/ liter; blood cultures were sterile; cerebrospinal fluid, skull, and sinus roentgenograms were normal. An

Received May 11, 1962; accepted for publication May 29, 1962.
* From the Pathologic Anatomy Department, Clinical Center, and Cardiology Branch, National Heart Institute, National Institutes of Health, Bethesda, Maryland.
Requests for reprints should be addressed to William C. Roberts, M.D., Department of Medicine, The Johns Hopkins Hospital, Baltimore 5, Maryland.

DOI: 10.1201/9781003409342-4

electrocardiogram (Figure 1) disclosed a vertical upright electrical axis, first degree atrioventricular block, and right ventricular hypertrophy. A chest roentgenogram (Figure 2) showed a slightly enlarged heart, diminished pulmonary vascularity, and a concavity in the region of the pulmonary artery. A phonocardiogram (Figure 3) revealed a complex first sound at the base, which contained an atrial sound, an atrioventricular valve closure sound, and an aortic ejection sound. The second sound at

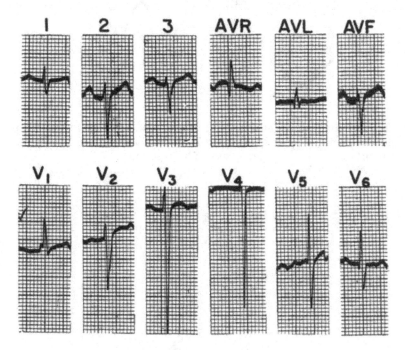

Figure 1 Electrocardiogram.

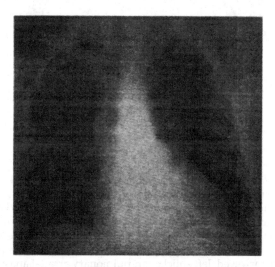

Figure 2 Anteroposterior roentgenogram.

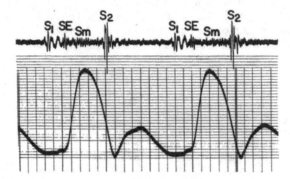

Figure 3 Phonocardiogram recorded in the second right intercostal space and simultaneous indirect carotid pulse tracing. S_1, first heart sound; SE, systolic ejection sound; Sm, systolic murmur; S_2, second heart sound.

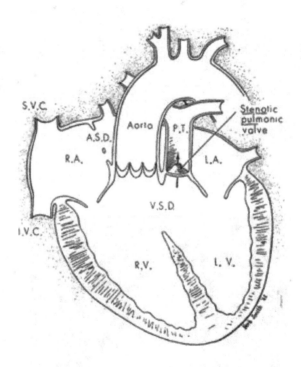

Figure 4 Diagram depicting the multiple cardiac anomalies in this patient. There is complete transposition of the great vessels, with the aorta arising entirely from the right ventricle, and the pulmonary trunk exclusively from the left ventricle. Several defects are present in the atrial septum, and one large defect is present in the basal portion of the ventricular septum. The pulmonic valve is stenotic, and the pulmonary trunk, relatively hypoplastic. All cardiac chambers are dilated. The patent, although narrowed, left subclavian-pulmonary arterial anastomosis and the bronchial arterial collateral circulation are not shown in this diagram.

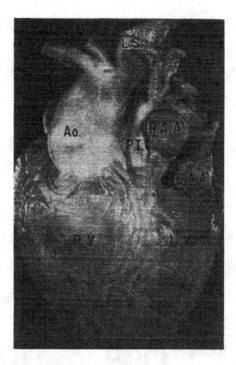

Figure 5 Anterior view of the heart (550 g). The ascending aorta (Ao) arises to the right of, and anterior to, the pulmonary trunk (P.T.). The left subclavian (L.S.)—left pulmonary arterial anastomosis is intact. Both atrial appendages lay to the left of the pulmonary trunk and adjacent to one another. The right appendage (R.A.A.) is the larger one and lies to the right of the left atrial appendage (L.A.A.). Both ventricles (R.V. and L.V.) are dilated and hypertrophied.

the base was single in all phases of respiration, and appeared to be produced by aortic valve closure. A long systolic murmur which reached aortic valve closure was recorded at the base, and a continuous murmur was recorded over the left sternal border.

The life-threatening neurological complications prevented definitive evaluation of the patient's cyanotic congenital heart disease. His condition progressively deteriorated, and on the ninth hospital day he had a generalized seizure and became semicomatose. During the next 3 days additional seizures occurred, and, despite large doses of anticonvulsants, he became comatose and died.

PATHOLOGIC FINDINGS

The pathologico-anatomic features of the heart and great vessels are described in Figures 4–8. There was complete transposition of the great vessels; also, there were atrial and ventricular septal defects, valvular pulmonic stenosis, juxtaposition of the atrial appendages, and collateral bronchial arterial circulation. Vascular thrombi were widespread. There were both old and recent thrombi occluding the superior sagittal sinus, the left middle cerebral and mesenteric arteries, and right iliac, femoral, and splenic veins. Multiple infarcts were present in the liver, spleen, and left lung. The lungs and viscera were acutely and chronically congested. The right adrenal gland was normal, but the left one contained a large, well-circumscribed

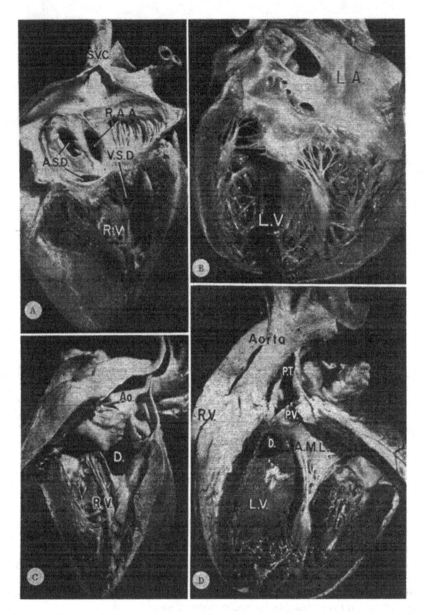

Figure 6 Photographs showing the interior of the cardiac chambers. *A*. The right atrium and right ventricle (R.V.) are opened. Defects (A.S.D.) are present in both the mid and lowermost portions of the atrial septum. The opening into the right atrial appendage (R.A.A.) is located immediately anterior to the largest atrial septal defect. The ventricular septal defect (V.S.D.) is located behind the junction of the anterior and septal tricuspid valve leaflets. The superior vena cava (S.V.C.) is designated. *B*. The left atrium (L.A.) and left ventricle (L.V.) are opened. The multiple defects in the atrial septum are apparent. The mitral valve is normal. Many recent ante-mortem thrombi are interspersed among the trabeculae carneae muscles in the apex of the left ventricle. *C*. The ascending aorta (Ao.) and right ventricle (R.V.) are opened.

Figure 6 (Continued) Probes are placed in each of the ostia of the coronary arteries. Note that there is no connection between the tricuspid and aortic valves. The ventricular septal defect (D), which measures 2.5 × 3 cm in size, is located immediately below the aortic valve cusps and is bordered anteriorly, posteriorly, and caudally by ventricular myocardium. The right ventricular wall is greatly hypertrophied. *D.* The pulmonary trunk (P.T.), pulmonic valve (P.V.), and left ventricle (L.V.) are opened. The stenotic, dome-shaped pulmonic valve is continuous with the anterior mitral leaflet (A.M.L.). The pulmonary trunk (P.T.) is small and the ascending aorta, dilated. There is a rim of myocardium between the pulmonic valve and the cephalic margin of the ventricular septal defect (D). Both atrial appendages are visible to the left of the pulmonary trunk.

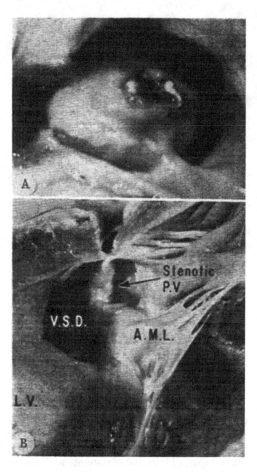

Figure 7 Photographs demonstrating the pulmonic valve before it was opened. *A.* The domeshaped pulmonic valve, which is fibrotic and partially calcified, as viewed from above. *B.* The stenotic pulmonic valve (P.V.) as seen from the left ventricular (L.V.) aspect. The ventricular septal defect (V.S.D.) and the anterior mitral leaflet (A.M.L.) are apparent.

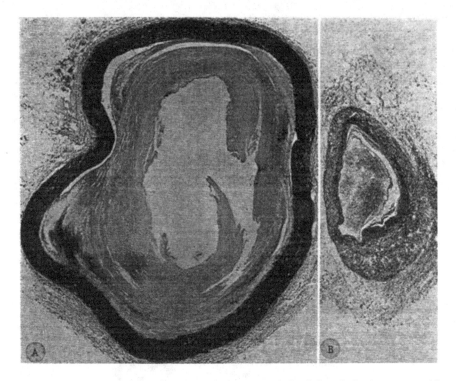

Figure 8 Photomicrographs of cross-sections of the left subclavian artery (*A*), which was anastomosed to the left main pulmonary artery (Blalock-Taussig procedure), and closed ductus arteriosus (*B*). In A, note the marked intimal fibrous proliferation. The intima of the adjoining aorta and main left pulmonary artery, in contrast, was free of fibrosis. The fibrous proliferation on the intimal surface is believed to be the result of a "jet lesion." In B, note the large number of elastic fibers (stained black) in the occluded lumen. Verhoeff-van Gieson elastic tissue stain; original magnification of each, × 17.

nodule, which weighed 36 grams, and which showed histologically a pleomorphic collection of cells which invaded the capsule (Figure 9). No metastases, however, were found.

COMMENTS

This patient represents the longest survival of an individual whose major cardiovascular anomaly was complete transposition of the great vessels. This 21-year-old man, however, had had a Blalock-Taussig anastomosis at the age of 10 years, and this procedure apparently lengthened his life span. Previous reports record only 4 instances, proven by autopsy, of survival of patients with this malformation to the age of 10 years or longer[1-4]; the oldest of these cases lived for 18 years.[3] Other patients, who have been described as having complete transposition and who lived into adulthood, should be classified instead under their major cardiac defect (usually tricuspid atresia or single ventricle).[5-8] The 44-year-old patient reported by Carns, Ritchie, and Musser[9] probably had corrected transposition of the great vessels, rather than the complete ("uncorrected") variety. The 38-year-old patient reported by Messeloff

42

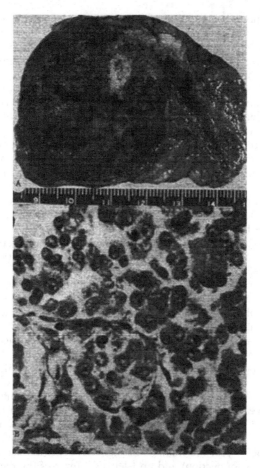

Figure 9 A. Photograph of the left adrenal gland containing a well-circumscribed adrenal-cortical tumor. There is considerable focal hemorrhagic necrosis of the tumor. B. Photomicrograph of the adrenal tumor shown in A. Original magnification, × 610.

and Weaver[10] also had partial anomalous pulmonary venous connection. Since this anomaly provided partial physiologic "correction," this case probably should be excluded from a consideration of patients with complete transposition of the great vessels in which the venous connections of the heart are normal.

Of the 5 patients with complete transposition who survived to the age of 10 years or longer, only 2 possessed more than one communication between the 2 circulations. In addition to the present case, Keith's patient[4] also had ventricular and atrial septal defects, as well as pulmonic stenosis. Hanlon and Blalock[11] showed that the length of survival in complete transposition is related to the number of defects present, namely, ventricular and atrial septal defects, patent ductus arteriosus, and collateral bronchial arterial circulation. In their series, the single compensating abnormality associated with the longest life expectancy was a ventricular septal defect; an atrial defect was the next most favorable isolated defect, and the combination of these 2 provided the best prognosis of all.

Pulmonic stenosis is also a favorable lesion in patients with complete transposition, since it prevents excessive pulmonary blood flow, allows more left to right shunting through the intracardiac communications, and, consequently, more saturated blood enters the systemic circuit. In a review of complete transposition of the great vessels, pulmonic stenosis was found in more than a third of the cases.[12] Lev, Alcalde, and Baffes[13] mention that the pulmonic stenosis in complete transposition "is almost, if not always, some distance from the pulmonary orifice and may be so-called 'subpulmonary' or 'left infundibular.'" The stenosis in the present patient, however, clearly involved only the valve.

The occurrence of both atrial appendages on the same side of the great vessels (juxtaposition) is more than an anatomical curiosity. Although this anomaly is of no functional significance, it may be interpreted on angiocardiography as an atrial aneurysm or pathologic diverticulum. During open heart surgery, the absence of a normally situated right atrial appendage might present the surgeon with considerable technical difficulty at cannulation. At least 20 examples of juxtaposition of the atrial appendages have been recorded; both appendages lay to the left of the great vessels in 18 (left juxtaposition), and both to the right (right juxtaposition), in 2.[14–16] All 20 had transposition of the great vessels and, frequently, tricuspid atresia or pulmonic stenosis.

In 1960, Bartter and associates[17] reported a cyanotic 25-year-old man who died with congenital heart disease and an endocrine tumor. This patient, who presented with the clinical picture of Cushing's syndrome, had total anomalous pulmonary venous connection, pituitary (? chromophobe) adenoma, and bilateral adrenal cortical hyperplasia. Since that time, 4 other patients with heart disease and an endocrine tumor have been autopsied at the Clinical Center. Three of these patients had unilateral adrenal cortical tumors, which were not apparent clinically. The patient described in this report had a pleomorphic adrenal cortical carcinoma, which invaded the capsule but did not metastasize; the other 2 patients, acyanotic men aged 57 and 48 years with isolated calcific aortic stenosis, each had large (4 by 3 centimeters and 2 by 2 centimeters, respectively), histologically uniform adrenal cortical adenomas which neither invaded the capsule nor metastasized. The fifth patient, a cyanotic 46-year-old man, had congenital heart disease (total anomalous pulmonary venous connection) and an islet cell tumor of the pancreas, not clinically apparent, which metastasized to the peripancreatic lymph nodes. In summary, of nearly 300 patients with congenital or rheumatic heart disease autopsied at the Clinical Center, 5 had associated endocrine tumors. All of these cases were adults; 3 had congenital malformations of the heart and great vessels leading to cyanosis, 2 had isolated calcific aortic stenosis of uncertain etiology, and in 4 the tumors involved the pituitary-adrenal axis. This association appears to be more than mere coincidence. Four patients in whom pheochromocytoma was associated with cyanotic congenital heart disease have been observed at The Johns Hopkins Hospital.[18] This association of adrenal tumors with cyanotic congenital heart disease conceivably could be related to the stress produced by prolonged hypoxemia.

SUMMARY

A man is described who lived for 21 years with complete transposition of the great vessels. He is believed to represent the oldest pathologically proven instance of complete transposition. Associated abnormalities included valvular pulmonic stenosis, ventricular and atrial septal defects, and collateral bronchial arterial circulation. A Blalock-Taussig anastomosis, in combination with these associated defects, may have been responsible for the patient's long survival. Left juxtaposition of the atrial appendages was an additional anomaly. An unilateral adrenal-cortical carcinoma was found at autopsy, and the association of endocrine tumors with heart disease, particularly of the cyanotic variety, may be more than mere coincidence.

SUMMARIO IN INTERLINGUA

Es describite un homine qui viveva 21 annos con transposition complete del grande vasos. Es opinate que iste patiente representa le plus perdurative, pathologicamente verificate caso de transposition complete. Le associate anormalitates includeva stenosis pulmono-valvular, defactos septal ventricular e atrial, e circulation broncho-arterial collateral. Un anastomosis Blalock-Taussig in combination con le mentionate associate defectos esseva possibilemente responsabile pro le longe superviventia del patiente. Juxtaposition sinistre del appendice atrial esseva un anormalitate additional. Un unilateral carcinoma adreno cortical esseva trovate al necropsia. Le association de tumores endocrin con morbo cardiac, particularmente morbo cardiac de typo cyanotic, es possibilemente plus que un coincidentia. Inter quasi 300 patientes con congenite o rheumatic morbo cardiac qui esseva necropsiate al Centro Clinic, 5 habeva associate tumores endocrin. In omne iste casos il se tractava de adultos. Tres habeva malformationes congenite del corde o del grande vasos con resultante cyanosis; 2 habeva isolate calcific stenosis aortic de incerte etiologia; e in 4 le tumores afficeva le axe pituitarioadrenal.

REFERENCES

1. DORNING, J.: A case of transposition of the aorta and pulmonary artery, with patent foramen ovale; death at ten years of age. *Trans. Amer. Pediat. Soc.* 2: 46, 1890.
2. ALEXANDER, F., WHITE, P. D.: Four important congenital cardiac conditions causing cyanosis to be differentiated from the tetralogy of Fallot: tricuspid atresia, Eisenmenger's complex, transposition of the great vessels, and a single ventricle. *Ann. Intern. Med.* 27: 64, 1947.
3. PUNG, S., GOTTSTEIN, W. K., HIRSCH, E. F.: Complete transposition of the great vessels in a male aged 18 years. *Amer. J. Med.* 18: 155, 1955.
4. KEITH, A.: Six specimens of abnormal heart. *J. Anat. Physiol.* 46: 211, 1911–1912.
5. NASSE, F.: *Leichenöffnungen: zur Diagnostik und Pathologischen Anatomie. Bildungsfehler des Herzens in Einem Falle von Blauer Krankheit*, Adolph Marchus, Bonn, 1821, pp. 162–194.
6. HEDINGER, E.: Transposition der grossen Gefässe bei rudimentärer linker Herzkammer bei einer 56 jährigen Frau. *Zbl. Allg. Path.* 26: 529, 1915.
7. MARCHAND: Cited by Hedinger (6).
8. LEWIS, F. T., ABBOTT, M.: Reversed torsion of the human heart. *Anat. Rec.* 9: 103, 1915.
9. CARNS, M. L., RITCHIE, G., MUSSER, M. J.: An unusual case of congenital heart disease in a woman who lived for forty-four years and six months. *Amer. Heart J.* 21: 522, 1941.
10. MESSELOFF, C. R., WEAVER, J. C.: A case of transposition of the large vessels in an adult who lived to the age of 38 years. *Amer. Heart J.* 42: 467, 1951.
11. HANLON, C. R., BLALOCK, A.: Complete transposition of the aorta and the pulmonary artery. Experimental observations on venous shunts as corrective procedures. *Ann. Surg.* 127: 385, 1948.
12. BECKER, M. C., BRILL, R. M.: Complete transposition of the great vessels; report of three cases and a review of the literature. *Arch. Pediat.* 65: 249, 1958.
13. LEV, M., ALCALDE, V. M., BAFFES, T. G.: Pathologic anatomy of complete transposition of the arterial trunks. *Pediatrics* 28: 293, 1961.
14. DIXON, A. ST. J.: Juxtaposition of the atrial appendages: two cases of an unusual congenital cardiac deformity. *Brit. Heart J.* 16: 153, 1954.
15. SMYTH, N. P. D.: Lateroposition of the atrial appendages. A case of levoposition of the appendages. *Arch. Path.* 60: 259, 1955.

16. FRAGOYANNIS, S. G., NICHERSON, D.: An unusual congenital heart anomaly. Tricuspid atresia, aortic atresia, and juxtaposition of atrial appendages. *Amer. J. Cardiol.* 6: 678, 1960.

17. BARTTER, F. C., LIDDLE, G. W., BELL, N. H., BRAUNWALD, E., HILBISH, T. G., CORNELL, W., HICKLIN, M.: Problem in differential diagnosis: clinical pathological conference at the National Institutes of Health. *Ann. Intern. Med.* 52: 1289, 1960.

18. ROSS, R. S., CARPENTER, C. C. J., GLANCY, D. L.: Personal communication.

Case 16 Combined Congenital Pulmonic and Mitral Stenosis*

William C. Roberts, MD†, Allan Goldblatt, MD‡, Dean T. Mason, MD§ and Andrew G. Morrow, MD¶
Bethesda, Maryland

IN AN OCCASIONAL patient with rheumatic mitral stenosis tricuspid stenosis is present as well. In the combined lesion the usual symptoms and signs of mitral stenosis may be absent since the obstruction in the right side of the heart tends to prevent pulmonary vascular congestion. The occurrence of a right-sided stenotic lesion in a patient with congenital mitral stenosis, on the other hand, has not previously been described. Such a case was seen, however, in a three-year-old, poorly developed girl who fatigued easily and periodically had signs of right-sided cardiac failure. Examination disclosed a loud (Grade 4 of 6) ejection-type systolic murmur over the pulmonic area, but no precordial diastolic murmur was either audible or recordable. An electrocardiogram showed right-axis deviation and hypertrophy of the right ventricle and atrium, and a roentgenogram of the chest disclosed enlargement of the left atrium as well as the right atrium and ventricle. Cardiac catherization (Figure 1) and a cineangiogram of the right ventricle confirmed the clinical impression of congenital pulmonic stenosis but also aroused suspicion of a left-sided cardiac lesion since the pressure in the left atrium was elevated (Figure 2). After direct measurement of the pressure in the left ventricle, which was normal, a pulmonary valvulotomy was performed. After release of the right-sided obstruction no immediate change was observed in the already elevated pressure in the left atrium (Figure 2), but the pulmonary arterial systolic pressure was noted to be considerably elevated (Figure 3). The patient died suddenly one day after operation, and at autopsy the mitral valve was also found to be congenitally stenotic (Figure 4).

This case (Figure 5) demonstrates the possible consequences of releasing the right-sided cardiac obstruction without also relieving the left-sided valvular stenosis. The lungs are suddenly overfilled with blood since the runoff from the lungs is unable to keep pace with the inflow to the lungs. In a review of 43 patients with congenital mitral stenosis none had an associated pulmonic stenosis, and only 1 lived for more than three years.[1] The right-sided cardiac obstruction in the patient described above appears to have allowed considerably longer

* From the Pathologic Anatomy Department, Clinical Center and Cardiology Branch and Clinic of Surgery, National Heart Institute, National Institutes of Health, United States Public Health Service.

† Assistant resident, Osler Medical Service, Johns Hopkins Hospital, Baltimore, Maryland; formerly, resident, Pathologic Anatomy Department, Clinical Center, National Institutes of Health, Bethesda, Maryland.

‡ Resident, Children's Hospital Medical Center, Boston, Massachusetts; formerly, pediatric associate, Cardiology Branch, National Heart Institute, Bethesda, Maryland.

§ Clinical associate, Cardiology Branch, National Heart Institute.

¶ Chief, Clinic of Surgery, National Heart Institute.

DOI: 10.1201/9781003409342-5

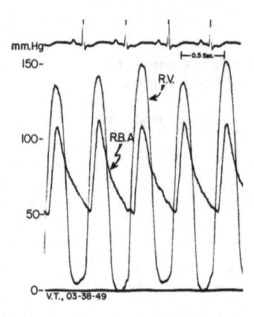

Figure 1 Simultaneously recorded pressure pulses in the right ventricle (R.V.) and brachial artery (R.B.A.), demonstrating ventricular hypertension secondary to pulmonic-valve stenosis. The pulmonary trunk could not be entered by the catheter.

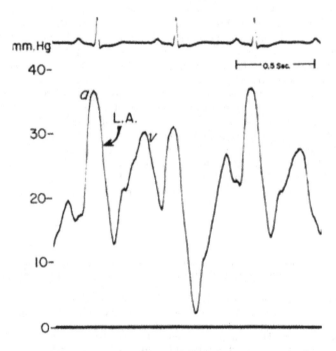

Figure 2 Preoperative pressure tracing of the left atrium (L.A.). The pressure by direct puncture after the pulmonic valvulotomy was identical to this preoperative recording; the mean pressure is 25 mm. of mercury.

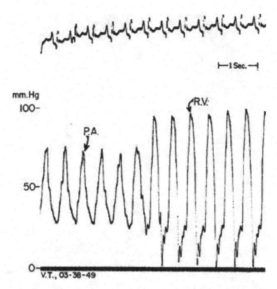

Figure 3 Continuous pressure tracing of the pulmonary artery (P.A.) and right ventricle (R.V.) by direct puncture after operation. A residual pulmonic-valve systolic gradient is evident, as well as pulmonary hypertension.

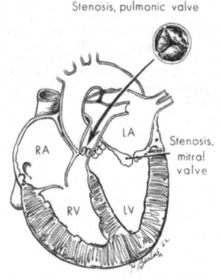

Figure 4 Diagram of the heart in the patient described. The mitral-valve leaflets are fibrotic, thickened and shortened and insert at times directly into the papillary muscles. The remaining chordae tendineae are fused, thickened and shortened. The left atrium is dilated, and its endocardium diffusely thickened. The pulmonic valve is stenotic. Three distinct pulmonic-valve cusps are identified. Each is thickened and fibrotic, but the commissures are not fused. The orifice of the pulmonic valve is centrally located. (It is unusual for a tricuspid pulmonic valve to produce stenosis, but this clearly occurred in the present patient; in most patients with valvular pulmonic stenosis the valve has a dome shape without distinct commissures.) The wall of the right ventricle is greatly hypertrophied, being thicker than that of the left ventricle. The aortic and tricuspid valves are normal. RA = right atrium; RV = right ventricle; LA = left atrium; and LV = left ventricle.

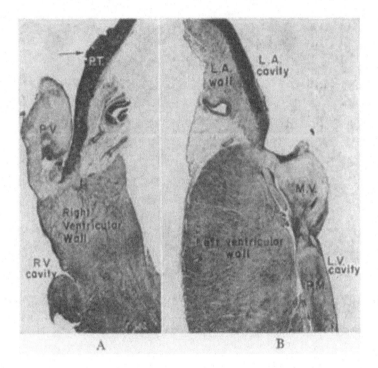

Figure 5 Photomicrographs (Verhoeff—Van Gieson elastic-tissue stains; original magnification X6 for A and X5 for B) of sections through the pulmonic (*A*) and mitral valves (*B*). The leaflets of each valve are markedly thickened by fibrous proliferation. The arrow (left) points to a jet lesion on the intima of the pulmonary trunk (P.T.) just above the pulmonicvalve cusp (P.V.). The posterior leaflet of the mitral valve (M.V.) inserts directly into the papillary muscle (P.M.). There is secondary endocardial fibro-elastosis of the left atrium (L.A.).

survival than would have resulted if the stenosis of the mitral valve had been an isolated lesion.

REFERENCE

1. Ferencz, C., Johnson, A. L., and Wiglesworth, F. W. Congenital mitral stenosis. *Circulation* **9**:161–179, 1954.

Case 17 The Significance of Asplenia in the Recognition of Inoperable Congenital Heart Disease

William C. Roberts, MD, William B. Berry, MD, and Andrew G. Morrow, MD

SPLENIC AGENESIS in association with congenital heart disease implies the presence of multiple and complex malformations of the heart and great vessels,[1-3] and consequently inoperable cardiac disease.[3] Such was the case in an extremely cyanotic and dyspneic 3-month-old male infant with no cardiac murmur. The electrocardiogram showed right axis deviation, and suggested right atrial enlargement, right ventricular hypertrophy, and abnormal positioning of the ventricles. Chest roentgenogram (Figure 1) disclosed a normal-sized, normally located heart and a right-sided gastric air bubble. Selective angiocardiography (Figure 2) showed transposition of the great vessels, a single ventricle, a right aortic arch, and probable pulmonic valvular and subvalvular stenosis. Necropsy following sudden death revealed additional malformations (Figures 3 and 4).

This patient demonstrates the syndrome of splenic agenesis, partial situs inversus, and multiple congenital cardiovascular anomalies. Approximately 100 patients with this entity have been reported. All of the more common malformations of the heart and great vessels associated with this syndrome are illustrated in the patient described herein. The complexity of the cardiac disorders can be determined only by intracardiac catheterization and usually by angiocardiography. The diagnosis of asplenia, on the other hand, frequently may be made simply by study of the peripheral blood smear. Howell-Jolly bodies or siderotic granules in the erythrocytes of the peripheral blood for practical purposes indicate an absent spleen.[3] The presence of situs inversus, which often suggests that asplenia also exists, can usually be determined by routine radiographic examination. The gastric air bubble on the right means situs inversus. The upright abdominal roentgenogram is extremely helpful in determining the presence or absence of the spleen and will frequently demonstrate the anteroinferior margin of the liver on the left, and also flattening of this margin.[4]

From the Pathologic Anatomy Department, Clinical Center, and the Clinic of Surgery, National Heart Institute, National Institutes of Health, Bethesda, Maryland.

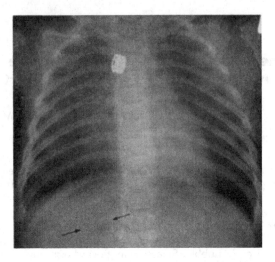

Figure 1 Chest roentgenogram in the patient (A59–151) presented. The prominent shadow at the left upper cardiac border is produced by the dilated, transposed ascending aorta, and not by the pulmonary trunk, which is small and lies to the right of the ascending aorta. The gastric air bubble on the right is designated by the arrows.

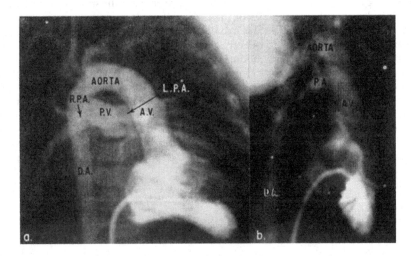

Figure 2 Angiocardiograms. The contrast material is injected into the systemic ventricle. *a.* Anteroposterior projection showing that the aortic valve (A.V.) lies directly to the left of the pulmonic valve (P.V.), and that the two semilunar valves are on the same frontal plane. The rudimentary chamber proximal to the pulmonic valve appears to be filled in a retrograde fashion, since no contrast material is seen entering this subvalvular outflow tract from the systemic ventricle. The aorta descends (D.A.) on the right and the great arteries arising from the arch have a mirror-image reverse of normal. The patent ductus arteriosus is not clearly identified. *b.* Lateral view. The aorta arises anteriorly, indicating transposition of the arterial trunks. In this view the pulmonary trunk is apparent directly behind the proximal portion of the ascending aorta.

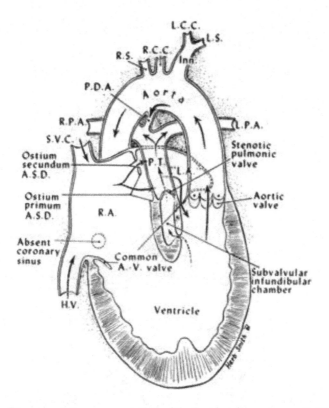

Figure 3 Diagrammatic representation of the heart and great vessels. Blood enters the right atrium (R.A.) through the superior vena cava (S.V.C.) and the hepatic vein (H.V.). The termination of the inferior vena cava was not determined at the time of the original dissection, but it is apparent that this vessel did have an abnormal course. The coronary sinus is absent. Blood in the right atrium either enters the left atrium ("L.A.") through defects in the lowermost and midportions of the atrial septum, or enters the systemic ventricle directly through a common atrioventricular valve. No vessels are connected to the left atrium, although a small protrusion on its surface suggests a rudimentary vascular bud. The right and left pulmonary veins drain into a common pulmonary vein (shown in figure 4), which in turn terminates by dividing into two branches: the larger one connects to the "left" gastric vein; the smaller one, to the portal vein. The left-sided atrium is anatomically a right atrium in that its wall is composed entirely of pectinate muscles. The systemic ventricle, which is large and thick-walled, functions as a single ventricle. The leaflets of the common AV valve are not continuous with those of either the aortic or pulmonic valves. An intramural opening (0.3 cm. in diameter) below the aortic valve connects the systemic ventricle to a rudimentary, smooth-walled chamber below a stenotic dome-shaped, unicuspid, unicommissural pulmonic valve. The pulmonary trunk is hypoplastic. The aortic valve is located on the same plane and directly to the left of the pulmonic valve. The aorta arises anteriorly and does not cross the pulmonary trunk in its ascent. A small patent ductus arteriosus, which is connected to the right pulmonary artery, is present. The pressure in the systemic ventricle was recorded as 70/5 mm. Hg and the peripheral arterial oxygen saturation was 58 per cent. In summary, there is total anomalous pulmonary and systemic venous drainage, persistent common atrioventricular canal, common ventricle, transposition of the great vessels, stenotic subpulmonary outflow tract with pulmonic valvular stenosis, patent ductus arteriosus, right aortic arch, absent coronary sinus, and anatomic double right atrium.

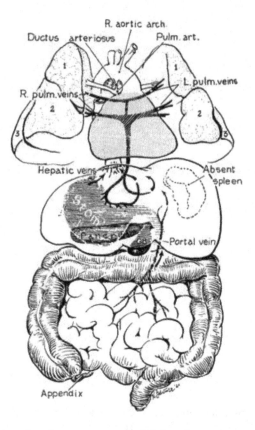

Figure 4 This drawing demonstrates partial situs inversus, symmetrically lobed lungs, and abnormal systemic and pulmonary venous connections in the patient described. The largest lobe of the liver is on the left, the stomach and tail of the pancreas, on the right. The gallbladder is in the midline, and the spleen is absent. The colon and appendix are normally located but the mesenteric attachments of the small intestine are abnormal.

SUMMARY AND CONCLUSION
The finding of asplenia and situs inversus in a patient with congenital heart disease virtually precludes the presence of cardiac lesions which would be benefited by corrective or even palliative surgical procedures.[3]

REFERENCES
1. IVEMARK, B. I.: Implications of agenesis of the spleen on the pathogenesis of cono-truncus anomalies in childhood: An analysis of the heart malformations in the splenic agenesis syndrome, with fourteen new cases. *Acta Paediat.* Suppl. 104, **44**: 110, 1955.
2. PUTSCHAR, W. G. J., AND MANION, W. C.: Congenital absence of the spleen and associated anomalies. *Am. J. Clin. Path.* **26**: 429, 1956.

3. LYONS, W. S., HANLON, D. G., HELMHOLZ, H. F., DUSHANE, J. W., AND EDWARDS, J. E.: Cardiac Clinics. CXLVIII. Congenital cardiac disease and asplenia: Report of seven cases. *Proc. Staff Meet. Mayo Clin.* **32**: 277, 1957.
4. LUCAS, R. V., NEUFELD, H. N., LESTER, R. G., AND EDWARDS, J. E.: The symmetrical liver as a roentgen sign of asplenia. *Circulation* **25**: 973, 1962.

Case 18 Spontaneous Closure of Ventricular Septal Defect*

Anatomic Proof in an Adult with Tricuspid Atresia

William C. Roberts, MD, Andrew G. Morrow, MD, Dean T. Mason, MD, and Eugene Braunwald, MD

SPONTANEOUS CLOSURE of ventricular septal defect has been suspected on the basis of clinical examinations by physicians caring for children with congenital cardiac disease. Confirmative clinical and hemodynamic evidence documenting spontaneous closure of such lesions also have been presented in several recent reports.[1-6] In only one patient, however, has anatomic proof of spontaneous closure of a ventricular septal defect been recorded.[7]

We recently studied an adult patient in whom the diagnosis of tricuspid atresia was established and who died after operation. At autopsy, there was unequivocal evidence that a functional ventricular septal defect had been present and had subsequently closed. The clinical and pathologic observations leading to this concluion are summarized in this report,

CLINICAL SUMMARY

A. H. (No. 03-87-02), a 27-year-old man, had had cyanosis, clubbing, and a precordial murmur since infancy. During childhood and adolescence, fatigue, dyspnea, and repeated upper respiratory infections prevented him from attending school. At the age of 17 a left subclavian-pulmonary arterial anastomosis was performed at another hospital. The cyanosis and dyspnea, however, were only transiently improved, and his physical activity became progressively limited.

On examination he was cyanotic, and there was marked clubbing of the fingers and toes. The heart was enlarged, and a left ventricular thrust was palpable. The second sound at the base was single, and a grade II/VI ejection-type systolic murmur and a faint continuous murmur were heard at the upper left sternal border. The electrocardiogram revealed left ventricular hypertrophy, left axis deviation, left atrial enlargement, and abnormal initial forces indicative of an old anteroseptal myocardial infarct. Fluoroscopic and radiographic examinations disclosed enlargement of the left ventricle and hypoplasia of the pulmonary arterial segment. The hematocrit value was 82 per cent.

At right heart catheterization the catheter passed across an interatrial communication into the left atrium and then into a ventricular chamber, where a pressure of 116/12 mm. Hg and an oxygen saturation of 83 per cent were recorded. Simultaneously, the systemic arterial pressure was 112/66 mm. Hg and systemic arterial oxygen saturation was 88 per cent. Neither the pulmonary artery nor the right ventricle was entered by the catheter. Indicator-dilution curves indicated a

* From the Pathologic Anatomy Department, Clinical Center, and the Clinic of Surgery and Cardiology Branch, National Heart Institute, National Institutes of Health, Bethesda, Maryland.

Dr. Roberts present address is Department of Medicine, The Johns Hopkins Hospital, Baltimore, Maryland.

DOI: 10.1201/9781003409342-7

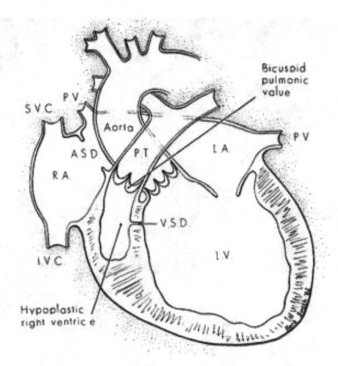

Figure 1 Diagram summarizing the multiple cardiac anomalies in the patient herein described. There is atresia (agenesis) of the tricuspid valve, a large atrial septal defect (A.S.D.), a large left ventricle (L.V.) (functional single ventricle), a ventricular septal defect (V.S.D.) which has closed, and a hypoplastic right ventricle. The pulmonic valve is bicuspid. S.V.C., superior vena cava; I.V.C., inferior vena cava; R.A., right atrium; L.A., left atrium; P.V., pulmonary vein; and P.T., pulmonary trunk.

large right-to-left shunt at the atrial level. A selective angiocardiogram with right atrial injection confirmed the clinical diagnosis of tricuspid atresia.

At operation an anastomosis was created between the distal end of the right pulmonary artery and the proximal end of the superior vena cava. The procedure was complicated by the presence of an extensive collateral circulation between the lung and chest wall, and the patient died in the early postoperative period of massive and uncontrollable bleeding into the pleural space.

PATHOLOGIC FINDINGS

The pertinent patho-anatomic features of the heart are summarized in figure 1 and illustrated in figures 2 through 4. A closed defect was present in the basal portion of the muscular ventricular septum. The gross and microscopic appearance of this lesion is shown in figure 3.

DISCUSSION

In this patient the evidence provided by both gross and microscopic study furnishes proof not only that a ventricular septal defect had been present but that prior to its spontaneous closure it had been of functional significance. This is indicated by the prominent jet lesion still evident in the right ventricle and also by the size of

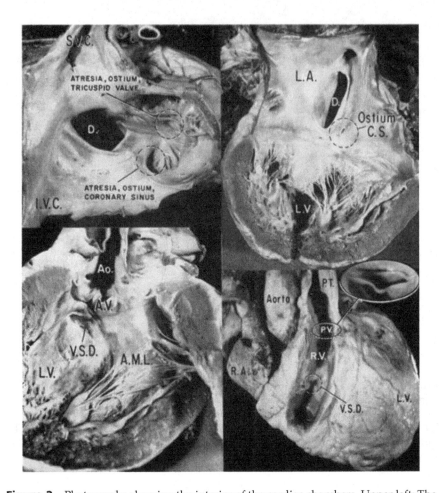

Figure 2 Photographs showing the interior of the cardiac chambers. Upper left: The right atrium. No remnant of the tricuspid valve is present. The ostium of the coronary sinus is also atretic. The atrial septal defect (D.), which measures 3.5 by 2.0 cm., is of the foramen ovale type. The superior (S.V.C.) and inferior (I.V.C.) venae cavae are connected normally to the right atrium. Upper right: The left atrium (L.A.), mitral valve and left ventricle (L.V.). The valve guarding the foramen ovale is totally incompetent resulting in the large atrial septal defect (D.). The dashed circle depicts the communication between the coronary sinus (C.S.) and the left atrium. The left ventricular chamber is considerably dilated and its wall thickened. Lower Left: The ascending aorta (Ao.), aortic valve (A.V.), and septal wall of the left ventricle (L.V.) are shown. The ventricular septal defect (V.S.D.), which has closed, is located immediately below the aortic valve. This view also illustrates the normal continuity between the anterior leaflet of the mitral valve (A.M.L.) and the aortic valve. The ostia of the coronary arteries are apparent. These vessels were widely patent and normally distributed. Lower right: The anterior wall of the hypoplastic right ventricle (R.V.) has been removed, exposing the site of the former defect (V.S.D.) in the muscular ventricular septum. Note the jet lesions on the endocardium of the right ventricle adjacent to the site of the former opening in the ventricular septum. The pulmonic valve (P.V.) and pulmonary trunk (P.T.) are only slightly smaller than normal. Note that the left ventricle (L.V.) accounts for most of the mass of the heart. The inset is the bicuspid pulmonic valve as seen from above. (R.A.) right atrium.

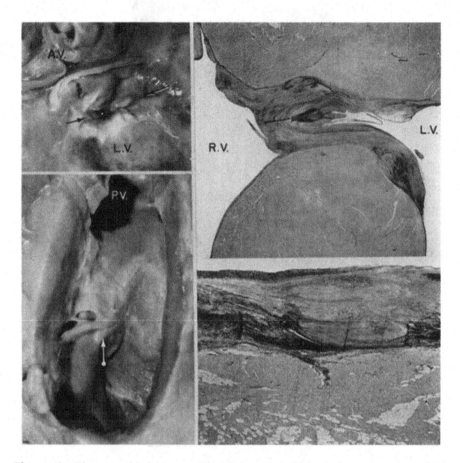

Figure 3 Photographs demonstrating the gross and histologic appearance of the closed ventricular septal defect. Upper left: The closed defect from the left ventricular (L.V.) aspect. The site of the former defect (designated by the arrows) is a linear indentation 1 cm. below the aortic valve (A.V.). The endocardium adjacent to the indentation is elevated, smooth, and pearly white. The endocardial thickening is probably the result of turbulent flow of blood in this area. Lower left: The site of the former defect as viewed from the right ventricular aspect. The anterior wall of the hypoplastic right ventricle has been removed. The depression between the muscle bands is the site of the former defect. The arrow points to the pearly white endocardial thickening, clearly the result of a jet lesion, on the lateral and superior walls of this chamber opposite the depression. (P.V.), pulmonic valve. Upper right: Photomicrograph of a section through the closed defect in the muscular ventricular septum. The entire area of the former defect was blocked, embedded in paraffin, and serially sectioned at intervals of 6 micra. In none of the sections was a residual opening apparent. A representative section is shown here. Note that the actual closure of the defect is produced by fibrous proliferation (jet lesion), and not by direct apposition of the myocardium. No lesions were found in the adjacent myocardium. (R.V.), right ventricle; (L.V.), left ventricle. Verhoeff-Van Gieson elastic tissue stain: original magnification, × 8. Lower right: Photomicrograph of the jet lesion on the laterosuperior aspect of the right ventricle. There is marked fibroelastic thickening of the endocardium. Verhoeff-Van Gieson elastic tissue stain: original magnification, × 21.

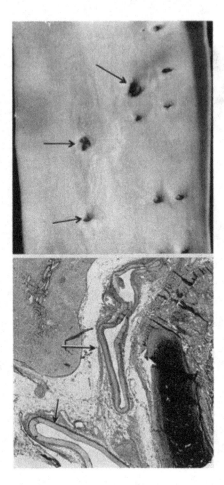

Figure 4 Photographs demonstrating the marked bronchial arterial collateral circulation in the patient described. This patient's relatively long life-span probably can be attributed to the enormous bronchial collateral blood flow which was further augmented by the subclavian-pulmonary arterial anastomosis. Upper: The descending thoracic aorta is opened. The dilated ostia of the bronchial arteries are designated (arrows). Lower: Photomicrograph of a section of lung demonstrating the dilated and thick-walled bronchial arteries (arrows). The bronchial cartilage is on the right. Verhoeff-Van Gieson elastic tissue stain: original magnification, × 16.

the right ventricle. For some time prior to the terminal operation and death, pulmonary blood flow was supplied entirely by systemic collateral vessels and by the subclavian-pulmonary arterial anastomosis. The right ventricle was functionless and received no blood except that minute amount which may have been returned to it from Thebesian vessels or retrograde through the pulmonic valve. Had this situation been present throughout the patient's life, the right ventricle would probably have been atretic. Instead, its cavity, although small, approximated the size of the pulmonary trunk, which was essentially normal. It seems clear, therefore, that the right ventricle attained its size as a result of ejecting blood that was shunted into it when the defect was patent.

Spontaneous closure of a ventricular septal defect is probably a relatively unusual occurrence, and it would appear likely that only those defects whose margins are entirely muscular can do so. Edwards[7] has suggested that the closure of defects of this type, which occur relatively infrequently, may be related to progressive elongation of the myocardial fibers bordering them. Initially the defect may be round or oval but with growth it becomes slit-like and finally its margins approximate each other as the myocardium hypertrophies and stretches. In the elderly patient reported by Edwards closure was apparently effected entirely by apposition of muscle. In the present patient this process also was operative but actual closure resulted from endocardial proliferation, probably stimulated by turbulent blood flow through the defect. In the usual type of ventricular septal defect, involving principally the membranous septum, muscle approximation is impossible and it would seem unlikely that closure of a defect in this location could occur without the superimposition of an active inflammatory process, such as bacterial endocarditis. In this regard, it should be noted that the patient described gave no history suggestive of endocarditis and there were no lesions in the myocardium bordering the closed defect that suggested previous inflammation.

Of additional interest is the prolonged survival of the present patient. Recently Fontana and Edwards[8] reported 125 cases of tricuspid atresia confirmed at autopsy, 119 of which were collected from the literature. Two thirds of these patients died within the first year of life and only eight lived for more than 10 years. Probably the main factor allowing such a long survival in our patient was the extensive bronchial collateral circulation. The left subclavian-pulmonary arterial anastomosis, which was performed when the patient was 17 years old, further augmented the collateral blood flow to the lungs. The decrease in pulmonary blood flow during his latter years, as evidenced by increasing cyanosis and disability, no doubt was caused by progressive closing of the ventricular septal defect.

REFERENCES

1. AZEVEDO, A. DE C., TOLEDO, A. N., CARVALHO, A. A. DE, ZANIOLO, W., DOHMANN, H., AND ROUBACH, R.: Ventricular septal defect; an example of its relative diminution. *Acta Cardiol.* 13: 513, 1958.
2. HARNED, H. S., AND PETERS, R. M.: Spontaneous closing of ventricular septal defects: Two cases reported. *Abstract, Circulation* 22: 760, 1960.
3. EVANS, J. R., ROWE, M. B., AND KEITH, J. D.: Spontaneous closure of ventricular septal defects. *Circulation* 22: 1044, 1960.
4. NADAS, A. S., SCOTT, L. P., HAUCK, A. J., AND RUDOLPH, A. M.: Spontaneous functional closing of ventricular septal defects. *New England J. Med.* 264: 309, 1961.
5. AGUSTSSON, M. H., GASUL, B. M., ARCILLA, R. A., BICOFF, J. P., AND MONCADA, R.: Spontaneous closure of ventricular septal defect in eight children demonstrated by serial cardiac catherization and by angiocardiography. *Abstract, Circulation* 24: 874, 1961.
6. BLOOMFIELD, D. K.: Spontaneous closure of ventricular septal defect: Clinical and pathologic correlations. *Abstract, Circulation* 24: 890, 1961.
7. EDWARDS, J. E.: Congenital malformations of the heart and great vessels. In Gould, S. E.: *Pathology of the Heart.* Springfield, IL, Charles C. Thomas, 1953, p. 266.
8. FONTANA, R. S., AND EDWARDS, J. E.: *Congenital Cardiac Disease: A Review of 357 Cases Studied Pathologically.* Philadelphia, PA, W. B. Saunders Company, 1962, p. 291.

Case 30 Aortico-Left Ventricular Tunnel*

A Cause of Massive Aortic Regurgitation and of Intracardiac Aneurysm

William C. Roberts, MD, and Andrew G. Morrow, MD
Bethesda, Maryland

AMONG the unusual causes of aortic regurgitation is an accessory vascular channel which originates in the ascending aorta, bypasses the aortic valve and communicates with the left ventricle through the upper ventricular septum. Although isolated reports of clinical and necropsy findings in patients with this lesion had appeared previously,[1-4] Levy and his associates,[5] in 1963, presented the first definitive characterization of the entity, and termed it "aortico-left ventricular tunnel."

This report describes the clinical, roentgenographic, hemodynamic and pathologic findings in an additional patient in whom an aortico-left ventricular tunnel not only caused aortic regurgitation, but also gave rise to an intracardiac aneurysm which was responsible for severe right ventricular outflow obstruction.

CASE REPORT

W. M. (01-21-10), a fourteen year old school boy, was found to have a precordial murmur at three months of age. He grew slowly, and at the age of five years, after cardiac catheterization and angiocardiography were performed at another hospital, his parents were told that he had aortic regurgitation. He was first seen at the National Heart Institute at the age of eight years. He was asymptomatic and played football, baseball, and swam without experiencing discomfort. On examination he was poorly developed and appeared undernourished. The heart was grossly enlarged to palpation, and there was a prominent left ventricular lift. Both systolic and diastolic thrills were present. At the base of the heart a grade 5/6 systolic ejection-type murmur was audible, and was immediately followed by a grade 5/6 high-pitched, blowing diastolic murmur which was transmitted along the left sternal border. The peripheral pulses were bounding, both systolic and diastolic murmurs were audible over the femoral arteries, and the blood pressure in the arm was 120/0 mm. Hg.

Chest roentgenograms disclosed marked enlargement of the left ventricle and ascending aorta; the electrocardiogram demonstrated normal sinus rhythm, biventricular hypertrophy and ventricular premature contractions. Retrograde arterial catheterization was performed and simultaneous measurements of left ventricular and femoral arterial pressures were 117/10 and 189/37 mm. Hg, respectively.

In the ensuing two years the patient remained asymptomatic; he was readmitted at the age of ten years for further study. At right heart catheterization the pulmonary arterial and pulmonary capillary wedge pressures were normal, but a large systolic pressure gradient was demonstrated within the right ventricle; high in the outflow tract the pressure was 22/1 mm. Hg while near the tricuspid valve it was 120/4 mm. Hg. No intracardiac shunts were demonstrated by the inhaled nitrous oxide test. A retrograde aortogram (Figure 1) showed marked dilatation of the ascending aorta

---

* From the Clinic of Surgery, National Heart Institute, National Institutes of Health, Bethesda, Maryland. Manuscript received February 2, 1965.

   DOI: 10.1201/9781003409342-8

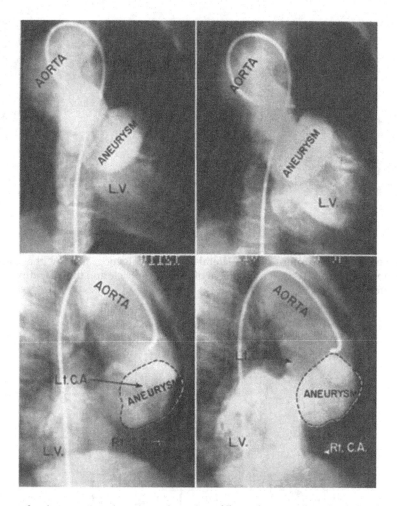

Figure 1 Anteroposterior views (*upper*) and lateral views (*lower*) of the thoracic aortogram. Following injection of contrast material into the ascending aorta the aneurysmal intracardiac portion of the aortico-left ventricular tunnel opacifices immediately, and is well outlined before radiopaque material enters the left ventricular cavity. The ascending aorta and sinuses of Valsalva are dilated. L.V. = left ventricle. Rt. C.A. = right coronary artery. Lt. C.A. = left coronary artery.

and regurgitation of dye, initially into a smooth-walled subaortic chamber and subsequently into the left ventricular cavity. The aortic sinuses of Valsalva also were dilated. It was considered that the patient had either an aneurysm of the sinus of Valsalva with rupture into the left ventricle, or cystic medial necrosis of the aorta; because of the latter possibility, and because he was asymptomatic, operative treatment was not undertaken.

The patient remained well, continued to participate in sports, despite advice to the contrary, and never experienced syncope, precordial pain, troublesome dyspnea or other symptoms of cardiac failure. His heart increased in size only in proportion to his growth (Figure 2), but electrocardiograms (Figure 3) showed progressive deepening of the T waves in the precordial leads. When the boy was fourteen years

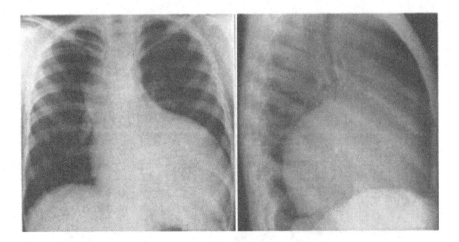

Figure 2 Posteroanterior and lateral chest roentgenograms of the patient described. There is striking enlargement of the left ventricle and the ascending aorta is dilated.

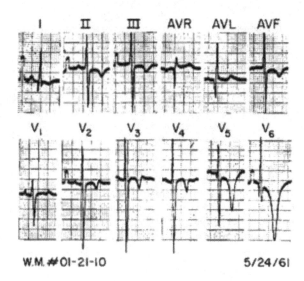

Figure 3 Electrocardiogram. Leads II, III and V_2 through V_6 are at half-standardization. The T wave deflection in lead V_6 exceeds 50 mm.

old a corrective operation was scheduled, but he died suddenly at home before it was performed.

Necropsy (A63–139) disclosed that the aortic regurgitation was due to a large accessory communication, an aortico-left ventricular tunnel, between the markedly dilated ascending aorta and the left ventricle. The pathologic aspects of this communication are illustrated in detail in Figures 4 through 6. Immediately below its origin

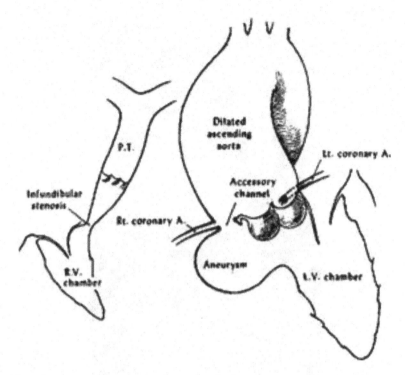

Figure 4 Diagram illustrating the essential anatomic features of the aortico-left ventricular tunnel in the patient described. The right and left sides of the heart are shown separately for simplicity, but the comparative size of each is correct. The right ventricular (R.V.) chamber is much smaller than the left ventricular (L.V.) one. A localized area of stenosis is present at the beginning of the right ventricular out-flow tract. The remainder of the infundibular chamber is of normal size as is the pulmonary trunk (P.T.). The ascending aorta is diffusely dilated. A wide open accessory channel lies between the aorta and the subaortic aneurysm and left ventricular chamber. The aneurysm is actually the tunnel located immediately behind the right ventricular infundibulum. The aortic valve is bicuspid. The ostium of the right coronary artery is located immediately above the aortic ostium of the accessory channel.

from the aorta the tunnel was aneurysmally dilated, and the mass of the aneurysm displaced the upper portion of the ventricular septum into right ventricular outflow tract. (Figure 7.) The coronary arteries were normal on both gross and microscopic examinations and neither was compressed by the aneurysm. Multiple sections of the left ventricular wall revealed hypertrophy of the myocardial fibers and rare foci of interstitial and replacement fibrosis. In sections of the ascending aorta, the configuration of the elastic fibers was normal and no excessive amount of mucopolysaccharide material was evident.

COMMENTS

The basic anatomic malformation in aortico-left ventricular tunnel is an abnormal vascular channel which begins in the aortic root, passes through the upper portion of the ventricular septum and enters the outflow tract of the ventricle. Aortico-left

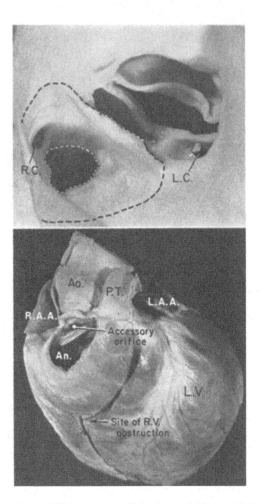

Figure 5 Photographs of the aortic root area from above and below. *Top,* the aortic valve and ostium of the accessory channel as viewed from the aorta. The aortic valve contains only two cusps. A thick band separates the aortic valve orifice from the orifice of the accessory channel. If the top of this ridge and the surrounding aorta at this level (large black-dashed area) are considered the origin of the tunnel, then the right (R.C.) and left (L.C.) coronary arteries arise below this level. If on the other hand the actual opening into the heart (small white-dashed circle) is considered the origin of the tunnel, then the coronary arteries arise above it. *Bottom,* the heart as it appears from the anterior view. The anterior wall of the intracardiac aneurysm (An.), which is a thin fibrous membrane, has been removed allowing visualization of the accessory orifice from below. Ao. = ascending aorta. P.T. = pulmonary trunk. R.A.A. = right atrial appendage. L.A.A. = left atrial appendage. R.V. = right ventricle. L.V. = left ventricle.

ventricular tunnel must be distinguished from an aneurysm of the sinus of Valsalva which has ruptured into the left ventricle, and Levy et al.[5] made this distinction by pointing out that in ruptured sinus aneurysm the orifice of the aneurysm is *below* the level of the ostia of the coronary arteries. In contrast, in each of the three patients

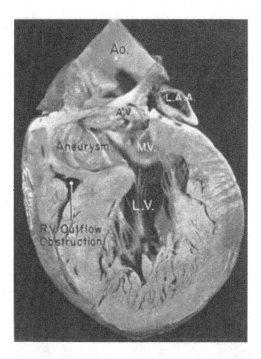

Figure 6 Sagittal section of heart transecting the accessory aortic orifice. The intracardiac aneurysm is located between the aorta and left ventricular cavity. The tunnel penetrates the portion of the muscular ventricular septum which also forms the posterior wall of the right ventricular infundibulum. The aneurysmal dilatation of the tunnel caused the posterior wall of the infundibulum to bulge into the right ventricular cavity with resulting obstruction to right ventricular outflow. The left ventricular wall is massively hypertrophied. The ostium into the left atrial appendage (L.A.A.) is congenitally atretic. A.V. = aortic valve cusps. M.V. = anterior mitral leaflet.

with aortico-left ventricular tunnel which he described, and in the one reported by Edwards,[4] the tunnel was considered to originate *above* the level of the aortic sinuses and coronary ostia. To some extent, however, the above-or-below relationship of the tunnel to the origins of the coronary arteries is a matter of semantics. In the present patient, those cited and in the patient described by Morgan and Mazur,[6] the orifice of the tunnel was separated from the aortic valve by a thick ridge, the upper margin of which was on the same horizontal plane as the upper margins of the aortic valve leaflets and commissures. If the top of the ridge and the surrounding aorta at this level are designated as the origin of the tunnel, then the coronary arteries arise below it. If, on the other hand, the orifice of the tunnel is considered to be the actual opening into the heart, then the coronary arteries arise above it (Figure 5).

Between the aorta and the heart, the tunnel may be tubular in shape or, more frequently, it may be dilated and appear as a discrete enlargement of the anterior portion of the aortic root.[5] In this case the angiographic appearance of the tunnel is that of a supracardiac saccular aneurysm and permits a precise diagnosis. In the present patient, however, although the tunnel was aneurysmal, the aneurysm was entirely within the heart and the dilated ascending aorta was of uniform configuration.

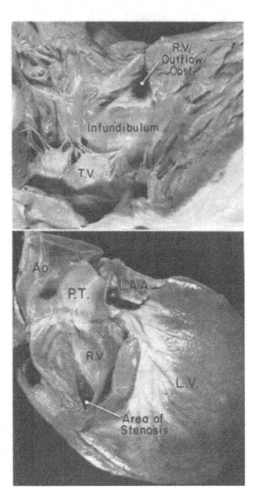

Figure 7 The area of right ventricular obstruction from below and above. *Top*, the obstruction (Obst.) is located at the beginning of the right ventricular outflow tract and is due to the infundibulum bulging anteriorly and inferiorly. There is endocardial thickening at the site of narrowing. *Bottom*, the right ventricular (R.V.) out-flow tract is opened and the area of stenosis is again seen, The wall of the right ventricular outflow tract is thin, but the wall of the inflow portion (upper) is thick. Ao. = ascending aorta. P.T. = pulmonary trunk. L.A.A. = left atrial appendage, L.V. = left ventricle.

The tunnel enters the heart through the muscular portion of the ventricular septum, directly below the aortic root, and terminates in the left ventricle immediately below the aortic valve. The area of the ventricular septum traversed by the tunnel constitutes the posterior wall of the right ventricular outflow tract. In this patient the aneurysmal intracardiac portion of the tunnel was so large that it displaced the posterior wall of the infundibulum into the right ventricular cavity and caused obstruction to right ventricular outflow. Right ventricular outflow obstruction by this mechanism has not been documented previously, although Levy and associates postulated that such might occur.

The available evidence indicates that aortico-left ventricular tunnel is a congenital rather than an acquired malformation, and signs of cardiac disease are usually present from an early age. The patient described by Morgan and Mazur,[6] for example, had aortic regurgitation from birth and died at fifteen days of age. At autopsy there was dilatation of the ascending aorta and the appearance of the aortic root was quite similar to that shown in Figure 5. The association of aortico-left ventricular tunnel with other congenital cardiovascular anomalies also lends support to a congenital basis for this lesion. The aortic valve was bicuspid in each of the autopsy cases reported by Edwards[4] and by Levy et al., and also in the present case. In the case of Morgan and Mazur[6] the aortic valve as illustrated, although described as being tricuspid, appears malformed. In the present case there was also absence of an ostium into the left atrial appendage. Levy and associates demonstrated histologically in one of their patients that the aortic media was continuous with the wall of the tunnel, and suggested that the tunnel represented an anomalous vessel rather than an acquired tract. In the present patient, microscopic sections of the ridge separating the aortic valve from the ostium of the tunnel disclosed that this structure had the same appearance as the media of the ascending aorta, consisting predominantly of elastic fibers. The anterior wall of the intracardiac portion of the tunnel, however, was composed of dense collagenous tissue containing only an occasional elastic fibril. Thus, in this patient, if the intracardiac portion of the tunnel originally had the structure of a blood vessel, it was not apparent at the time of necropsy. It is possible, of course, that the structure of the tunnel may have been altered by the trauma of systolic and diastolic blood flow through it during the fourteen years of the patient's life.

Patients with aortico-left ventricular tunnel present physical findings indistinguishable from those observed in patients with aortic regurgitation resulting from valvular abnormalities. A congenital malformation may be suggested by an early history of a precordial murmur, but the results of conventional roentgenographic examinations, electrocardiography and cardiac catheterization are not specific. It would appear that the correct diagnosis can be established only when the origin of the tunnel from the ascending aorta, as well as regurgitant flow into the left ventricle, can be demonstrated at thoracic aortography. Even this study may not be conclusive if, as in the present patient, the tunnel is dilated only within the roentgenographic silhouette of the heart, and resembles a ruptured aneurysm of the sinus of Valsalva.

Aortic regurgitation resulting from an aortico-left ventricular tunnel may be abolished by closure of the aortic ostium, and successful surgical treatment of this type has been reported in several patients.[5, 7, 8] This form of aortic regurgitation would thus appear to be a relatively favorable one, particularly in a child, since the insertion of a prosthetic aortic valve, virtually always necessary in valvular aortic regurgitation, is not required.

SUMMARY

The clinical, roentgenographic, hemodynamic and pathologic findings in a fourteen year old boy with aortico-left ventricular tunnel are presented. The accessory channel between the aorta and left ventricle resulted in massive aortic regurgitation, and the portion of the tunnel which traversed the ventricular septum was aneurysmal, displaced the posterior wall of the right ventricle and caused severe obstruction to right ventricular outflow. The presence of associated cardiovascular anomalies, in this and previously reported cases, suggests that the malformation is congenital rather than acquired.

The clinical and hemodynamic manifestations of aortico-left ventricular tunnel are indistinguishable from those observed with the more common forms of aortic regurgitation, and the correct diagnosis can be established only by thoracic aortography. The malformation is usually recognized in childhood; since aortic regurgitant flow can be abolished by simple closure of the aortic ostium, and without aortic valve replacement, the indications for operative treatment differ from those which apply in aortic regurgitation due to a valvular anomaly.

ADDENDUM

Since this manuscript was submitted for publication, Cooley et al.[9] described another patient with aortico-left ventricular tunnel. The unusual features in the sixteen month old boy were the presence of associated valvular aortic stenosis and deposits of mucopolysaccharide material in the ascending aorta. The latter suggested to these workers the possibility of a relationship between aortico-left ventricular tunnel and the Marfan syndrome.

REFERENCES

1. HART, K. Uber das Aneurysma des rechten Sinus Valsalvae der Aorta und seine Beziehungen zum oberen Ventrikelseptum. *Virchow's Arch. Path. Anat.*, 182: 167, 1905.
2. WARTHEN, R. O. Congenital aneurysm of the right anterior sinus of Valsalva (interventricular aneurysm) with spontaneous rupture into the left ventricle. *Am. Heart J.*, 37: 975, 1949.
3. TASAKA, S., YOSHITOSHI, Y., SEKI, K., KOIDE, K., OGATA, E. and NAKAMURA, K. Congenital aneurysm of the right coronary sinus of Valsalva with rupture into the left ventricle. *Jap. Heart J.*, 1: 106, 1960.
4. EDWARDS, J. E. *Atlas of acquired diseases of the heart and great vessels.* 3rd vol, p. 1142, Philadelphia, 1961, W. B. Saunders Co.
5. LEVY, M. J., LILLEHEI, C. W., ANDERSON, R. C., AMPLATZ, K. and EDWARDS, J. E. Aortico-left ventricular tunnel. *Circulation*, 27: 841, 1963.
6. MORGAN, R. I. and MAZUR, J. H. Congenital aneurysm of aortic root with fistula to left ventricle. A case report with autopsy findings. *Circulation*, 28: 589, 1963.
7. SHUMACKER, H. B., JR. and JUDSON, W. E. Rupture of aneurysm of sinus of Valsalva into left ventricle and its operative repair. *J. Thoracic & Cardiovasc. Surg.*, 45: 650, 1963.
8. SCOTT, H. W., JR., COLLINS, H. A. and SINCLAIR-SMITH, B. Surgical repair of congenital aneurysm of the right coronary sinus of Valsalva with rupture into the left ventricle. *J. Cardiovasc. Surg.*, 5: 231, 1964.
9. COOLEY, R. N., HARRIS, L. C. and RODIN, A. E. Abnormal communication between the aorta and left ventricle. Aortico-left ventricular tunnel. *Circulation*, 31: 564, 1965.

Case 51 Complex Congenital Cardiac Malformation

Corrected Transposition, Origin of Both Great Vessels From the Anatomic Right Ventricle, Common Ventricle, and Dextroversion[1]

William C. Roberts,[2] Joseph C. Eggleston and J. O'Neal Humphries

Departments of Pathology and Medicine, The Johns Hopkins University School of Medicine and Hospital

In the entity "corrected transposition of the great vessels" the pulmonary trunk and ascending aorta are transposed, and the ventricles, ventricular septum, atrioventricular (A-V) valves and coronary arteries are inverted in a mirror image of normal. This arrangement of the great arteries and ventricles (in contrast to the entity "complete or uncorrected transposition") permits functional correction, so that systemic venous blood passes into the pulmonary trunk while arterialized pulmonary venous blood flows into the aorta. Corrected transposition infrequently is the sole cardiac anomaly, and the associated malformations are the ones usually responsible for the clinical cardiac signs and symptoms. The most frequently associated lesions are ventricular septal defect and deformities of the left-sided (arterial) atrioventricular valve, most often the Ebstein-type malformation.[1,2] Other commonly associated anomalies include atrial septal defect, patent ductus arteriosus, valvular and subvalvular pulmonic stenosis, accessory valve-like tissue in the subpulmonary area, and dextroversion (right-sided apex in situs solitus).[1-7] Rarer associated malformations described in association with "corrected transposition" include common or single ventricle, persistent atrioventricular canal, pulmonary or left-sided (arterial) A-V valve atresia, anomalous muscle bundle in the arterial left-sided (anatomically right) ventricle, the "parachute mitral valve syndrome" and origin of both great vessels from the same ventricle.[1-3, 8-13]

None of the several reviews in recent years on the entities "corrected transposition",[1-3] or "origin of both great arteries from the right ventricle"[14-16] have described patients having these two malformations associated with one another, and only four patients to our knowledge have been described with such a combination of lesions.[10-13] It was therefore deemed worthwhile to describe the following patient.

REPORT OF PATIENT

R.R. (JHH # 53 72 38), a 21-year-old man with known cyanotic congenital heart disease, died on February 15, 1966. He had appeared normal at birth, but at 8 months of age cyanosis was noted during and shortly after episodes of crying. Examination at age 1 year disclosed slight cyanosis, and a harsh continuous murmur over the lower left sternal border with wide transmission of the systolic component. Chest

Received for publication November 3, 1960

[1] Supported in part by Graduate Cardiovascular Training Grant #2 T1 HE 5159 and Undergraduate Cardiovascular Training Grant #5 T2 HE 260 from the National Heart Institute.

[2] Present Address: Laboratory of Pathology, Clinic of Surgery, National Heart Institute, National Institutes of Health, Bethesda, Maryland.

DOI: 10.1201/9781003409342-9

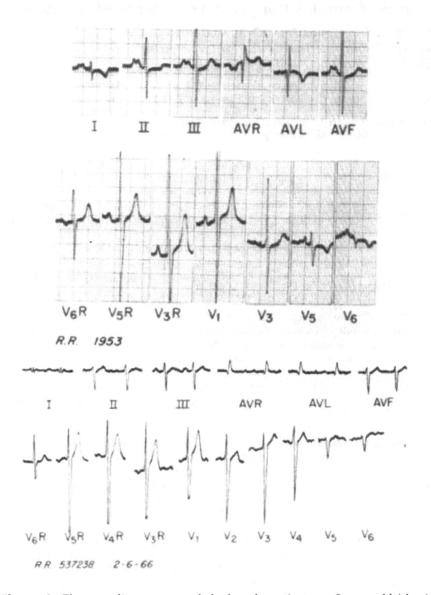

Figure 1 Electrocardiograms recorded when the patient was 8 years old (*above*), and nine days before death when he was 21 years old (*below*). The upright P wave in lead I (*above*) indicates that the malrotation of the heart is dextroversion rather than dextrocardia. The atrial fibrillation (*below*) began 18 months before he died.

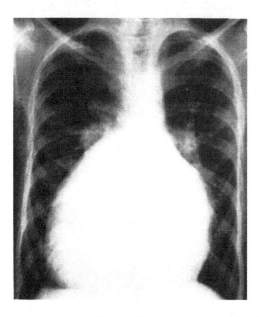

Figure 2 Chest roentgenogram. The cardiac apex points to the right.

roentgenogram showed an enlarged and dextrorotated heart. At age 20 months signs of cardiac failure appeared; he was digitalized and remained on digitalis the rest of his life. He was followed closely in the Harriet Lane Home Cardiac Clinic and over the years the heart murmur separated into a harsh, loud, pansystolic component best heard at the right sternal border, but widely transmitted, and a softer diastolic component heard at the apex. The cardiac apex moved laterally to the right anterior axillary line, and a systolic thrill was palpated widely over the active right anterior chest. Slight cyanosis and clubbing were occasionally described. At cardiac catheterization at age 8 (1953) the pressure in the "right ventricle" was 92/6, and in the femoral artery, 102/64 mm. Hg. The pulmonary trunk was not entered. The systemic arterial oxygen saturation was 90 per cent. The cardiac output was 3.4 L./min.

Except for slight dyspnea and cyanosis on strenuous exertion, he was asymptomatic until about one and a half years before death. He completed high school and one year of college, played and marched with his high school band and worked in the summers. In August, 1964 he noted a rapid pulse and decreased exercise tolerance and was found to have atrial fibrillation. This arrhythmia persisted until his death despite conversion attempts with quinidine. Paroxysms of rapid tachycardia occurred during his last year.

He was hospitalized on February 7, 1966, because of increasing fatigability, exertional dyspnea, reduced exercise tolerance, insomnia and nervousness. The liver was enlarged, the pretibial regions edematous, the digits moderately clubbed and the nail beds quite cyanotic. The hematocrit was 63 per cent; the electrocardiogram (Figure 1) showed atrial fibrillation, and ventricular hypertrophy, and the chest roentgenogram (Figure 2) showed marked cardiomegaly, dextrocardia, enlarged pulmonary vessels, and a narrowed "vascular pedicle." The hematocrit was lowered to 59 per cent by the removal of 500 ml. of blood. On February 15, he developed severe pain in his right eye, and three hours later ventricular fibrillation appeared and he died.

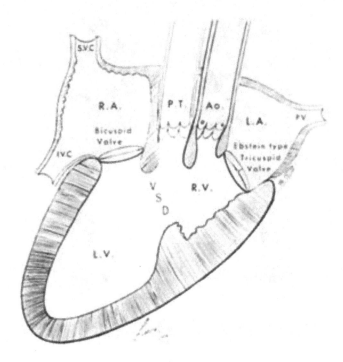

Figure 3 Diagram of the heart. The right (R.A.) and left atria (L.A.), vena cavae (S.V.C. and I.V.C.) and pulmonary veins (P.V.) are normally situated. The right sided atrioventricular valve is bicuspid, and the left sided one is tricuspid. The large ventricular cavity, with its apex pointing to the right (dextroversion), is for practical purposes a single ventricle with remnants of ventricular septum (below the ventricular septal defect) serving as the point of separation between right and left halves of the common ventricle. The interior lining of the right sided ventricle is smooth and is typical of that of a normal left ventricle (L.V.). The wall of the left sided ventricle is thicker, its interior lining is coarser, and it contains an infundibulum. The latter two features are characteristic of an anatomic right ventricle (R.V.). Both pulmonary trunk (P.T.) and aorta (Ao.) arise from the anatomic right ventricle, and both pulmonic and aortic valves are separated from the A-V valves and from one another by infundibulum. Since both great arteries arise from the anatomic right ventricle, the only outlet for blood from the anatomic left ventricle is via the huge ventricular septal defect (V.S.D.). Both pulmonic and aortic valves are on the same horizontal plane, and these arteries ascend parallel to one another.

The cardiac findings at autopsy (#34437) are summarized in Figure 3, and described in detail in Figures 4 to 6. He had *corrected transposition of the great vessels*, a huge *ventricular septal defect* (functionally single ventricle), *origin of both great vessels from the anatomic right ventricle* (double outlet right ventricle), and *dextroversion*.

The pulmonary arteries and veins were dilated. Microscopically, the pulmonary arteries showed medial hypertrophy and focal narrowing of the lumens by fibrous intimal proliferation.

COMMENTS

Confusion may arise when the more or less contradictory terms "corrected transposition of the great arteries," "origin of both great vessels from the right ventricle"

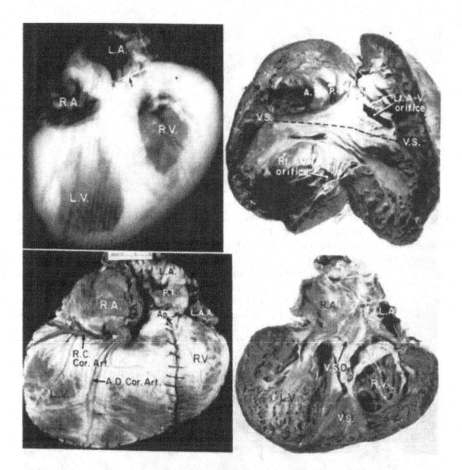

Figure 4   Various views of the heart. *Upper left:* Radiograph of the heart specimen. A large deposit of calcium is present in the left atrium (L.A.), and it extends down one portion of the left A-V valve to the base of a papillary muscle of the anatomic right ventricle (R.V.). Before this radiograph was taken pins (arrows) were placed laterally (right to left) across the superior margins of each of the semilunar valves. On this radiograph the two pins arc virtually superimposed on one another, indicating that one valve lies directly behind the other and that each is on the same horizontal plane. The latter is a characteristic feature of the entity "origin of both great vessels from the right ventricle." (16) R.A. = right atrium. L.V. = anatomic left ventricle. *Lower left:* Anterior view of the heart. The apex points to the right. The coronary arteries have a mirror image of normal: the anterior descending (A.D.) branch arises from the right circumflex (R.C.) coronary artery. The left coronary artery is not shown. The aorta (Ao.) is anterior to the pulmonary trunk (P.T.). Abbreviations as in upper left; L.A.A. = left atrial appendage. *Upper right:* The ventricular cavity is opened along its entire inferior (caudal) border. From this view the orifices of both A-V valves are seen and each of these valves is continuous with one another across the dashed line which represents the circumference of the huge ventricular septal defect. The remnant of the ventricular septum (V.S.) is shown. Both aorta (A.) and pulmonary trunk (P.) arise from the anatomic right ventricle. *Lower right:* The anterior half of the heart has now been removed. The interior lining of both anatomic left ventricle (L.V.) and anatomic right ventricle (R.V.) are well seen. The arrows designate the large communication (V.S.D.) between the two ventricles.

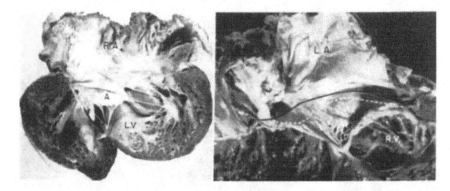

Figure 5 The atrioventricular valves. *Left:* Opened right atrium (R.A.), right A-V valve and anatomic left ventricle (L.V.). This valve has the configuration of a mitral valve. A = anterior leaflet. *Right:* Opened left atrium (L.A.), left A-V valve and anatomic right ventricle (R.V.). The large calcium deposits extending from the left atrium to the base of a papillary muscle may be seen. The solid black line designates the mitral valve annulus, and the dashed white line, the basal attachment of the valve leaflets. The basal attachment of the valve leaflets is not to the mitral annulus, but to the left ventricular wall, and this malformation constitutes the Ebstein-type anomaly.

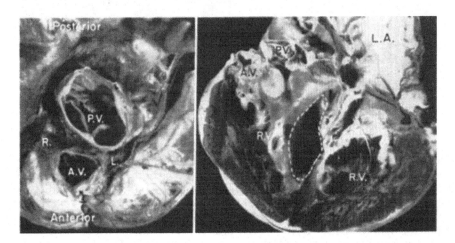

Figure 6 The semilunar valves. *Left:* From above. The aortic valve (A.V.) is smaller and anterior to the pulmonic valve (P.V.). The left (L) and right (R) coronary arteries arise from the aorta. *Right:* Opened anatomic right ventricle (R.V.) showing that the semilunar valves (A.V. and P.V.) are separated from one another by one limb of infundibular myocardium and from the A-V valves by another limb of infundibulum. The circumference of the ventricular septal defect is designated by the dashed white line. LA. = left atrium.

and "common ventricle" are employed to describe the same heart. Each term is applicable, however, in the case of the patient presented herein. The aorta arose anterior to the pulmonary trunk (transposition of the great vessels), and the ventricles, A-V valves, and coronary arteries were inverted in a mirror image of normal (inversion). The anatomic left ("venous") ventricle was located on the right side of the heart and the anatomic right ("arterial") ventricle was located on the left side of the heart. In contrast to the typical "corrected transposition" heart, however, the pulmonary trunk was not attached to the venous ventricle, but both great arteries arose from the anatomic right ventricle (double outlet right ventricle), and neither semilunar valve was continuous with an A-V valve. The only outlet for blood from the anatomic left ventricle was through the huge ventricular septal defect. Since only a remnant of a ventricular septum was present, it appears best to consider this defect as absent ventricular septum or single ventricle.

The patient described above is very similar to the 47-year-old man reported by Rawson and Doerner.[13] Their patient also had "corrected transposition," "origin of both great vessels from the anatomic right ventricle," "common ventricle," "dextroversion," but in addition had valvular pulmonic stenosis. Most patients with virtually absent ventricular septa die during the first few months or years of life, and survival to adulthood is rare. It is well recognized that obstruction to pulmonary blood flow (by valvular or subvalvular pulmonic stenosis) increases the length of survival of patients with common ventricle. It is remarkable that the present patient survived so long since he also had a common ventricle, but no obstruction of flow of blood to the lungs.

SUMMARY

The clinical and pathologic findings are described in a 21-year-old man who died of a complex cardiac malformation consisting of "corrected transposition," "origin of both great vessels from the anatomic right ventricle," single ventricle, and dextroversion.

REFERENCES

1. SCHIEBLER, G. L., EDWARDS, J. E. BURCHELL, H. B., DUSHANE, J. W., ONGLEY, P. A. AND WOOD, E. H.: Congenital corrected transposition of the great vessels: A study of 33 cases. *Pediatrics* (Suppl.), 1961, **27**: 851.
2. BERRY, W. B., ROBERTS, W. C., MORROW, A. G. AND BRAUNWALD, E.: Corrected transposition of the aorta and pulmonary trunk. *Amer. J. Med.*, 1961, **36**: 35.
3. LEV, M. AND ROWLATT, U. F.: The pathologic anatomy of mixed levocardia. A review of thirteen cases of atrial or ventricular inversion with or without corrected transposition. *Amer. J. Cardiol.*, 1961, **8**: 216.
4. LEVY, M. J., LILLEHEI, C. W., ELLIOTT, L. P., CAREY, L. S., ADAMS, P., JR. AND EDWARDS, J. E.: Accessory valvular tissue causing subpulmonary stenosis in corrected transposition of great vessels. *Circulation*, 1963, **27**: 494.
5. ESPINO-VELA, J.: On a variety of the "corrected" type of transposition of the great vessels associated with dextrocardia: A study of two cases with autopsy report. *Amer. Heart J.*, 1959, **58**: 250.
6. MORGAN, A. D., KROVETZ, L. J., BARTLEY, T. D., GREEN, J. R., SHANKLIN, D. R., WHEAT, M. W. AND SCHIEBLER, G. L.: Clinical features of single ventricle with congenitally corrected transposition. *Amer. J. Cardiol.*, 1966, **17**: 379.
7. RATNER, B., ABBOTT, M. E. AND BEATTIE, W. W.: Rare cardiac anomaly: Cortriloculare biventriculare in mirror-picture dextrocardia with persistent omphalo-mesenteric bay, right aortic arch and pulmonary artery forming descending aorta. *Amer. J. Dis. Child.*, 1921, **22**: 508.

8. ANSELMI, G., MUNOZ, S., MACHADO, L., BLANCO, P. AND ESPINO-VELA, J.: Complex cardiovascular malformations associated with the corrected type of transposition of the great vessels. *Amer. Heart J.*, 1963, **66**: 614.

9. TODD, D. B., ANDERSON, R. C. AND EDWARDS, J. E.: Inverted malformations in corrected transposition of the great vessels. *Circulation*, 1965, **32**: 298.

10. LOCHTE: Ein Fall von Situs Viscerum Irregularis, nebst eincm Beitrag zur Lehre von der Transposition der arteriellen grossen Gefässstämme des Herzens. *Beitr. path. Anat.*, 1898, **24**: 187.

11. ROYER, B. F. AND WILSON, J. D.: Incomplete heterotaxy, with usual heart malformations. Case report. *Arch. Pediat.*, 1908, **25**: 881.

12. ROSLER, H.: Beiträge zur Lehre von den angeborenen Herzfehlern. VI. Über die angeborene isolierte Rechtslage des Herzens. *Wien. Arch. Inn. Med.*, 1930, **19**: 505.

13. RAWSON, F. L., JR. AND DOEKNER, A. A.: Functional cortriloculare. *Amer. Heart J.*, 1953, **46**: 779.

14. NEUFELD, H. N., DUSHANE, J. W., WOOD, E. H., KIRKLIN, J. W. AND EDWARDS, J. E.: Origin of both great vessels from the right ventricle. I. Without pulmonary stenosis. *Circulation*, 1961, **23**: 399.

15. NEUFELD, H. N., DUSHANE, J. W. AND EDWARDS, J. E.: Origin of both great vessels from the right ventricle. II. With pulmonary stenosis. *Circulation*, 1961, **23**: 603.

16. NEUFELD, H. H., LUCAS, R. V., JR., LESTER, R. G., ADAMS, P., JR., ANDERSON, R. C. AND EDWARDS, J. E.: Origin of both great vessels from the right ventricle without pulmonary stenosis. *Brit. Heart J.*, 1962, **24**: 393.

Case 79 Aneurysmal Dilatation of the Coronary Arteries in Cyanotic Congenital Cardiac Disease*

Report of a Forty Year Old Patient with the Taussig-Bing Complex

Joseph K. Perloff, MD, Charles W. Urschell, MD, William C. Roberts, MD, and Walter H. Caulfield, Jr., MD
Washington, D. C.

Clinical, hemodynamic, angiocardiographic and autopsy observations are described in a forty year old woman with right ventricular origin of the aorta and biventricular origin of the pulmonary trunk. She lived longer than any previously described patient with this congenital malformation. At angiography and at autopsy the extramural coronary arteries were found to be aneurysmally dilated and tortuous. Coronary arterial ectasia has been described once before in patients with cyanotic congenital cardiac disease, but the remarkable degree of dilatation and tortuosity found in our patient has not been recorded.

MARKED dilatation and tortuosity of the coronary arteries in patients with cyanotic congenital heart disease has been commented upon only once before.[1] This report describes the clinical, hemodynamic, angiographic and necropsy findings in a forty year old cyanotic woman in whom the aorta arose entirely from the right ventricle, whereas the pulmonary trunk arose from both ventricles. She survived longer than any known patient with this malformation. In addition, she exhibited a degree of coronary arterial dilatation and tortuosity that is without precedent in the literature.

CASE REPORT

The patient, a white housewife, was first evaluated by us when she was thirty-eight years of age. She was the product of a normal pregnancy and apparently had been cyanotic from birth. Effort dyspnea, fatigue and orthopnea had been present from childhood. These symptoms lessened in the teens; she ultimately married and was able to do light housework. Mild exertional chest pain began at about twenty years of age and recurred intermittently thereafter. Between ages thirty-three and thirty-eight years, hemoptysis occurred three times. Two episodes were sudden and severe, each lasting a day. Increased fatigability began at age thirty-six, and there was a 15 pound weight loss between the ages of thirty-six and thirty-eight years.

* From the Department of Medicine, Georgetown University School of Medicine, Division of Cardiology, Georgetown University Hospital, Washington, D. C. and the Section of Pathology, National Heart Institute, National Institutes of Health, Bethesda, Maryland. This work was supported by U. S. Public Health Service Grant HE-09093, by Public Health Service Career Program Award HE-14,009, and by the Eric T. Paglin Memorial Fund for Cardiovascular Teaching and Research. Requests for reprints should be addressed to Joseph K. Perloff, M.D., at the Georgetown University Hospital, Washington, D. C. Manuscript received November 8, 1967.

DOI: 10.1201/9781003409342-10

When initially seen the patient complained of breathlessness, chest pain and fatigue but she was still able to do much of her shopping and was moderately active. On examination, she was a thin, small woman with distinct cyanosis and clubbing of the fingers but with much less cyanosis and little or no clubbing of the toes. The arterial pulses were normal, and the blood pressure was similar in the arms and legs (92/65 mm. Hg). The jugular venous pulse was normal in height and contour. The lungs were clear. A right ventricular impulse was readily appreciated, and a moderate left ventricular impulse was identified near the mid-clavicular line. The sound of pulmonary valve closure was palpable in the second left interspace. Auscultatory signs included a normal first heart sound, a pulmonic ejection sound, a grade 3/6 mid-systolic murmur maximal in the second and third left interspaces, a loud, single second sound in the second left interspace, and a soft, inconstant mid-diastolic murmur at the site of the left ventricular impulse. The liver was not enlarged and there was no edema.

The hematocrit was 60 per cent. On chest roentgenogram (Figure 1) the lung fields were plethoric, especially the middle and inner thirds. The pulmonary trunk was dilated. The atria were normal in size, and the right and left ventricles were only slightly enlarged. The electrocardiogram (Figure 2) showed a P-R interval of 0.20 second with P waves of right atrial and perhaps biatrial hypertrophy. Depolarization appeared to be clockwise with a frontal plane QRS axis directed inferiorly and to the right. Precordial leads confirmed the presence of right ventricular hypertrophy with tall R waves in lead V_1 and deep S waves in leads V_5 and V_6. Coexisting left ventricular hypertrophy was suggested by the relatively high R waves in leads V_5 and V_6 although Q waves of volume overload were not present.

Cardiac catheterization data are summarized in Table 1. A right saphenous venous catheter entered the right atrium, right ventricle and pulmonary artery in normal fashion. The descending aorta was easily entered via a patent ductus arteriosus. The atrial septum was crossed through a patent foramen ovale. Retrograde femoral arterial catheterization showed that the right ventricle communicated directly with the aorta which was in a relatively rightward position. Peak systolic pressures were identical in right ventricle, pulmonary trunk and aorta. The concentration of inhaled krypton[85] was greater in the pulmonary trunk than in the brachial artery

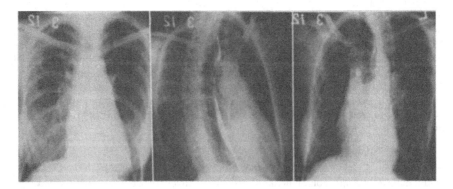

Figure 1 Anteroposterior, right oblique and left oblique chest roentgenograms. Pulmonary blood flow is increased, especially in the middle and inner thirds of the lung fields (anteroposterior projection). The position of the great vessels appears normal. The pulmonary trunk is moderately enlarged. The cardiac dimensions are relatively unimpressive.

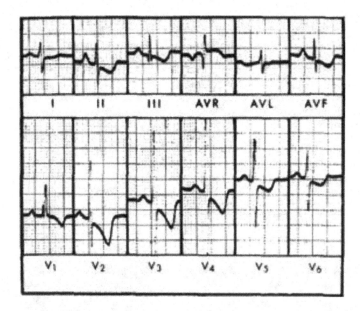

Figure 2 The P waves show hypertrophy of the right atrium and perhaps of the left atrium as well. There is distinct right ventricular hypertrophy. Coexisting left ventricular hypertrophy is suggested by the relatively tall left precordial R waves. Q waves of volume overload are absent.

(index 178 per cent). The oxygen content of pulmonary arterial blood was 22.4 volumes per cent and of aortic root blood 19.7 volumes per cent. Indocyanine green dye dilution curves showed the following patterns. With injection into the right atrium and right ventricle, the appearance time was five seconds, the primary curves large and the early recirculation peaks (left to right shunt) small. With injection into the left atrium, the appearance time was five and a half seconds, the primary curve relatively lower and the early recirculation peak (left to right shunt) larger. Right ventricular angiocardiograms (Figure 3) showed opacification of both great arteries. The aorta arose entirely from the right ventricle and the dilated pulmonary trunk arose from both ventricles (biventricular in origin). The aortic root was in a relatively anterior position and the aortic and pulmonary valves were in the same horizontal plane. The patent ductus arteriosus was readily identified. Tortuous coronary arteries were indistinctly seen on the surface of the heart following the right ventricular angiocardiogram (Figure 3), but were strikingly evident following injection of contrast material into the aortic root (Figure 4). Both coronary arteries were remarkably dilated and tortuous. In addition, the lateral projection showed that the first portion of the aortic root rose vertically and the plane of the aortic valve was horizontal (Figure 4).

Following these studies the patient was not seen again for two years. She was then deeply cyanosed, dyspneic and semistuporous, and she died within twenty-four hours.

At necropsy the heart weighed 350 gm. The principal morphologic features are described in detail in Figures 5 through 9. In summary, the aorta arose solely from the right ventricle, and the pulmonary trunk arose from both ventricles but predominantly from the left (Figure 5). The pulmonary trunk was greatly dilated and

Table 1: Cardiac catheterization data

Site	Pressure (mm. Hg)	Oxygen Content (Vol. %)	Krypton Index (%)
Right atrium	A5, V2, M2	17.8	7
Coronary sinus	. . .	10.1	. . .
Right ventricle (inflow)	91/3	17.1	. . .
Pulmonary artery	91/58	22.4	178
Aortic root	91/56	19.7	. . .
Descending aorta (via patent ductus arteriosus)	91/68	22.5	. . .
Brachial artery	93/56	19.6	. . .
Left atrium	A6, V4, M3	24.8	. . .
Pulmonary vein	. . .	24.6	. . .

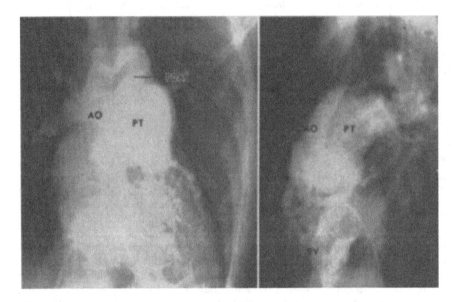

Figure 3 Biplane angiocardiograms with injection into the right ventricle (R.V.). The aorta is in a relatively rightward and anterior position, originating entirely from the right ventricle. The enlarged pulmonary trunk is biventricular in origin. The two semilunar valves are in the same horizontal plane (see Figure 5). The patent ductus arteriosus (P.D.A.) is readily identified. The coronary arteries are tortuous and dilated (see Figure 4).

straddled a large ventricular septal defect (2.2 cm. in diameter) that was situated just beneath the pulmonary valve (Figure 5). A large patent ductus arteriosus was present and there was hypoplasia of the transverse aorta (Figure 6). The foramen ovale was probe-patent but valvular-competent. The right and left coronary arteries and their branches were aneurysmally dilated and tortuous (Figure 6 through 8). Each contained an occasional yellow streak but their lumens were widely patent

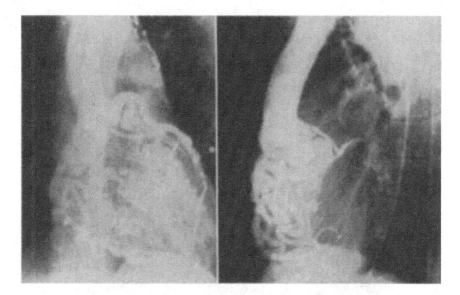

Figure 4 Biplane angiocardiograms with injection into the aortic root. There is enormous dilatation and tortuosity of both coronary arteries (compare with Figure 7). In the lateral projection, the first portion of the aortic root rises vertically and the plane of its valve is horizontal.

(Figure 8). The right ventricular wall was severely hypertrophied (Figure 5). The external diameters of several vessels were right coronary artery 0.7 cm., ascending aorta 2.0 cm., pulmonary trunk 3.8 cm., patent ductus arteriosus 1.5 cm., transverse aorta 1.0 cm. and proximal descending aorta 2.5 cm.

COMMENTS

The degree of coronary arterial dilatation and tortuosity in our patient was unique (Figures 4, 6, 7 and 8). In 1955 Aitchison et al.[2] published photographs of the heart of a thirty-four year old man with complete transposition of the great vessels. Unusually large, tortuous extramural coronary arteries were clearly visible but no comment was made about these vessels. In 1966 Bjork[1] reported "a rare and previously undescribed anomaly consisting of marked dilatation and tortuosity of the coronary arteries . . . in one adult and two children with tetralogy of Fallot." There were no abnormal communications between the coronary arteries or between them and the cardiac chambers or other vessels. Bjork called the anomaly "ectasia of the coronary arteries." Dr. Owings W. Kincaid and Dr. Jack L. Titus at the Mayo Clinic reviewed the coronary arteriograms shown in part in Figure 4. They commented upon their own experience in patients with cyanotic congenital heart disease of long duration together with dilated coronary arteries in the absence of other anomalies of these vessels[3]. They suggested that the findings in our patient appeared to be extreme dilatation of the coronary arteries secondary to prolonged congenital cardiac cyanosis with gradual progression of the dilatation over a period of years[3]. Bjork[1] had also remarked that the ectasia may become more pronounced with increasing age.

The cause of these morphologic changes in the coronary arteries is unknown, but the following speculation is offered. Nutritional requirements of myocardium normally demand maximal extraction of oxygen from coronary arterial blood,

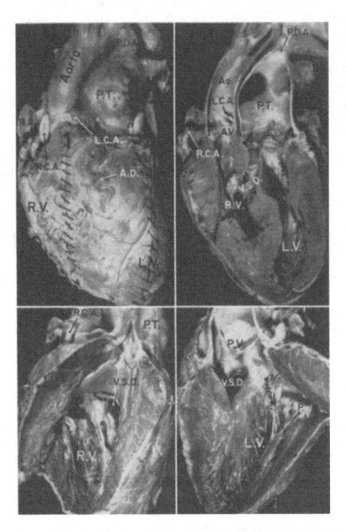

Figure 5 The exterior of the heart is shown in the *upper left*, and its interior (follow-ing removal of the anterior one-half) in the *upper right*. The pulmonary trunk (P.T.) is markedly dilated. The aorta (Ao.) arises entirely from the right ventricle (R.V.). The pulmonary trunk and pulmonic valve (P.V.) are so dilated and the ventricular septal defect (V.S.D.) so situated that this great vessel overrides both ventricles and receives blood from each of them, but mainly from the left (L.V.). The entrances into the great arteries are separated from one another by the septal band of the crista supraventric-ularis. The aortic (A.V.) and pulmonic (P.V.) valves are in the same horizontal plane. The patent ductus arteriosus (P.D.A.) is large but noncalcified. Both right (R.C.A.) and left (L.C.A.) coronary arteries are enormously dilated and tortuous, particularly the right one. The anterior descending (A.D.) branch of the left coronary is indicated. The right ventricular wall is severely hypertrophied (1.4 cm.) and thicker than the left ventricular wall (1.2 cm.). R.A. = right atrial appendage. *Lower left*, opened right ventricle (R.V.). *Lower right*, opened left ventricle (L.V.). The lower photographs show the location of the ventricular septal defect (V.S.D.). There is continuity between ele-ments of the anterior mitral leaflet (A.) and the pulmonic valve (P.V.). P = posterior mitral leaflet.

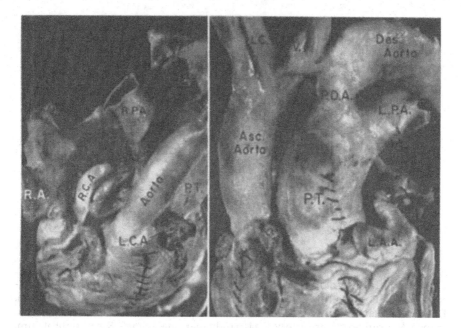

Figure 6 Coronary arteries, aorta and pulmonary trunk. *Left,* right (R.C.A.) and left (L.C.A.) coronary arteries as they arise from the aorta. The right one particularly is enormously dilated and tortuous. Two large tortuous arteries arise from it to supply the anterior and lateral walls of the right ventricle. P.A. = pulmonary trunk; R.P.A. = right pulmonary artery; R. A. = right atrial appendage. *Right,* note again the large size of the pulmonary trunk compared to the ascending (Asc.) aorta. The transverse aorta, particularly that portion between the origins of the left carotid, (L.C.) and vertebral artery (V.) is narrowed and considerably smaller than the lumen of the patent ductus arteriosus (P.D.A.). The vertebral artery (V.) arises anomalously directly from the aorta. The descending (Des.) aorta proximally is much larger than the transverse aorta as is the patent ductus arteriosus. L.P.A. = left pulmonary artery; L.A.A. = left atrial appendage.

which is high in oxygen content. When the aortic root saturation is low, as it is in the presence of a right to left intracardiac shunt, maximal extraction may not provide the heart with adequate oxygen. Under these circumstances, the deficit may be overcome by increased flow through the coronary bed. A large flow acting over a protracted period of time may result in dilatation and tortuosity of the coronary arteries found in some patients with cyanotic congenital heart disease of long-standing.

Right ventricular origin of both great vessels is a malformation in which the pulmonary trunk arises in its normal position but the aorta arises entirely from the right ventricle.[4-6] A ventricular septal defect provides the left ventricle with its only outlet. The position of the ventricular septal defect may be above the crista supraventricularis just beneath the pulmonic valve but some distance from the aortic valve.[5,7] Blood from the left ventricle is directed principally toward the pulmonary trunk, and from the right ventricle blood is directed toward the aorta so that cyanosis is invariable. The peak systolic pressures are the same in the right ventricle, aorta and pulmonary artery. The ventricular septal defect is generally large, and the anterior mitral leaflet usually lacks continuity with both aortic and pulmonic valves.[8] The

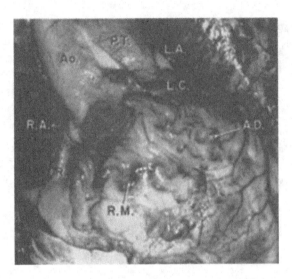

Figure 7 The external surface of the heart *in situ* showing the remarkable dilatation and tortuosity of the coronary arteries (compare with Figure 4). Ao. = aorta. P.T. = pulmonary trunk. L.C. = left circumflex branch. A.D. = anterior descending branch. R. = right coronary artery. R.M. = right marginal branch. R.A. = right atrium. L.A. = left atrium.

high location of the ventricular septal defect permits direct communication between the left ventricle and the pulmonary trunk, although the latter vessel originates wholly from the right ventricle. In some patients in whom the aorta arises entirely from the right ventricle, the pulmonary trunk straddles the ventricular septal defect to varying degrees and is therefore biventricular in origin.[7, 8] This condition of *right ventricular origin of the aorta and biventricular origin of the pulmonary trunk* is clinically similar to right ventricular origin of both great vessels with high ventricular septal defect. The internal architecture of the heart, however, has some features of *complete transposition of the great vessels*, especially when the pulmonary trunk arises principally from the left ventricle.[8] Under these circumstances there is continuity between elements of the mitral and pulmonary valves.[8] It has been argued that varying degrees of biventricular origin of the pulmonary trunk are part of a continuum, with right ventricular origin of both great vessels at one end of the spectrum and complete transposition of the great vessels at the other.[9] It is still debated as to whether the gradations in this continuum should be separately designated or whether they should merely be considered variations of each other.[9] Each of the two basic conditions, i.e. "right ventricular origin of both great vessels"[4, 7] and "right ventricular origin of the aorta with biventricular origin of the pulmonary trunk"[8] has been taken to represent the *"Taussig-Bing" complex.*[7, 10–13] The clinical and hemodynamic manifestations are much the same whether the pulmonary trunk originates entirely from the right ventricle or whether it straddles the ventricular septal defect and rises partially from the left ventricle, Accordingly, if the eponym "Taussig-Bing"[10] is used clinically, it should include both of these anatomic variations.

In the patient described in this report, the aorta arose entirely from the right ventricle, and the pulmonary trunk was biventricular in origin arising partially from the right ventricle but principally from the left (Figures 3 and 5). The peak systolic pressures were the same in the right ventricle and in both great arteries (Table 1).

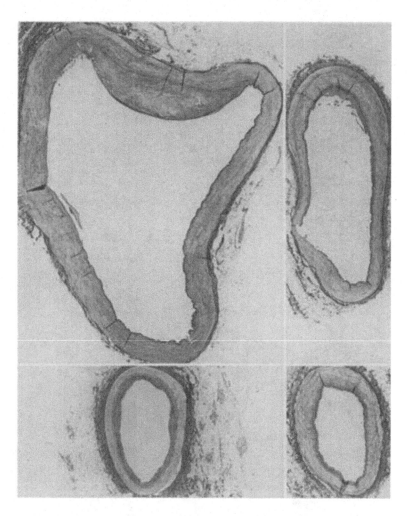

Figure 8 Photomicrographs of sections of right and left coronary arteries from our patient (*upper*) and from a thirty-five year old woman without cardiac disease (*lower*) for comparison. Each of the four sections is at the same magnification (× 18), and each is located 1 cm. from the coronary arterial ostia. The coronary arteries in our patient are severely dilated, particularly the right one (*upper left*). The coronary arteries in the lower panel are of normal size for comparison. *Lower left*, right coronary artery. *Lower right*, left coronary artery. Elastic van Gieson stain on each.

Pulmonary hypertension had apparently been present from birth since the configuration of elastic fibers in the pulmonary trunk was virtually indistinguishable from that in the ascending aorta[14] (Figure 9). The oxygen contents and krypton[85] concentrations were higher in the pulmonary artery than in the ascending aorta (Table 1) indicating that the left ventricle communicated directly with the pulmonary trunk which straddled the ventricular septal defect (Figures 3 and 5). The biventricular origin of the dilated pulmonary trunk and the right ventricular origin of the aorta were clearly shown in the angiocardiograms (Figure 3) and at necropsy (Figure 5).

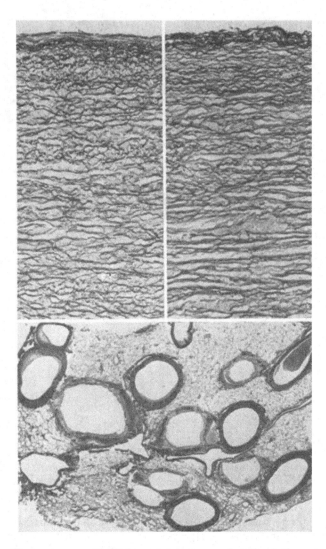

Figure 9 Photomicrographs of the pulmonary trunk (*upper left*), ascending aorta (*upper right*) and hilar pulmonary vessels (lower). The transverse sections of the pulmonary trunk and aorta were taken 1 cm. above the superior margins of the semilunar valves, each is taken at the same magnification (× 135), and each is stained for elastic fibers by the van Gieson method. The configuration of the elastic fibers of the pulmonary trunk indicates that pulmonary hypertension had been present from birth. Normally, after one year of age, the pulmonary trunk contains far less elastic fibers than the ascending aorta. *Lower*, section of hilar area of one lung showing that the pulmonary arteries are greatly dilated and that there is an insignificant amount of intimal proliferation. Multiple sections in the lungs themselves disclosed the muscular pulmonary arteries and arterioles to be dilated but their lumens to be virtually free of intimal proliferation. The media of some of the muscular arteries was mildly hypertrophied. Thus, despite pulmonary hypertension for forty years as evidenced by aortization of the pulmonary trunk, there were only insignificant changes of the muscular pulmonary arteries and arterioles. Elastic tissue stain, original magnification × 5.

Since the aorta arose wholly from the right ventricle (Figure 5), the position of its ascending portion differed from normal[15]. The aortic root was relatively rightward and anterior (Figure 3), the two semilunar valves were at the same body level (Figures 3 and 5), the root rose rather vertically (Figure 4) and the plane of its valve was horizontal rather than oblique[15] (Figure 4).

Anomalies of the aortic arch are commonly associated with either right ventricular origin of both great arteries[7] or with right ventricular aorta and biventricular pulmonary trunk.[8] In our patient three such anomalies were identified, namely, hypoplasia of the transverse aorta, patent ductus arteriosus and anomalous origin of the vertebral artery (Figure 6). The patent ductus arteriosus, together with the abnormal position of the great arteries, set the stage for an unusual form of differential cyanosis in which the toes were relatively pink and the fingers frankly blue. Recognition of this distribution of cyanosis is clinically useful in suspecting the basic malformation.[16] Oxygenated blood from the left ventricle entered the pulmonary trunk and flowed via the patent ductus arteriosus into the descending aorta. The toes, therefore, were relatively acyanotic and were clubbed little if at all. Unoxygenated blood from the right ventricle entered the ascending aorta so the fingers were obviously cyanosed and clubbed. These circulatory pathways are illustrated in Figure 5.

It is noteworthy that our patient's condition improved toward puberty. It may be postulated that in the early years of life, congestive cardiac failure occurred because pulmonary blood flow was excessive. As time went on, changes in pulmonary vascular resistance may have favorably regulated the amount of pulmonary blood flow so that even though adequate, it was not excessive. Under these circumstances the symptoms of cardiac failure may have been relieved and longevity improved. Patients with the Taussig-Bing complex have been known to live into the second, third or even fourth decades,[11, 12] but our patient is the oldest subject with right ventricular origin of the aorta and biventricular origin of the pulmonary trunk thus far reported.

The brisk bouts of hemoptysis appeared analogous to the hemoptysis occasionally observed in the pulmonary hypertension of Eisenmenger's complex[17]. The patient described by Eisenmenger in 1897 was a thirty-two year old man who died following a large hemoptysis.[17] Right ventricular aorta with biventricular pulmonary trunk differs clinically from Eisenmenger's complex in two respects. (1) In Eisenmenger's complex, cyanosis occurs with *normal or diminished* pulmonary blood flow whereas in our patient cyanosis occurred with *increased* pulmonary blood flow[11] (Figure 1). (2) In subjects with right ventricular aorta and biventricular pulmonary trunk, cyanosis is usually present from birth, but in Eisenmenger's complex cyanosis generally begins at a later date.[10]

REFERENCES

1. BJORK, L. Ectasia of the coronary arteries. *Radiology*, 87: 33, 1966.
2. AITCHISON, J. D., DUTHIE, R. J. and YOUNG, J. S. Palpable venous pulsations in a case of transposition of both arterial trunks and complete heart block. *Brit. Heart J.*, 17: 63, 1955.
3. KINCAID, O. W. and TITUS, J. L. Personal communication.
4. WITHAM, A. C. Double outlet right ventricle. *Am. Heart J.*, 53: 928, 1957.
5. NEUFELD, H. N., LUCAS, R. V., LESTER, R. G., ADAMS, P., JR., ANDERSON, R. C. and EDWARDS, J. E. Origin of both great vessels from the right venticle without pulmonary stenosis. *Brit. Heart J.*, 24: 393, 1962.
6. NEUFELD, H. N., DUSHANE, J. W., WOOD, E. H., KIRKLIN, J. W. and EDWARDS, J. E. Origin of both great vessels from the right ventricle. I. Without pulmonic stenosis. *Circulation*, 23: 399, 1961.

7. EDWARDS, J. E., CAREY, L. S., NEUFELD, H. N. and LESTER, R. G. *Congenital Heart Disease*, p. 306. Philadelphia, W. B. Saunders Co., 1965.

8. ELLIOTT, L. P., ADAMS, P., JR., LEVY, M. J. and EDWARDS, J. E. Right ventricular aorta and biventricular pulmonary trunk, an uncommon form of transposition. *Am. Heart J.*, 66: 478, 1963.

9. LEV, M., RIMOLDI, H. J. A., ECKNER, F. A. O., MELHUISH, B. P., MENG, L. and PAUL, M. H. The Taussig-Bing heart. Qualitative and quantitative anatomy. *Arch. Path.*, 81: 24, 1966.

10. TAUSSIG, H. B. and BING, R. J. Complete transposition of the aorta and a levoposition of the pulmonary artery. *Am. Heart J.*, 37: 551, 1949.

11. CAMPBELL, M. and HUDSON, R. E. B. A case of Taussig-Bing transposition with survival for 34 years. *Guy's Hosp. Rep.*, 107: 14, 1958.

12. BEUREN, A. Differential diagnosis of the Taussig-Bing heart from complete transposition of the great vessels with a posteriorly overriding pulmonary artery. *Circulation*, 21: 1071, 1960.

13. MARINI, A. Clinical features in the Taussig-Bing syndrome. *Ann. Paediat.*, 197: 19, 1961.

14. ROBERTS, W. C. Histologic structure of the pulmonary trunk in patients with primary pulmonary hypertension. *Am. Heart J.*, 65: 230, 1963.

15. CAREY, L. S. and EDWARDS, J. E. Roentgenographic features in cases with origin of both great vessels from the right ventricle without pulmonic stenosis. *Am. J. Roentgenol.*, 93: 269, 1965.

16. TAUSSIG, H. B. *Congenital Malformations of the Heart*, p. 162. Cambridge, Harvard University Press, 1960.

17. WOOD, P. The Eisenmenger syndrome. *Brit. M. J.*, 2: 701, 1958.

Case 84 Scimitar Syndrome Associated with Patent Ductus Arteriosus, Aortic Coarctation and Irreversible Pulmonary Hypertension

D. Luke Glancy, Nina S. Braunwald, Kevin P. O'Brien and William C. Roberts

The scimitar syndrome receives its name from the scimitar-like, roentgenographic appearance of an anomalous vein connecting most or all of the right pulmonary veins with the inferior vena cava[1]. The venous abnormality is usually associated with other anomalies of the right lung. Since it was first recognized[2] in 1836, this congenital malformation has been observed in over 70 patients,[3,4] but hemodynamic data together with detailed morphologic study at necropsy have been presented in only one of them[1]. This report describes the clinical, hemodynamic, and necropsy findings in a boy with patent ductus arteriosus and preductile aortic coarctation, a complex of malformations not previously found in association with the scimitar syndrome.

REPORT OF PATIENT

A seven-year-old boy (C.C. #07-39-01) entered the National Heart Institute for evaluation of cardiomegaly, first noted at age two months, and a precordial murmur, discovered at age three years. During infancy he had gained weight slowly, had frequent respiratory infections, and had developed dyspnea and cyanosis with exertion. At age three years he had been given digoxin, and thereafter his respiratory infections and symptoms had steadily decreased. Examination (age seven) revealed a bulging precordium, a prominent left parasternal lift, and a loud pulmonic closure sound. A grade 3/6 continuous murmur beneath the left clavicle, a grade 2/6 basal systolic ejection murmur, and a grade 2/6 mid-diastolic rumble at the lower left sternal border were heard. Femoral arterial pulsations were full, but delayed. The electrocardiogram and chest roentgenograms are shown in Figures 1 and 2, respectively.

At cardiac catheterization (Table I) oxygen step-ups were found high in the inferior vena cava and in the pulmonary artery. Pulmonary blood flow was calculated to be twice systemic flow, and the pulmonary resistance to be approximately one third of systemic resistance. A 13 mm Hg pressure gradient was measured across the junction of an anomalous right pulmonary vein with the inferior vena cava at the level of the diaphragm. Pressures in the pulmonary artery and descending aorta, entered from the pulmonary artery, were identical. Cinearteriograms following an aortic root injection showed narrowing of the aortic isthmus and filling of the pulmonary artery from the aorta distal to the coarctation. A 30 mm Hg peak systolic pressure gradient was measured across the coarctation.

On August 23, 1967, the aortic coarctation was resected; its lumen measured 1.5 mm in diameter (Figure 5). A patent ductus arteriosus, which was distal to the

The Section of Pathology and the Surgery and Cardiology Branches, National Heart Institute, National Institutes of Health, Bethesda, Maryland
Received for publication July 29, 1968

DOI: 10.1201/9781003409342-11

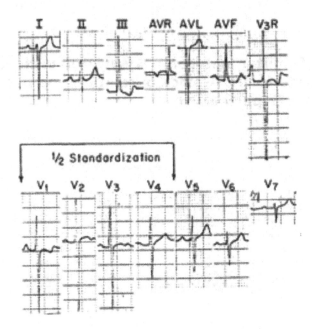

Figure 1 Electrocardiogram showing right axis deviation, right ventricular hypertrophy and right atrial enlargement.

coarctation and 0.75 cm in diameter, was closed with sutures and divided. At the end of the operation the pulmonary arterial pressure was 70/40 and systemic arterial pressure, 95/70 mm Hg. Postoperatively, the child developed respiratory distress, intermittent fever, anemia, leukocytosis, and changing pulmonary infiltrates. Despite antibiotics and adrenal corticosteroids, the dyspnea gradually worsened, and he died eight weeks after operation.

The pulmonary and cardiac findings at necropsy (A67–254) are illustrated in Figures 2–5. The left lung was of normal size, had two lobes, and its bronchi, arteries and veins had normal distributions and connections. In contrast, the right lung was small and had abnormalities of lobation, bronchial distribution, arterial supply, and venous connections. The right lung had no middle lobe. The lower lobe had an extra segment on its medial surface, which was partially separated from the rest of the lower lobe by pleura. A bronchus, arising from the main bronchus to the right lower lobe just distal to its origin, supplied both the extra segment and a portion of the upper lobe. The right pulmonary artery was of normal size and divided into three branches: large ones to the upper and lower lobes and a smaller one to the extra segment. A systemic artery arising from the aorta at the level of the diaphragm entered the posterior basal segment of the right lower lobe. Histologically, it was an elastic artery. The pulmonary venous connections are described in Figures 2 and 3.

All segments of both lungs were consolidated and hemorrhagic. Virtually every alveolus was filled with erythrocytes and/or edema fluid. Large mononuclear cells were present in most alveoli. Many contained hemosiderin, many had foamy cytoplasm, a few had phagocytosed erythrocytes, and an occasional multinucleated cell was seen. Pleural veins and lymphatics were dilated, and the interlobular septae were edematous.

In every segment of both lungs there were grade 4/6 [Heath and Edwards classification[5]] changes of hypertensive pulmonary arterial disease: medial hypertrophy;

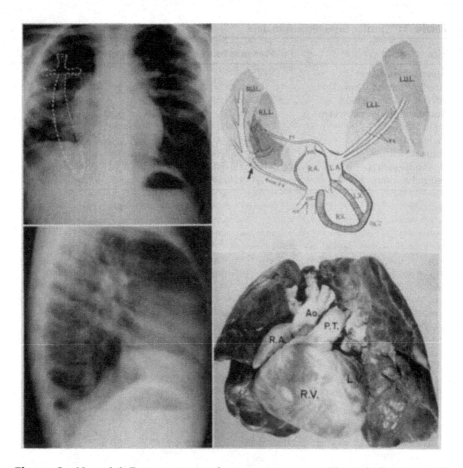

Figure 2 *Upper left:* Posteroanterior chest roentgenogram. The right lung is small; the right diaphragm is elevated; and the heart is shifted to the right. Within the blade of the scimitar (dashed lines) is a long, anomalous, pulmonary vein which descends in the interlobar fissure to connect with the inferior vena cava. The pulmonary trunk is prominent. *Lower left:* Lateral roentgenogram showing the elevated right hemidiaphragm and the retrosternal space filled by the large right ventricle. *Upper right:* Diagram of the heart, lungs, and pulmonary veins (P.V.). The right lung has no middle lobe, but the right lower lobe (R.L.L.) has an extra segment (dark stippling) on its medial surface. All veins from the left upper (L.U.L.) and left lower (L.L.L.) lobes and a small vein from the R.L.L. connect with the left atrium (L.A.) normally. All right upper lobe (R.U.L.) and most R.L.L. veins connect with an anomalous vein (Anom. P.V.) which empties into the inferior vena cava (I.V.C.) just below the right atrium (R.A.) and above the hepatic veins (H.V.). The anomalous vein appears to be compressed (arrow) as it emerges through a notch on the inferomedial surface of the lung, and its extra-pulmonary segment is narrower than its intrapulmonary segment. L.V. = left ventricle; R.V. = right ventricle; S.V.C. = superior vena cava. *Lower right:* Anterior view of the heart and lungs at necropsy. The left lung is larger than the right. The right ventricle (R.V.) is massively hypertrophied and forms the apex of the heart. A white fibrous plaque, so-called soldier's patch, is on its epicardial surface. The right atrial appendage (R.A.) and pulmonary trunk (P.T.) are dilated. Ao. = aorta; L.V. = left ventricle.

Table 1: Cardiac catheterization data

Site	Pressure (mm Hg)	Oxygen Saturation (%)
Superior vena cava		67
Inferior vena cava, low		73
Inferior vena cava, high		79
Anomalous pulmonary vein	17	93
Right atrium	4	77
Right ventricle	96/4	78
Pulmonary artery	96/60	83
Descending aorta	96/60	92
Left radial artery	126/69	94

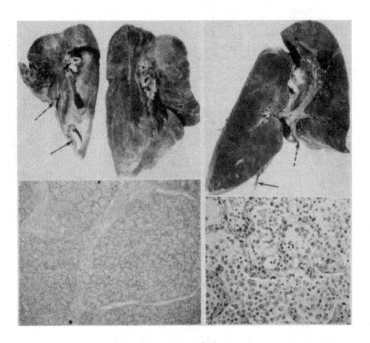

Figure 3 The lungs. *Upper left:* Medial surface of the lungs. The right lung is much smaller than the left. The solid arrow indicates the systemic artery which enters the posterior basal segment of the right lower lobe; and the dashed arrow, the notch through which the anomalous vein left the lung to connect with the inferior vena cava. The extra right lower lobe segment is between the two arrows. *Upper right:* The lateral portion of the right lung has been cut away. The parenchyma of both lobes is consolidated and hemorrhagic. The anomalous pulmonary vein and several of its larger branches lie in the interlobar fissure. The solid arrow indicates the systemic artery; and the dashed arrow, the anomalous vein where it is compressed as it leaves the lung. *Lower left:* Histologic section of lung in which every alveolus is filled with blood and/or edema fluid. Many alveoli also contain large mononuclear cells. Two dilated lymphatics are on the right, and an edematous interlobular septum is in the middle of the field (H and E; × 19). *Lower right:* A higher power photomicrograph (periodic acid-Schiff; × 147) showing alveoli containing numerous large mononuclear cells, occasional multinucleated forms, and a few polymorphonuclear neutrophils.

intimal proliferation, which was most severe in the medium-sized muscular arteries; numerous plexiform lesions; and occasional dilatation lesions. Small infarcts were present in both lungs. The configuration of the elastic fibers in the media of the pulmonary trunk and ascending aorta were identical, suggesting that pulmonary hypertension had been present from birth[6].

Most of the cardiac mass was right ventricle. Although hypertrophied, the left ventricle was much smaller than the right ventricle. The right atrium and pulmonary trunk were dilated; their walls were thicker than normal; and the intima of the pulmonary trunk contained small deposits of lipid. The aortic valve was congenitally bicuspid, but otherwise normal. The aortic lumen at the site of anastomosis measured 6.5 mm in diameter.

COMMENTS

The essential component of the scimitar syndrome is an anomalous vein which connects most or all of the right pulmonary veins with the inferior vena cava. Other components which are frequently present are listed in Table II. Almost one fourth of the patients have had other congenital cardiovascular anomalies. Atrial septal defect has been the most common, and coarctation of the aorta has been reported only once previously[7]. Congenital anomalies outside the cardiopulmonary system, such as hemivertebrae, double ureter, uterine duplication, and omphalocele, have occasionally been observed[1, 3]. Two thirds of the patients have been females.

In the absence of other cardiovascular anomalies, patients with the scimitar syndrome usually have normal or only mildly elevated pulmonary arterial pressures, and 56/26 mm Hg is the highest recorded[8]. This finding is not surprising since the left-to-right shunt occurs proximal to the tricuspid valve as in atrial septal defect, is usually small, and in some patients cannot be detected by oxygen series[3]. Only one reported patient has had a shunt greater than 50% of pulmonary blood flow[4], and in him coexisting mitral stenosis, by elevating the pressure in the normally draining pulmonary veins, probably encouraged flow through the anomalous vein. Four patients, including ours, have had moderate or severe pulmonary hypertension[1, 9, 10], and each of them had patent ductus arteriosus. In our patient and two others[1, 9] with patent ductus and pulmonary hypertension, a pressure gradient was measured between the anomalous vein and the inferior vena cava. Venous obstruction of one lung can cause pulmonary arterial hypertension[11] and may have contributed to the pulmonary hypertension in these patients. At least one reported patient with the scimitar syndrome and obstruction of the anomalous vein, however, did not have pulmonary arterial hypertension[12]. Pulmonary parenchymal disease, hypoplasia or absence[13] of the right pulmonary artery, or multiple pulmonary arterial branch stenoses[9] could potentiate pulmonary hypertension in patients with the scimitar syndrome.

In our patient the large patent ductus arteriosus probably was the most important factor in the development of severe pulmonary hypertension and obliterative arterial disease. When he was catheterized at age seven, a moderate-sized left-to-right shunt was demonstrated, but most of this was probably obligatory shunting via the anomalous vein. Bidirectional shunting may have been present through the ductus, and indicator dilution curves from the right side of the heart with sampling from the femoral artery might have been the best method for uncovering the right-to-left component, which at the time of catheterization must have been small since the oxygen saturation was only 2% higher in radial arterial blood than in simultaneously obtained descending aortic blood. Despite overall pulmonary/systemic flow and resistance ratios which seemed favorable for operation, the patient had irreversible obliterative pulmonary arterial disease. Like most patients with Eisenmenger's syndrome, he did not tolerate closure of the communication between systemic and pulmonary circulations, and extensive intra-alveolar hemorrhage resulted in death.

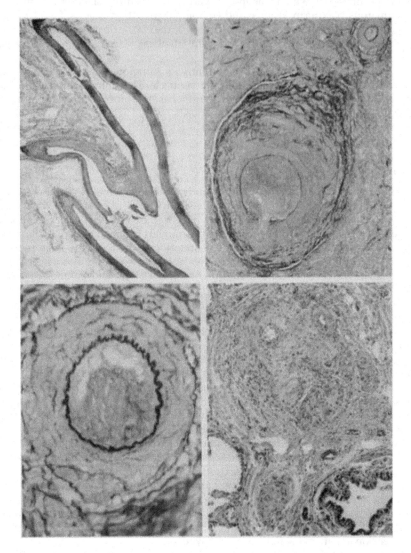

Figure 4 Photomicrographs of arteries in the lungs. *Upper left:* Elastic tissue stain (× 22) of the systemic artery as it branches on entering the right lower lobe. The arterial media is composed primarily of elastic tissue. *Upper right:* A medium-sized, muscular, pulmonary artery. The adventitia is thickened by fibroelastic tissue; the media is hypertrophied; and the lumen, including the orifice of a small branch, is completely obliterated by fibrous intimal proliferation. A small muscular artery with medial hypertrophy and intimal proliferation is seen in the upper right corner of the field (elastic tissue stain; × 83). *Lower left:* A small, muscular, pulmonary artery with marked medial hypertrophy and a lumen almost completely obliterated by fibro-cellular intimal proliferation (elastic tissue stain; × 356). *Lower right:* A plexiform lesion with marked medial hypertrophy and cellular intimal proliferation of both the parent muscular artery (upper left) and its branches (H and E; × 88).

Table 2: Scimitar syndrome

1. Connection of most or all of the right pulmonary veins to the inferior vena cava via an anomalous vein.
2. Small right lung associated with:
   a. Deficient or abnormal lobation.
   b. Anomalous distribution of bronchi.
   c. Bronchial diverticula or cysts.
   d. Diaphragmatic elevation or anomaly.
   e. Rightward cardiac displacement.
3. Hypoplasia of the right pulmonary artery.
4. Branches of the upper abdominal or lower thoracic aorta supply part of the right lung.
5. Congenital cardiac disease (20–25%):
   a. Atrial septal defect.
   b. Patent ductus arteriosus.
   c. Tetralogy of Fallot.
   d. Ventricular septal defect.
   e. Coarctation of the aorta.

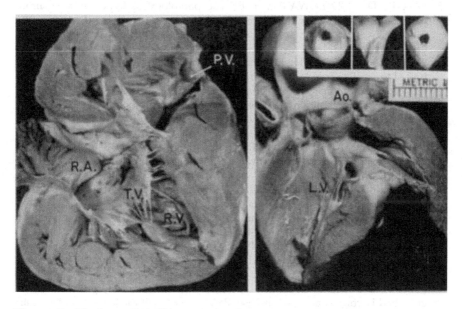

Figure 5   The heart. *Left:* The opened right atrium (R.A.), tricuspid (T.V.) and pulmonic (P.V.) valves, and massively hypertrophied right ventricle (R.V.). *Right:* The opened left ventricle (L.V.), aortic valve, and aorta (Ao.). Although its wall is thicker (1.5 cm) than normal, the left ventricle is dwarfed by the right. (Both pictures were taken from the same distance.) The aortic valve is congenitally bicuspid. The posterior cusp is intact; the anterior cusp has been cut. *Inset:* The resected aortic coarctation: proximal (left), lateral and distal (right) aspects. The lumen measures 1.5 mm in diameter. The ruler measures only the coarctation specimen.

SUMMARY

The clinical, hemodynamic and necropsy findings are presented in a seven-year-old boy with the scimitar syndrome, patent ductus arteriosus, preductile aortic coarctation and severe pulmonary hypertension, and hemodynamic findings in patients with the scimitar syndrome are discussed.

REFERENCES

1. NEILL, C. A., FERENCZ, C., SABISTON, D. C. AND SHELDON, H.: The familial occurrence of hypoplastic right lung with systemic arterial supply and venous drainage "scimitar syndrome." *Bull. Hopkins Hosp.*, 107: 1, 1960.
2. COOPER. G.: Case of malformation of the thoracic viscera: Consisting of imperfect development of right lung, and transposition of the heart. *London Med. Gaz.*, 18: 600, 1836.
3. KIELY, B., FILLER, J., STONE, S. AND DOYLE, E. F.: Syndrome of anomalous venous drainage of the right lung to the inferior vena cava. A review of 67 reported cases and three new cases in children. *Amer. J. Cardiol.*, 20: 102, 1967.
4. KALKE, B. R., CARLSON, R. G., FERLIC, R. M., SELLERS, R. D. AND LILLEHEI, C. W.: Partial anomalous pulmonary venous connections. *Amer. J. Cardiol.*, 20: 91, 1967.
5. HEATH, D. AND EDWARDS, J. E.: The pathology of hypertensive pulmonary vascular disease. A description of six grades of structural changes in the pulmonary arteries with special reference to congenital cardiac septal defects. *Circulation*, 18: 533, 1958.
6. HEATH, D., WOOD, E. H., DU SHANE, J. W. AND EDWARDS, J. E.: The structure of the pulmonary trunk at different ages and in cases of pulmonary hypertension and pulmonary stenosis. *J. Path. Bact.*, 77: 443, 1959.
7. STEINBERG, I.: Roentgen diagnosis of anomalous pulmonary venous drainage of right lung into inferior vena cava. Report of three new cases. *Am. J. Roentgen.*, 81: 280, 1959.
8. FRYE, R. L., MARSHALL, H. W., KINCAID, O. W. AND BURCHEL, H. B.: Anomalous pulmonary venous drainage of the right lung into the inferior vena cava. *Brit. Heart J.*, 24: 696, 1962.
9. YONEHIRO, E. G., HALLMAN, G. L. AND COOLEY, D. A.: Anomalous pulmonary venous return from a hypoplastic right lung to the inferior vena cava (scimitar syndrome): Report of successful correction and review of surgical treatment. *Cardiov. Res. Cent. Bull. (Houston)*, 4: 106, 1965–1966.
10. JUE, K. L., AMPLATZ, K., ADAMS, P., JR. AND ANDERSON, R. C.: Anomalies of the great vessels associated with lung hypoplasia. The scimitar syndrome. *Amer. J. Dis. Child.*, 111: 35, 1966.
11. FERENCZ, C. AND DAMMANN, J. F., JR.: Significance of the pulmonary vascular bed in congenital heart disease. Part V. Lesions of the left side of the heart causing obstruction of the pulmonary venous return. *Circulation*, 16: 1046, 1957.
12. KAPLAN, S.: quoted by Neill, C. A., et al. in reference 1.
13. HOLLIS, W. J.: The scimitar anomaly with absent right pulmonary artery. *Amer. J. Cardiol.*, 14: 262, 1964.

Case 92 Anomalous Left Ventricular Band
*An Unemphasized Cause of a Precordial Musical Murmur**

William C. Roberts, MD, F.A.C.C.
Bethesda, Maryland

CONDITIONS that temporarily increase the speed of blood flow through the heart or great vessels are usually the cause of transient precordial murmurs. The states generally listed as responsible for "functional," "innocent," "hemic" or "benign" murmurs are nervousness, anemia, fever, tachycardia, exercise, hyperthyroidism and pregnancy. Transient dilatation of the cardiac ventricles from any cause resulting in stretching of the atrioventricular rings and papillary muscles may be responsible for a precordial systolic murmur that may subsequently disappear. Likewise, transient papillary muscle dysfunction is now recognized as a cause of a transient as well as a permanent precordial systolic murmur. Another but hitherto unemphasized cause of a transient precordial murmur is an anomalous band in the left ventricle. This report briefly describes a patient in whom this band appeared to be the cause of a transient precordial murmur and reviews the pathologic features of these bands and previous reports describing them.

CASE HISTORY
A 68 year old man[†] was hospitalized because of severe congestive cardiac failure secondary to coronary atherosclerosis. On examination, in addition to severe pitting subcutaneous edema and pulmonary rales, a musical grade 3/6 systolic murmur was audible over the precordium. After the patient lost 8 kg. in weight in two days, the cardiac silhouette was smaller on chest roentgenogram, and the precordial murmur was no longer present. Several days later the patient unexpectedly died.

At necropsy, the heart was of normal size, the cardiac valves and rings were normal, but the major coronary arteries were considerably narrowed. A fibrous cord, approximately 2 mm. in diameter (Figure 1), stretched from the endocardium of the ventricular septum across the left ventricular cavity to the endocardium of its lateral wall.

COMMENTS
The mechanism of the transient, precordial murmur in this patient is uncertain, but the anomalous left ventricular cord may have been the cause. The sequence of events leading to the murmur and to its transient nature may have been the following. When the patient was first hospitalized, he was in severe cardiac failure, and the left ventricular cavity was dilated. The anomalous cord was pulled taut by the dilated

* From the Section of Pathology, National Heart Institute, National Institutes of Health, Bethesda, Md. Manuscript received October 17, 1967.
† This patient was examined clinically and at necropsy in 1962 at The Johns Hopkins Hospital, Baltimore, Md., when I was an assistant resident on the Osler Medical Service.
Address for reprints: William C. Roberts, M.D., Section of Pathology, National Heart Institute, National Institutes of Health, Bethesda, Md. 20014.

DOI: 10.1201/9781003409342-12

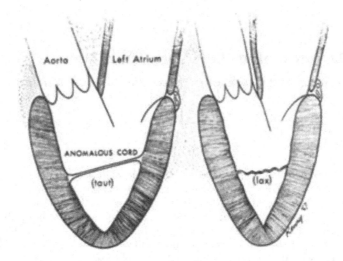

Figure 1 Diagrammatic representation of the anomalous left ventricular cord observed in the patient described. When the chamber is dilated, the cord is pulled taut, and a murmur is produced. When the left ventricular cavity becomes smaller, the cord becomes lax and the murmur disappears.

left ventricle and, therefore, blood ejected across it produced localized turbulence and a murmur. When the patient lost excessive body fluid after bed rest, digitalis and diuretic therapy, the size of the left ventricular cavity returned to normal. When this chamber was no longer stretched, the anomalous cord became lax, and the murmur disappeared (Figure 1).

It is possible that the anomalous cord was not a factor in the production of the murmur, which was simply the result of dilatation of the mitral annulus or stretching of the left ventricular papillary muscles, both consequences of left ventricular dilatation from any cause. Obviously, the larger the mitral annulus and the greater the tension on the left ventricular papillary muscles produced by stretching, the less likely it is that the mitral orifice may have been closed completely by the leaflets during ventricular systole. The circumference of the mitral annulus and the "tautness" of the papillary muscles would decrease with the restoration of cardiac compensation.

Anomalous left ventricular cords, such as that illustrated, are not rare. (I have seen them in a number of hearts during the past seven years, and Turner observed them at necropsy in 4 patients during a five year period.[1-4]) The anomalous bands may be located transversely within the left ventricular cavity, stretching from the septum to the lateral wall (Figure 2) or to a papillary muscle,[5] or from one papillary muscle to another,[5] or from one free wall to the other.[6] More commonly, however, the bands are located in a more vertical or longitudinal axis within the chamber (Figure 3); often they extend from one papillary muscle to the free or septal ventricular wall or to one or more of the trabeculae carnae in the apex of this chamber. These anomalous bands, which occasionally are multiple,[1] may consist of myocardium surrounded by endocardium (Figure 2), but more commonly they consist of dense fibrous tissue similar to a chorda tendinea (Figure 3).

The production of musical murmurs by anomalous left ventricular bands has been summarized by McKusick.[7] Huchard[6] in 1893 apparently was the first to describe the clinical findings associated with such bands, which he called "aberrant tendons."

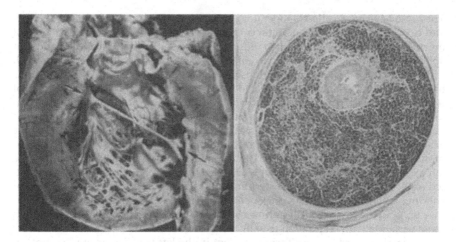

Figure 2   A large muscular band (**between the arrows**) in the left ventricular outflow tract of a 40 year old man who died of cardiac failure secondary to aortic regurgitation. He had loud nonmusical precordial systolic and diastolic murmurs, which were attributed to the dysfunctioning aortic valve. *The photomicrograph on the right* is of a cross section of the anomalous left ventricular band, which consisted primarily of myocardium. The overlying endocardium is thickened, the fibrous tissue in the interstitial myocardial areas is increased, and a thick-walled artery runs through the entire length of the anomalous band. (Hematoxylin and eosin × 28, reduced by 25 per cent.)

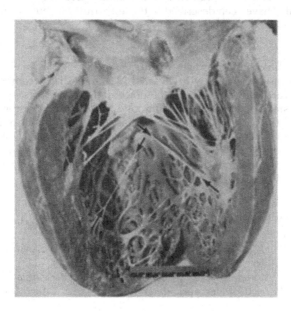

Figure 3   Opened left atrium, mitral valve and left ventricle of a 34 year old man who died after aortic valve replacement for severe aortic regurgitation. At necropsy, two anomalous left ventricular cords (between the arrows), each extending from a papillary muscle to the outflow tract, were found.

They also have been called "moderator bands" since they were believed to "moderate" or "checkrein" dilatation of the ventricle.[8] The main feature is that the musical murmur is not present from birth, despite the congenital nature of the band, but appears when the ventricle becomes dilated because of some unrelated strain such as heart failure or systemic hypertension. To produce a murmur, the anomalous band must be pulled taut and be located more or less perpendicular to the stream of flow in the left ventricle. McKusick compared the murmur produced by the anomalous cords to the musical vibration produced by an Aeolian harp. Huchard's first observation[6] of this lesion was in a 49 year old man who had signs of severe systemic arterial hypertension with cardiomegaly and congestive failure. A murmur typical of mitral regurgitation was audible in this patient over the cardiac apex and in the left axilla. More medially, maximal in the area of the xiphoid and widely transmitted especially to the right of the sternum and to the cardiac base, was a purring or snoring systolic murmur. McKusick pointed out that extracardiac musical murmurs may occur in the same clinical setting and display the same characteristics, although more variation with respiration usually can be demonstrated.

Anomalous cords are uniformly present in the left ventricular outflow tract in patients with persistent common atrioventricular canal, and occasionally in subjects with isolated ventricular septal defect. McKusick has suggested that these anomalously inserted chordae tendineae may rarely produce unusual harmonics, which have been demonstrated in the Roger murmur. Chiari's network in the right atrium, a common anatomic finding (2 to 3 per cent of necropsies),[9] apparently is a very rare cause of a musical precordial murmur, although 2 such cases have been described.[10, 11] It is probable that, as with the ventricular bands and anomalous chordae tendineae, not only does the Chiari network need to be properly oriented in relation to the venae cavae, but also dilatation of the atrium with tensing of the network favors development of such a murmur. Anomalous bands stretching from the septum to the free wall also have been described in the left atrium,[12, 13] but murmurs resulting from them have not been reported.

SUMMARY

The pertinent clinical and necropsy features are described in an elderly man who had a loud precordial murmur when he was in severe cardiac decompensation. With restoration of cardiac compensation the precordial murmur disappeared and the heart became smaller. At necropsy, a fibrous cord was found in the left ventricle, stretching from the septum to the free wall. It is suggested that the murmur was the result of this band's being stretched taut when the left ventricular cavity was dilated. When the left ventricular chamber returned to normal size, the anomalous band became lax and the murmur disappeared. Other reports describing anomalous left ventricular bands are briefly reviewed.

REFERENCES

1. TURNER, W. Heart with moderator band in left ventricle. *J. Anat. & Physiol.*, 27 (n.s. 7):19, 1893.
2. TURNER, W. Heart with moderator band in left ventricle. *J. Anat. & Physiol.*, 30 (n.s. 10):568, 1896.
3. TURNER, W. Moderator band in left ventricle. *J. Anat. & Physiol.*, 32:373, 1898.
4. TURNER, W. Tricuspid left auriculo-ventricular valve. *J. Anat. & Physiol.*, 32:374, 1898.
5. ROLLESTON, H. D. Heart showing a muscular band passing between the two ventriculi papillares of the left ventricle and capable of acting as a moderator band. *J. Anat. & Physiol.*, 32:21, 1897.

6. HUCHARD, H. *Traité Clinique des Maladies du Coeur et de L'aorte*, ed. 3, Vol. III, pp. 640 and 641. Paris, O. Doin, 1905.

7. MCKUSICK, V. A. *Cardiovascular Sound in Health and Disease*, pp. 209–211. Baltimore, Williams & Wilkins, 1958.

8. KING, T. W. An essay on the safety-valve function in the right ventricle of the human heart, and the gradations of this function in the circulation of warm-blooded animals. *Guy's Hosp. Rep.*, 2:104, 1837.

9. YATER, W. M. The paradox of Chiari's network. Review and report of a case of Chiari's network ensnaring a large embolus. *Am. Heart J.*, 11:542, 1936.

10. ALVAREZ, J. A. and HERRMANN, G. Unusual signs from an expansive Chiari network along with signs of a syphilitic aortic regurgitation, *Am. J. Syph.*, 15:532, 1931.

11. WILSON, R. A case of Chiari's network associated with a murmur resembling the bruit de Roger. *J.A.M.A.*, 111:917, 1938.

12. ROLLESTON, H. D. Band in left auricle of heart. *J. Anat. & Physiol.*, 30 (n.s. 10):5, 1896.

13. TURNER, W. Moderator band in left auricle. *J. Anat. & Physiol.*, 30:582, 1896.

Case 93 Rocks in the Right Ventricle

A Complication of Congenital Right Ventricular Infundibular Obstruction Associated With Chronic Pulmonary Parenchymal Disease

David C. Dean, MD,[†] Thomas Pamukcoglu, MD,[‡]
and William C. Roberts, MD, F.A.C.C.[§]
Buffalo, New York and Bethesda, Maryland

CALCIUM IN THE HEART is most frequently located in coronary arteries or in aortic or mitral valve leaflets or "rings." Occasionally, however, it is found in left atrial or left ventricular mural thrombi, thickened pericardia, intracardiac neoplasms and myocardium. The occurrence of calcific deposits in mural thrombi indicates that thrombosis occurred in the distant past. In contrast to calcific deposits located in left atrial thrombi, left ventricular deposits are usually small and rarely protrude into the cavity of the chamber. Calcific material in either of these two chambers nearly always is attached to the endocardium over a broad base. Localized protruding deposits of calcium in a cardiac ventricle is indeed rare, and to our knowledge there are no reported instances of multiple focal intracardiac masses of calcium in the right ventricle. Such was the case, however, in a patient we recently studied.

CASE REPORT

A 56 year old white man, who died on May 15, 1967, had been well until age 33 when bronchial asthma developed during his service in the Army. Because of the development of continuous wheezing, associated with exertional dyspnea, nonproductive cough, substernal chest pain, and frequent episodes of cough syncope, he was examined at the Buffalo Veterans Administration Hospital in March 1962 at age 51. The blood pressure was 142/90 mm. Hg, and rhonchi and wheezes were audible over the chest. A grade 1/6 precordial pansystolic murmur was present. The chest roentgenogram revealed slight enlargement of the left ventricle and the major pulmonary arterial branches. Numerous calcific densities were visible in the cardiac silhouette at this time. A repeat roentgenogram three years later (Figure 1) was unchanged. The electrocardiogram disclosed incomplete right bundle branch block and an electrical axis of +90°.

The patient carried on his usual activities until four hours before death, when severe, crushing pain in the chest developed, radiating down both arms. On admission to the hospital he was cyanotic and sweating profusely. The neck veins were severely distended. Wheezes, rhonchi and rales were audible over both lungs.

From the Departments of Medicine and Pathology, State University of New York at Buffalo,
[†] The Veterans Administration Hospital, Buffalo, New York
[‡] and the Section of Pathology, National Heart Institute, National Institutes of Health, Bethesda, Md.
[§] Manuscript received January 31, 1968.
Address for reprints: David C. Dean, M.D., Veterans Administration Hospital, Buffalo, N. Y. 14215, or William C. Roberts, M.D., Section of Pathology, National Heart Institute, National Institutes of Health, Bethesda, Md. 20014.

DOI: 10.1201/9781003409342-13

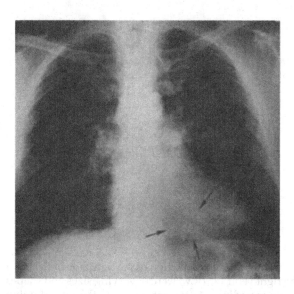

Figure 1 Chest roentgenogram, taken in February 1965. Numerous cardiac calcific densities (**arrows**) are present.

A quadruple gallop rhythm was present. The blood pressure was 130/70 mm. Hg on admission, but was not recordable thereafter. The hematocrit was 52 per cent. The electrocardiogram, which had shown incomplete right bundle branch block 19 days earlier (Figure 2), now showed complete right bundle branch block. The patient failed to respond to antihypotensive medication and died three hours after admission.

At necropsy, the heart weighed 480 gm. Eleven calcified nodules (rocks or stones), ranging in diameter from 0.6 to 2.1 cm., were present in the right ventricle (Figures 3 to 6). Each stone was attached to the right ventricular endocardium by a small (less than 0.2 cm.) fibrous stalk. The right ventricular stones consisted primarily of calcified material, but dense fibrous tissue surrounded the calcific deposits. Biochemical examination of one of the right ventricular stones disclosed that it consisted of 32 per cent hydroxyapatite, 56 per cent tricalcium phosphate and 12 per cent protein. The endocardium of the right ventricle, both beneath and between the stones, was extensively but focally thickened. The entrance into the infundibulum was narrowed by thickened endocardial fibrous tissue, hypertrophied myocardium and

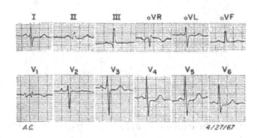

Figure 2 *Electrocardiogram* recorded 19 days before death.

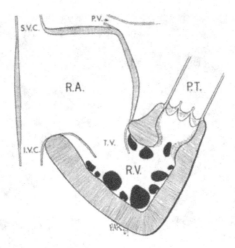

Figure 3 Diagrammatic representation of the right side of the heart. The 11 stones (in black) in the right ventricle (R.V.) were of varying sizes and shapes, and each was attached to the endocardium. At the entrance into the infundibulum there was an area of discrete narrowing produced by thickened myocardium, endocardial fibrosis and a stone at this site. Distal to the area of right ventricular outflow obstruction, the endocardium was thickened, the result almost surely of turbulent flow. The ventricular aspects of the pulmonic valve cusps also were thickened by the same mechanism. The wall of the body of the right ventricle, that portion proximal to the area of infundibular obstruction, was thicker than that portion distal to the obstruction. The right atrium (R.A.) was dilated. (I.V.C. = inferior vena cava; P.T. = pulmonary trunk; S.V.C. = superior vena cava; T.V. = tricuspid valve.)

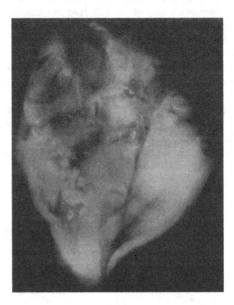

Figure 4 Radiogram of the excised heart at necropsy demonstrating the right ventricular stones and the calcified plaques in the coronary arteries. The specimen had been opened before the radiogram was taken.

106

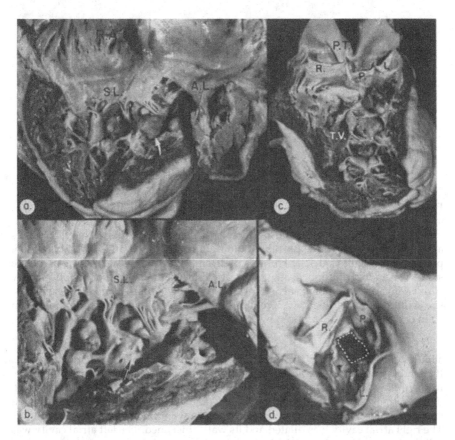

Figure 5   The opened right side of the heart. **a,** opened right atrium (R.A), tricuspid valve and right ventricle. The stones in the right ventricle are apparent. The **arrow** points to the stone upon which the biochemical analysis was performed. The septal (S.L.), anterior (A.L.) and posterior tricuspid valve leaflets and chordae tendineae are thickened. **b,** close-up view of the inflow portion of the right ventricle following removal of the stone designated by the arrow in **a.** The endocardium is extensively thickened. The **arrow** points to the previous site of attachment of the excised stone. **c,** opened pulmonary trunk (P.T.), pulmonic valve and right ventricle again exposing the stones. The right (R.), left (L.) and posterior (P.) cusps of the pulmonic valve are thickened. (T.V. = tricuspid valve orifice.) **d,** pulmonic valve from above demonstrating the area of narrowing (enclosed by the dashes) at the entrance into the infundibulum.

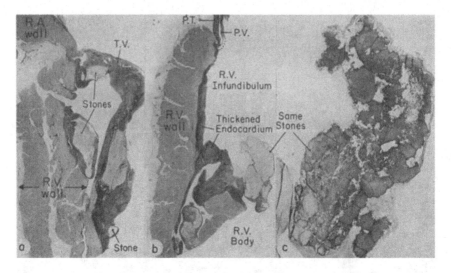

Figure 6 Photomicrographs of the right ventricular wall and of several stones. **a,** section includes right atrial (R.A.) and right ventricular (R.V.) walls and tricuspid valve (T.V.) leaflet. The latter is considerably thickened by fibrous tissue. The stones are designated. The inflow portion of the right ventricular wall is thick. **b,** outflow portion of the right ventricle. The area of discrete narrowing is at the site of a large stone. The endocardium beneath it is greatly thickened. The wall of the pulmonary trunk (P.T.) and a pulmonic valve (P.V.) cusp are shown. (Both a and b are elastic tissue stains, each magnified × 2.5, reduced by 28 per cent.) **c,** hematoxylin and eosin stain of one stone. (× 18, reduced by 28 per cent.)

stones located at this site. The pulmonic valve was wide open, although each of its three cups was diffusely thickened by fibrous tissue. The wall of the right ventricle in the inflow tract measured up to 0.9 cm. in thickness, and in the outflow tract, distal to the area of obstruction, up to 0.5 cm. in thickness. The leaflets of the tricuspid valve and most of its chordae tendineae were thickened by fibrous tissue. The right atrial cavity was dilated and its walls thickened. The left atrial cavity was mildly dilated. The left ventricular wall was of normal thickness and its cavity of normal size. No scars or areas of softening were present in the left ventricular myocardium. The mitral and aortic valves were normal. The lumens of the right, left and left circumflex coronary arteries were narrowed between 25 and 75 per cent by focal, fibrous and calcified plaques.

The lungs were congested and edematous and, focally, emphysematous and fibrotic. Two laminated nodules were in the lung parenchyma, and on histologic examination each contained large numbers of organisms consistent with Histoplasma capsulatum.

COMMENT

The origin of the stones in the right ventricle is uncertain, but at least two possibilities exist. First, they may represent the end stage of organized mural thrombi. The patient presumably had mild right ventricular hypertension during his entire life, the result of the infundibular narrowing. In later life this ventricular hypertension was further aggravated by pulmonary parenchymal disease. The endocardial thickening in the right ventricle may represent organization of flat thrombi. However, it may have resulted from trauma to this chamber by the right ventricular rocks and by the turbulent flow produced by the infundibular obstruction. A second but unlikely possibility is that the stones may represent calcified endocardial granulomas secondary to histoplasmosis. This possibility is suggested by the presence of histoplasma granulomas in the lung, although no organisms were found in any of the right ventricular stones or in other portions of the heart. Histoplasma organisms, however, have been known to cause pericarditis, myocarditis and valvular endocarditis.

No reports describing deposits of calcium in the heart similar to those observed in the patient described have appeared to our knowledge.

SUMMARY

Clinical and necropsy findings are described in a 56 year old man who was found to have multiple rocks in the right ventricular cavity and a congenitally narrowed infundibulum. The size, distribution and location of the rocks in the right ventricle appear unique. Possible causes of the rocks in the heart are speculated upon.

Case 94 The Angiographic Features of a Case of Parachute Mitral Valve

Allan L. Simon, MD*, William F. Friedman, MD, William C. Roberts, MD
Baltimore, Md.

The parachute deformity is an uncommon variant of congenital mitral stenosis, consisting of the insertion of all of the chordae tendineae of the mitral valve into a single, large papillary muscle. In the initial description by Shone and associates,[1] and in other reports,[2, 3] the anomaly has been most often found as part of a developmental complex consisting of aortic coarctation, subaortic stenosis, and supravalvular ring in the left atrium. If diagnosed correctly, it is apparent that a corrective operation may be accomplished.[4] In this regard, the angiographic appearance of the parachute mitral valve per se has received scant attention, although the radiographic features of the associated cardiovascular malformations have been discussed recently.[5] A description of the characteristic angiographic appearance of the left ventricular cavity and mitral valve in a well-studied patient with the parachute deformity and a discussion of the mechanism of obstruction to left ventricular outflow in this disorder forms the basis of the present report.

CASE REPORT

Cyanosis and congestive heart failure were recognized shortly after the premature birth of J. L. H. (N.I.H. 06-50-00), a 4-year-old Caucasian girl. She was treated with oxygen and digitalis and was acyanotic when discharged from the hospital at 2 months of age. Her subsequent course was marked by retarded growth and frequent respiratory infections, and at 2½ years of age she underwent cardiac catheterization at another institution. The hemodynamic data (Table 1) were consistent with the diagnosis of valvular pulmonic stenosis and subaortic stenosis. Severe mitral regurgitation was seen on a left ventricular angiocardiogram. The risk of operation was considered prohibitive and the child was discharged from the hospital. The next 1½ years were characterized by chronic congestive heart failure and frequent episodes of acute pulmonary edema which responded initially to increased digitalis, diuretics, salt restriction, and oxygen. She had become refractory to these measures and was in pulmonary edema when first referred and admitted to the National Heart Institute.

Physical examination revealed a markedly cachectic, acyanotic girl (height 87 cm., weight 9.7 kilograms). The chest was barrel shaped and the heart greatly enlarged. A continuous thrill was prominent at the apex and a systolic thrill was palpable in the suprasternal notch. The first and second heart sounds were single; third and fourth heart sounds were audible at the lower left sternal border. A Grade

From the Radiology Department, Clinical Center, and the Cardiology Branch, Section of Pathology, National Heart Institute, National Institutes of Health, Bethesda, Md.

Received for publication March 25, 1968.

* Present address: Director, Cardiovascular Diagnostic Laboratory, CMSC-5–109, The Johns Hopkins Hospital. Baltimore, Md. 21205.

DOI: 10.1201/9781003409342-14

Table 1: Hemodynamic findings; pressure in millimeters of mercury

	Age 2½ yr.	Age 4 yr.	Intra-operative
RAm*	5	7	
RV	130/10	142/6	70/1
MPA	22/10	32/18	22/6
PCW		a 25	
		v 24	
		m 19	
LAm	20		7
LVb	160/–	168/15	95/1
LVo	90/–	86/15	
Aorta	90/50	86/42	70/30
LA-LV		9	
Post-PVC pulse pressure		5	

* Abbreviations: RAm, right atrial; RV, right ventricular; MPA, main pulmonary arterial; PCW, pulmonary capillary wedge; a, a wave; v, v wave; m, mean pressure; LAm, left atrial mean; LVb, body of left ventricle; LVo, outflow tract of left ventricle; PVC, premature ventricular contractions.

3/6 systolic ejection murmur radiated from the parasternal area at the third interspace into the neck and back. There was a Grade 4/6 decrescendo, holosystolic murmur and a Grade 3/6 diastolic rumbling murmur at the apex. The patient had a hypochromic, microcytic anemia (hemoglobin 8 grams per cent, hematocrit 26 per cent). The electrocardiogram showed right axis deviation, left atrial enlargement, and right ventricular hypertrophy. Chest roentgenograms demonstrated massive biventricular and left atrial enlargement and pulmonary venous congestion and edema.

The findings at cardiac catheterization are summarized in Table 1 and, on the basis of the hemodynamic findings, together with the left ventricular angiocardiogram discussed in detail below, the child was referred for operation, with a diagnosis of valvular pulmonic stenosis, subaortic stenosis, and parachute deformity of the mitral valve.

At operation, the mitral valve was found to be funnel shaped. Instead of normal leaflets, there was an extremely thick cone of fibrous tissue with a 4 mm. eccentric orifice. All of the mitral chordae tendineae inserted on a single large papillary muscle which occupied the apex of the left ventricle (Figures 1, A and 2). Endocardial thickening was noted in the left ventricular outflow tract, opposite the mitral annulus. The mitral valve and papillary muscle were excised and replaced with a low-profile Kay-Shiley prosthetic valve; a pulmonary valvotomy was also performed. The hemodynamic measurements determined immediately thereafter are presented in Table 1 and reveal marked reductions in the gradients across both the pulmonary valve and subaortic regions compared to the preoperative values. The absence of flow measurements, however, precludes estimation of changes in orifice size.

The postoperative period was characterized by marked respiratory distress and signs of insufficient cardiac output. The patient died 42 hours postoperatively, presumably of dysfunction of the prosthetic mitral valve.

At postmortem examination, the foramen ovale was patent. Both ventricles and the interventricular septum were markedly enlarged. The commissures of a dome-shaped pulmonic valve with a small central orifice had been separated at operation

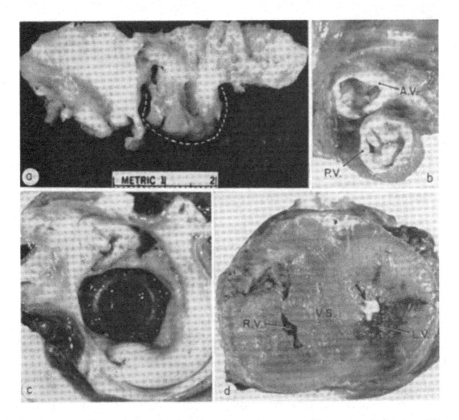

Figure 1 *a,* Opened mitral valve showing only one papillary muscle (enclosed by broken line). The leaflets are attached to the papillary muscle by very short chordae tendineae. The leaflets are diffusely and irregularly thickened but free of calcium deposits. *b,* Intact pulmonic (*P.V.*) and aortic valves (*A.V.*). The former is severely stenotic. *c,* Opened left atrium showing thrombus occluding the Kay-Shiley mitral orifice. The left atrial wall is thickened and the chamber is dilated but no supramitral ring is present. *d,* Transverse section showing that the cavities of both ventricles are small. The arrow points to thickened endocardium in the left ventricular outflow tract.

(Figure 1, *B*). A thin membrane of clot over the atrial aspect of the prosthetic mitral disc valve completely occluded its orifice (Figure 1, *C*).

DISCUSSION

In the present patient, the hemodynamic determination of pressure gradients across the left and right ventricular outflow tracts and the mitral valve localized 3 sites of obstruction within the heart (Table 1). Pulmonic valvular stenosis was clearly demonstrated by the pullback pressure recording across the right ventricular outflow tract, and by a right ventricular angiocardiogram. Mitral and subaortic stenosis were also demonstrated by catheter pullback. The decline in systemic arterial pulse pressure following a premature ventricular contraction suggested that functional rather than fixed orifice obstruction to left ventricular outflow existed at the subvalvular level.[6]

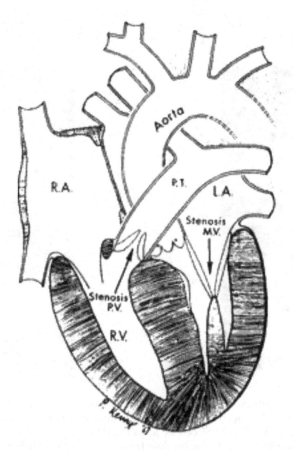

Figure 2 Diagrammatic representation of the cardiac lesions. The markedly thickened mitral leaflets insert almost directly into the single, large papillary muscle at the apex of the left ventricle. Obstruction to left ventricular ejection is caused by restriction of posterior motion of the leaflets which prevents their retraction from the outflow tract during systole, and contact between the mitral leaflets and hypertrophied muscular interventricular septum. Mitral regurgitation results from restricted leaflet motion which prevents occlusion of the mitral orifice.

Angiocardiography greatly facilitated the more precise assessment of the lesions responsible for obstruction at both the subaortic and mitral valve levels. Severe deformity of the mitral valve as well as marked thickening of its leaflets was observed in all phases of the cardiac cycle. The diastolic position of the mitral leaflets can be seen in lateral views of the opacified left ventricle (Figure 3, F); there was restriction of forward motion of the leaflets, leading to a funnel shape. During systole, in addition to the demonstration of mitral regurgitation, there was marked anterior concavity of the anterior mitral leaflet, and the leading edges of both leaflets were seen to be projecting into the left ventricular outflow tract well below the aortic valve (Figure 3, D). It was apparent that the leading edge of the anterior mitral leaflet formed the posterior component of the obstruction to left ventricular ejection. A markedly thickened interventricular septum formed the anterior and lateral components of the obstruction. Normally, during systole, the anterior mitral

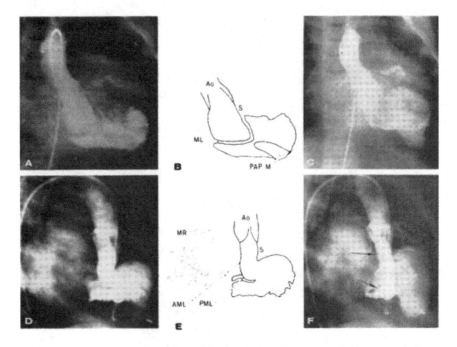

Figure 3 Left ventricular angiocardiograms and diagrams of the contracted ventricle, in the frontal projection after ejection (*A* and *B*), the hypertrophied muscular interventricular septum (*S*) can be seen bulging into the lateral aspect of the left ventricular outflow tract. The outflow tract obstruction is visible as a V-shaped radiolucent line, formed by the leading edges of the mitral leaflets (*ML*) as they come in contact with the area of the septal hypertrophy, about 2 cm. below the opened aortic valve (*A*). The single large papillary muscle (*PAP. M*) is seen as a radiolucent defect at the apex of the left ventricle. In diastole (*C*), the septal hypertrophy results in a deformity along the inferior surface of the outflow tract. The papillary muscle cannot be delineated, since it is surrounded by a large pool of contrast material. In the lateral projection, after ventricular contraction (*D* and *E*) the hypertrophied interventricular septum (*S*) protrudes into the anterior portion of the outflow tract. The thickened anterior mitral leaflet (*AML*) and posterior mitral leaflet (*PML*) are held forward in the outflow tract, several centimeters below the aortic valve, forming the posterior component of the subaortic obstruction. Mitral regurgitation (*MR*) is also demonstrated. There is superimposition of the body and apex of the left ventricle so that the papillary muscle is obscured. In diastole in the lateral projection (*F*), septal hypertrophy is visible along the anterior aspect of the left ventricular outflow tract, immediately below the aortic valve, and the indentation along the inferior aspect of the ventricle is also caused by hypertrophy of the muscular septum. The interface between the opacified left ventricular blood and less-opacified left atrial blood is formed by the mitral leaflets (arrows) and shows their restricted opening and a funnel deformity.

leaflet swings posteriorly out of the outflow portion of the ventricle and meets the posterior mitral leaflet to occlude the mitral orifice so that, in spite of contraction of the muscular interventricular septum, the outflow tract is widened.[7] In the frontal projection, during systole (Figure 3, A), contact between the leading edge of the deformed mitral valve and the anterior bulge of the hypertrophied interventricular septum was visible as a V-shaped, thick, radiolucent line several centimeters below the aortic valve. This location corresponds to the point of pressure change within the ventricle. The normal left ventricular outflow tract shows no such radiolucent defect in systole, since the mitral valve moves posteriorly away from the septum.[7]

Although chordae tendineae may not be visualized on a normal left ventricular angiogram, ordinarily two discrete papillary muscles are noted in both the frontal and lateral projections. The anterior muscle may be seen along the anterosuperior surface and the posterior muscle along the posteroinferior surface of the ventricle.[7] Both filling defects were not present in this patient. Rather, only a single, large filling defect was seen in an unusual position, occupying the cardiac apex (Figures 2 and 3, A).

It was of particular interest that the dynamics and the appearance of the left ventricular outflow obstruction in this patient resembled those shown to exist in idiopathic hypertrophic subaortic stenosis (IHSS). In the latter condition, the pressure gradient within the body of the left ventricle is thought by some authors to be caused by the abnormal systolic position of the leading edge of the mitral valve leaflets as it contacts the hypertrophied interventricular septum.[7] In IHSS, it is postulated that the abnormal position of these leaflets, which causes mitral regurgitation and subaortic obstruction, probably results from traction on the chordae tendineae due to dislocation of the left ventricular papillary muscles by the hypertrophied septum.

In this patient, the parachute deformity of the mitral valve (with shortening and fusion of the chordae tendineae as well as fibrosis of the mitral valve) prevents the normal systolic excursion of the mitral leaflets and is responsible for the subaortic stenosis and mitral regurgitation. For this reason, the diagnosis of parachute deformity of the mitral valve should be entertained whenever the angiocardiographic association of a single large papillary muscle at the apex coexists with abnormal systolic position of the mitral valve.

REFERENCES

1. Shone, J. D., Sellers, R. D., Anderson, R. C., Adams, P., Jr., Lillehei, C. W., and Edwards, J. E.: The developmental complex of "parachute mitral valve," supravalvular ring of left atrium, subaortic stenosis, and coarctation of aorta, *Am. J. Cardiol.* **11**:714, 1963.

2. Mehrizi, A., Hutchins, G. M., Wilson, E. F., Breckenridge, J. C., and Rowe, R. D.: Supravalvular mitral stenosis, *J. Pediat.* **67**:1141, 1965.

3. Swan, H., Trapnell, J. M., and Denst, J.: Congenital mitral stenosis and systemic right ventricle with associated pulmonary vascular changes frustrating surgical repair of patent ductus arteriosus and coarctation of the aorta, *Am. Heart J.* **38**:914, 1949.

4. Prado, S., Levy, M., and Varco, R. E.: Successful replacement of "parachute" mitral valve in a child, *Circulation* **32**:130, 1965.

5. Carey, L. S., Sellers, R. D., and Shone, J. D.: Radiologic findings in the development complex of parachute mitral valve, supravalvular ring of left atrium, subaortic stenosis, and coarctation of aorta, *Radiology* **82**:1, 1964.

6. Brockenbrough, E. C., Braunwald, E., and Morrow, A. G.: A hemodynamic technic for the detection of hypertrophic subaortic stenosis, *Circulation* **23**:189, 1961.

7. Simon, A. L., Ross, J., Jr., and Gault, J. H.: The angiographic anatomy of the left ventricle and mitral valve in idiopathic hypertrophic subaortic stenosis, *Circulation* **36**:852, 1967.

Case 108 Chronic Intravascular Hemolysis (Renal Hemosiderosis) After Incomplete Prosthetic Closure of a Ventricular Septal Defect and Noncalcific Aortic Regurgitation

Thomas J. Liddy, MD, and William C. Roberts, MD

Pathologic Anatomy Branch, National Cancer Institute and Section of Pathology, National Heart and Lung Institute, National Institutes of Health, Bethesda, Maryland 20014

Clinical and pathologic features of the case of an 11-year-old boy who underwent operative repair of tetralogy of Fallot nine months before death are described. Aortic regurgitation was produced inadvertently at operation during an unsuccessful patch closure of the ventricular septal defect. Postoperatively, the child developed severe cardiac failure and mild anemia. During a second operation seven days before death, aortic blood, which regurgitated through the aortic valve, was observed to contact the nonendothelialized ventricular septal patch, which only partially closed the septal defect. Erythrocytes were traumatized by the jet of blood contacting the nonendothelialized patch, liberating free hemoglobin, which was filtered by glomeruli and reabsorbed by renal tubules (renal hemosiderosis). Intravascular hemolysis after patch closure of ventricular septal defect has not been described previously.

CHRONIC INTRAVASCULAR HEMOLYSIS occurs occasionally in patients with severe calcific aortic valvular stenosis and regurgitation.[1] After replacement of aortic valves with a caged-ball or Teflon-leaflet prosthesis, however, intravascular hemolysis invariably occurs,[2-4] but it usually is not clinically significant. Chronic intravascular hemolysis also occurs occasionally in patients with partial atrioventricular canals after prosthetic closure of the atrial septal defects, with or without repair of the cleft anterior mitral leaflets.[5-7] The hemolysis in these patients has been attributed to contact of erythrocytes regurgitated from the left ventricle at high velocity and pressure against the prosthetic atrial septal patch. A review of the literature disclosed that intravascular hemolysis after operative closure of ventricular septal defect with prosthetic material has not been described. However, intravascular hemolysis did develop in a patient studied by us, in whom aortic valvular regurgitation was produced inadvertently while a ventricular septal defect was being closed incompletely. Clinical and autopsy findings in this patient are described.

REPORT OF A CASE

An 11-year-old boy had undergone repair of tetralogy of Fallot eight months before admission to the National Heart Institute. The ventricular septal defect allegedly had been closed by an Ivalon patch and the valvular and infundibular pulmonic stenosis was thought to be alleviated. During closure of the septal defect, a suture had caught an aortic valvular cusp and aortic regurgitation occurred. Severe right-sided congestive failure, evident immediately after operation, became progressively

Received April 10, 1969; accepted for publication May 27, 1969.
Dr. Liddy's present address is: St. Barnabas Medical Center, Livingston, N. J. 07039.
Requests for reprints should be directed to Dr. Roberts.

DOI: 10.1201/9781003409342-15

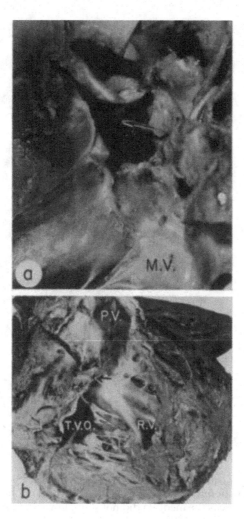

Figure 1 Opened heart of the patient. *a (upper)*, the aortic root, aortic valvular cusps, Ivalon patch *(arrow)*, anterior leaflet of the mitral valve *(M.V.)*, and the ventricular septum. The patch closing the ventricular septal defect is not covered by endothelium. The perforations in the noncoronary cusp are not seen in this view. *b (lower)*, the right ventricle *(R.V)*, tricuspid valvular orifice *(T.V.O.)*, ventricular septal patch *(arrow)*, and site of the surgically removed pulmonic valvular cusps *(P.V.)*.

more severe. Catheterization a month after operation disclosed a residual large left-to-right shunt at the ventricular level.

When admitted to the National Heart Institute for the first time eight months later (a month before death), the patient was severely ill (class IV). A grade 5/6 ejection-type systolic murmur was audible over the entire precordium and a grade 4/6 decrescendo diastolic blowing murmur was heard along the left sternal border. The hematocrit was 37%, hemoglobin 11.3 Gm. per 100 ml., platelet count 59,000 per cu. mm., and leukocyte count 6,000 per cu. mm. Serum iron was 86 μg. and the total iron-binding capacity, 330 μg. The direct Coombs' test proved negative. Total serum bilirubin was 2.7 mg. per 100 ml. and blood urea nitrogen, 10 mg. per 100 ml. Urine was normal. Repeat cardiac

117

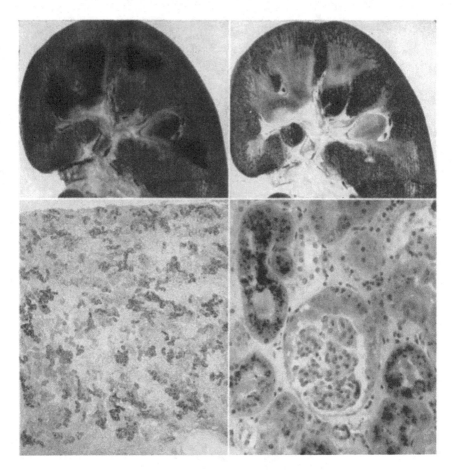

Figure 2 Kidney. *Upper left,* cut section. *Upper right,* same kidney after soaking in Prussian blue solution for 2 min. The cortex stained dark blue, indicating heavy deposits of iron, whereas the medulla did not stain. Lower left, photomicrograph of a section of kidney stained by the Prussian blue method. The dark-stained tubules indicate deposits of iron. The medulla (*bottom*) is free of iron deposits. × 20. Lower right, close-up showing that the iron deposits are situated predominantly in the cytoplasm of the proximal convoluted tubules, although some iron-positive material is present in Bowman's space and in the lumen of the proximal tubules. × 230.

catheterization disclosed a left-to-right shunt (1.5 to 1) at the ventricular level and elevated right ventricular (60/20 mm. Hg) and right atrial pressures (mean, 17; *a* wave, 23; *v* wave, 23 mm. Hg). The femoral arterial pressure was 110/48 mm. Hg. At reoperation (seven days before death), two perforations, each about 0.5 cm. in diameter, were found in the noncoronary aortic valvular cusp. The aortic valvular cusps were fibrotic, smooth, and free of calcific deposits; the two perforations, which were responsible for the severe aortic regurgitation, were closed by sutures. It was apparent that the regurgitant stream was in direct line with the ventricular septal patch, which was not covered by endothelium. The residual shunt resulted from partial detachment of the ventricular septal patch; the detached portion was reapproximated to the margin of the defect by sutures. Postoperatively, the patient had prolonged periods of hypotension, grand mal seizures, and hyperbilirubinemia (17 mg. per 100 ml.), and died.

At autopsy, the ventricular septal defect and the aortic valvular perforations were well closed (Figure 1). The erythroid elements in the bone marrow were hyperplastic and large deposits of iron were present in the cytoplasm of the proximal convoluted tubules of the kidney (Figure 2). No stainable iron was present in the liver or spleen.

COMMENTS

The intravascular hemolysis almost certainly resulted from damage to erythrocytes which contacted the nonendothelialized ventricular septal patch. Blood which regurgitated from the aorta through the perforated aortic valvular cusp and ejected from the left ventricle through the residual ventricular septal defect had direct contact with the prosthetic patch. Although few clinical tests for hemolysis were performed, there is unequivocal anatomic evidence, *i.e.*, renal hemosiderosis, that chronic intravascular hemolysis had occurred. Chronic intravascular hemolysis is the only condition which causes severe renal hemosiderosis without associated deposits of iron in the liver or spleen.[8] Acute hemolysis (resulting from cardiopulmonary bypass, for example) may cause glomerular filtration of hemoglobin, but hemosiderin in these patients is present only in the tubular lumens and in Bowman's spaces.[3] Prolonged periods of intravascular hemolysis are necessary before stainable iron can be detected in the cells of the proximal convoluted tubules. The amount of intravascular hemolysis required to produce severe renal hemosiderosis is not precisely known, but the extracorpuscular hemoglobin, at least initially, must exceed 100 to 140 mg. per 100 ml. plasma for hemoglobin to filter through renal glomeruli.[9] Prolonged intravascular hemolysis, however, depletes the serum haptoglobin, and this threshold falls accordingly.[10] The hemolysis in the patient described was well compensated, since he was only mildly anemic. The pronounced erythroid hyperplasia of the bone marrow in the presence of normal arterial oxygen saturation, however, indicates an active stimulus to erythropoiesis.

REFERENCES

1. Roberts, W. C.: Renal hemosiderosis (blue kidney) in patients with valvular heart disease. *Amer. J. Path.* **48**: 409–419, 1966.
2. Pirofsky, B., Sutherland, D. W., Starr, A., and Griswold, H. E.: Hemolytic anemia complicating aortic-valve surgery. An autoimmune syndrome. *New Eng. J. Med.* **272**: 235–239, 1965.
3. Roberts, W. C., and Morrow, A. G.: Renal hemosiderosis in patients with prosthetic aortic valves. *Circulation* **33**: 390–398, 1966.
4. Sears, D. A., and Crosby, W. H.: Intravascular hemolysis due to intracardiac prosthetic devices. Diurnal variations related to activity. *Amer. J. Med.* **39**: 341–354, 1965.
5. Sayed, H. M., Dacie, J. V., Handley, D. A., Lewis, S. M., and Cleland, W. P.: Haemolytic anaemia of mechanical origin after open heart surgery. *Thorax* **16**: 356–360, 1961.
6. Sigler, A. T., Forman, E. N., Zinkham, W. H., and Neill, C. A.: Severe intravascular hemolysis following surgical repair of endocardial cushion defects. *Amer. J. Med.* **35**: 467–480, 1963.
7. Verdon, T. A., Jr., Forrester, R. H., and Crosby, W. H.: Hemolytic anemia after open-heart repair of ostium-primum defects. *New Eng. J. Med.* **269**: 444–446, 1963.
8. Leonardi, P., and Ruol, A.: Renal hemosiderosis in the hemolytic anemias: Diagnosis by means of renal biopsy. *Blood* **16**: 1029–1038, 1960.
9. Lathem, W.: The renal excretion of hemoglobin: Regulatory mechanisms and the differential excretion of free and protein-bound hemoglobin. *J. Clin. Invest.* **38**: 652–658, 1959.
10. Veneziale, C. M., McGuckin, W. F., Hermans, P. E., and Mankin, H. T.: Hypohaptoglobinemia and valvular heart disease: Association with hemolysis after insertion of valvular prostheses and in cases in which operation had not been performed. *Mayo Clin. Proc.* **41**: 657–662, 1966.

Case 122 Congenital Atresia of the Left Main Coronary Artery

Nicholas J. Fortuin, MD,* and William C. Roberts, MD
Bethesda, Maryland

Clinical and pathologic features are described in a sixty-one year old man with long-standing clinical manifestations of ischemic heart disease. In addition to severe coronary atherosclerosis, congenital atresia of the left main coronary artery was present. Sudden death probably resulted from acute narrowing of the conus artery, the major collateral supplying the left ventricle.

The findings of angina pectoris, left bundle branch block, atrial fibrillation, systemic hypertension, hyperglycemia and hypercholesterolemia in an adult strongly suggest ischemic heart disease secondary to coronary atherosclerosis. A patient recently studied with these features died suddenly and at necropsy was found to have a congenitally atretic left main coronary artery in addition to extensive coronary atherosclerosis. A description of the coronary anomaly found in him and a discussion of its meaning and significance are presented.

CASE REPORT

A sixty year old physician (J.M.) died suddenly at home on March 8, 1969. He had been in good health until 1949 (age forty) when atrial fibrillation appeared. He was given digitalis for control of ventricular rate, and he continued to be asymptomatic until 1958 (age forty-nine) when he noted the onset of exertional, substernal chest pain which was typical of angina pectoris. Evaluation at this time disclosed moderate obesity and mild hypertension (blood pressure 150/100 mm Hg). An electrocardiogram (Figure 1) showed atrial fibrillation and nonspecific ST-T wave changes. A chest roentgenogram (Figure 2) showed the heart to be at the upper limits of normal in size. During the next ten years the angina did not worsen and occurred only with heavy exertion. Routine yearly examinations documented the persistence of mild systemic hypertension, but no changes in chest roentgenogram or electrocardiogram were noted. When seen on March 12, 1968, (one year before death) the patient had no new complaints. Blood pressure was 160/90 mm Hg. The heart was enlarged by palpation, and a grade 2/6 mid-systolic ejection murmur heard maximally at the base but well transmitted to neck and apex was described for the first time. An electrocardiogram (Figure 1) showed atrial fibrillation and left bundle branch block. On chest roentgenogram (Figure 2) the heart was enlarged. The two-hour postprandial blood glucose level was 258 mg per cent, serum cholesterol 317 mg per cent and serum uric acid 8.6 mg per cent. In January 1969 the patient consulted a physician complaining of a clear-cut change in the pattern of his angina. Chest pain occurred more frequently, with less provocation, occasionally after heavy meals and at rest.

From the Section of Pathology, National Heart and Lung Institute, National Institutes of Health, Bethesda, Maryland 20014. Requests for reprints should be addressed to Dr. William C. Roberts, National Heart and Lung Institute, National Institutes of Health, Bethesda, Maryland 20014. Manuscript received February 16, 1970.

* Present address: 1004 Columbia Street, Chapel Hill, North Carolina 27514.

DOI: 10.1201/9781003409342-16

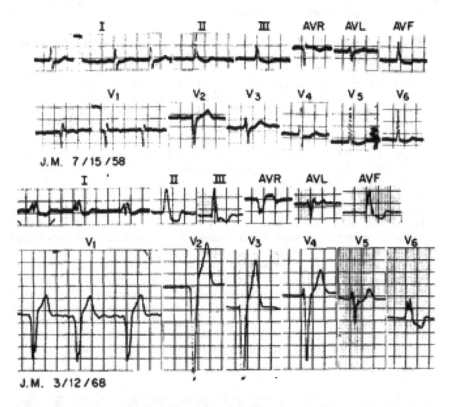

Figure 1 Electrocardiograms recorded nearly ten years apart.

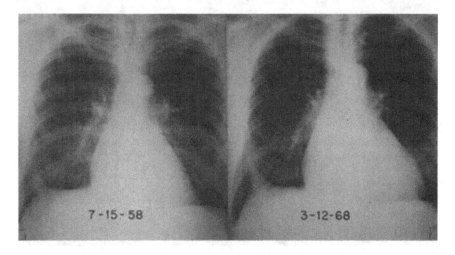

Figure 2 Chest roentgenograms taken nearly ten years apart.

The findings on physical examination, chest roentgenogram and electrocardiogram were unchanged from March 1968. The administration of long-acting vasodilators afforded some improvement. The patient died during sleep at home three months later.

At autopsy (A69–61), the heart weighed 800 gm. All chambers were dilated, hypertrophied, and the subepicardial adipose tissue was excessive. Focal deposits of calcium were present in the left and noncoronary cusps of the aortic valve, but the cusps were freely movable, competent and not stenotic. The other valves were normal. No foci of myocardial necrosis were present histologically, but focal fibrous scars were present in the anterolateral wall and papillary muscles of the left ventricle (Figure 3).

The altered anatomy of the coronary arteries is depicted in Figure 4. A tiny dimple, approximately 0.1 cm in diameter, was the only remnant of the left coronary arterial orifice in the left coronary sinus of the aorta. The right coronary orifice was normal. In the position of the normal left coronary artery a cord, 0.2 cm thick and 1.5 cm in length and composed of smooth muscle, was found (Figure 4). There was no lumen in the cord but five minute vessels containing erythrocytes were present. Distal to the atretic left main coronary artery, the circumflex and anterior descending branches arose and pursued normal courses. The circumflex branch terminated at the obtuse margin of the heart by dividing into three marginal branches. The anterior descending artery traversed the anterior interventricular sulcus terminating at the cardiac apex. The right coronary artery was a large vessel which also pursued a normal course in the atrioventricular groove, terminating just short of the obtuse margin of the inferior left ventricular surface. The anterior descending and circumflex branches were supplied by two large collaterals of the right coronary artery. The first, the conus branch (Figure 4), arose from the proximal right coronary artery and joined the atretic left main coronary artery, giving rise at this point to

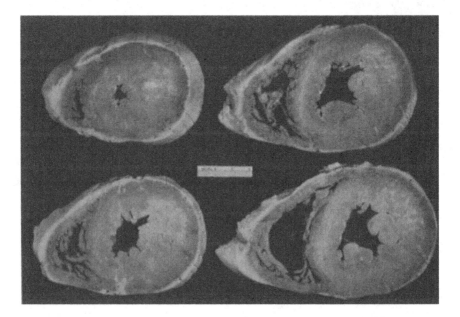

Figure 3 Transverse sections of cardiac ventricles showing multiple fibrous scars, severe left ventricular hypertrophy but no left ventricular dilatation.

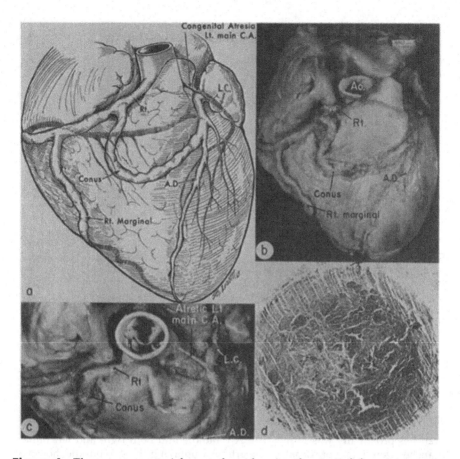

Figure 4   The coronary arterial anomaly. *a*, showing the atretic left main coronary artery and the large collaterals from the right coronary artery. L.C. = left circumflex; A.D. = anterior descending. *b*, heart from anterior view. *c*, coronary arteries and aorta from above. Focal calcific deposits are present in the aortic valve cusps. C.A. = coronary artery. *d*, photomicrograph of cross-section of congenitally atretic left main coronary artery. Hematoxylin and eosin stain, original magnification × 56.

both anterior descending and circumflex arteries. At the acute margin of the heart a marginal branch arose from the right coronary artery and connected with the anterior descending artery at the cardiac apex.

All extramural coronary arteries were rigid, tortuous and calcified (Figures 5 and 6). There were focal luminal narrowings throughout the coronary arterial tree by calcific and fibrous plaques. The lumen of the first portion of the conus artery was severely narrowed by hemorrhage into an old atherosclerotic plaque.

An attempt was made to determine the cause of the left bundle branch block in this patient. A large block of tissue which included the penetrating and bifurcating portions of the atrioventricular (A-V) bundle and the proximal right and left bundle branches was processed, embedded in paraffin and serially sectioned at 6 μ intervals. Of the 3,020 sections cut, each tenth was stained and examined histologically (odd numbered slides were stained by hematoxylin and eosin and even numbered slides by the elastic Van Gieson method). No anatomic interruption of the left bundle

123

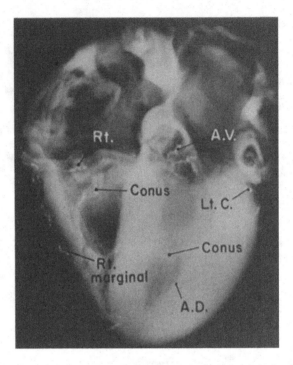

Figure 5 Roentgenogram of the heart at autopsy showing calcific deposits in the coronary arteries and in the aortic valve (A.V.).

branches proximally was found. The A-V bundle and both right and left bundle branches were intact proximally. The arteries supplying the A-V bundle, however, showed severe (up to >75 per cent) luminal narrowing by fibrous tissue proliferation.

COMMENTS

Congenital anomalies of the coronary arteries have been classified by Edwards[1] into those of minor and those of major functional significance. Included in the former are anomalies in which the coronary arteries arise from the aorta and in which no abnormal arteriovenous communication is present. Single coronary artery is an example of this type. This is a rare anomaly, only seventy-nine such cases having been reported through 1966.[2] It has long been appreciated that in the absence of other major congenital cardiovascular abnormalities, with which there is a high association, single coronary artery is compatible with a normal life expectancy.[3] This is so because major collateral channels develop which connect the single artery with the vascular bed lacking an aortic orifice, or the "missing" coronary artery is merely displaced and arises as a branch of the single coronary artery.[4] Functionally, these two situations are similar, but it is likely that they represent different abnormalities of embryogenesis.

In patients who survive to adulthood, atherosclerosis may complicate single coronary artery.[5, 6] One would expect that the consequences would be more severe in this situation. Allen and Snider,[5] however, found that the average age at death in nine recorded cases of single coronary artery with myocardial infarction was identical with the average age at death of all patients with myocardial infarction.[5] In our patient the course of ischemic heart disease was slow. The first manifestation

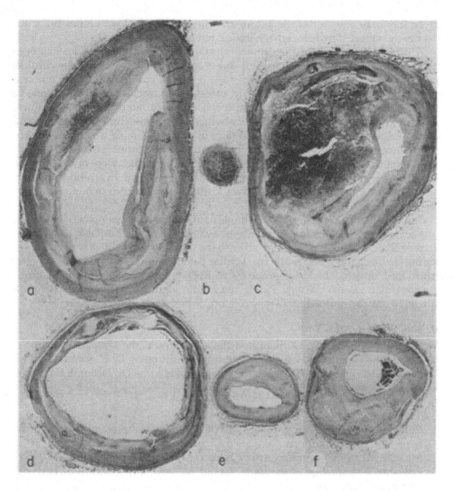

Figure 6 Photomicrographs of cross-sections of the major extramural coronary arteries, all taken at the same magnification (× 11.5). a, right coronary artery in first 1 cm. b, congenitally atretic left main coronary artery; c, first 1 cm of the conus artery showing a large hemorrhage into an old atherosclerotic plaque. The lumen is narrowed by the extravasated blood. d, proximal 1 cm of anterior descending vessel. e, proximal 1 cm of left marginal branch. f, proximal 1 cm of left circumflex branch. All sections stained with hematoxylin and eosin.

appeared twenty years before death, with the onset of atrial fibrillation. Angina pectoris occurred ten years later and remained of mild severity for the ensuing ten years. The development of cardiomegaly without signs or symptoms of congestive heart failure and the development of left bundle branch block on electrocardiogram preceded death by one year. Sudden death in this patient was heralded three months earlier by a change in the pattern of his previously stable angina pectoris. It is apparent that the branches of the left coronary artery, which were normally positioned, were adequately supplied by the two large collateral branches of the right coronary artery. Diffuse coronary atherosclerosis involving his entire coronary arterial tree was responsible for the manifestations of ischemic disease. The presence of a single coronary arterial orifice probably had little effect on his course until the conus artery, the main supplier of the left anterior descending and circumflex branches, was nearly occluded by hemorrhage into an old plaque.

A dimple at the site of the "absent" aortic coronary arterial orifice has been described in several recorded cases of single coronary artery,[4, 6, 7] but the cordlike structure which occupied the position of the left main coronary artery in our case has been reported only twice previously. Maddox and Isbister[8] briefly mentioned a similar structure replacing the main left coronary artery, but the histologic features were not described and the presence or absence of an aortic dimple was not noted. Murphy[2] described a patient similar to ours in whom a dimple was present in the aortic sinus, and a cord composed of cardiac muscle and fibrous tissue was the only remnant of the left main coronary artery. The distal branches were normally positioned. He believed that the structure most likely represented an atretic remnant of the left main coronary artery. The histologic findings of the cord in our case resembled those described by Murphy.

Smith[9] considered two embryologic mechanisms for the development of a single coronary artery: (1) congenital absence of a coronary arterial anlage, and (2) displacement of an anlage so that it fused with the normal vessel which remained. The findings in our patient and in the two similar patients previously described suggest a third mechanism, which was proposed by Roberts and Loube[6]: congenital atresia of a proximal coronary artery. Rarely the atretic segment may remain, as in our patient, or only an aortic dimple may remain, or perhaps neither may persist.[10]

ACKNOWLEDGMENT

We thank Dr. Charles M. Gillikan and his associates at the Outpatient Clinic of the U.S. Public Health Service, South Building, Washington, D. C., for making this patient's records available to us. Also, the help provided by Dr. Deborah Carpenter is gratefully acknowledged.

REFERENCES

1. Edwards JE: Anomalous coronary arteries with special reference to arteriovenous-like communications. *Circulation* 17: 1001, 1958.
2. Murphy ML: Single coronary artery. *Amer Heart J* 74: 557, 1967.
3. Edwards JE: *Pathology of the Heart* (Gould SE, ed), Springfield, IL, Charles C. Thomas, 1960, p. 426.
4. Blake HA, Manion WC, Mattingly TW, Barotch G: Coronary artery anomalies. *Circulation* 30: 927, 1964.
5. Allen GL, Snider TH: Myocardial infarction with a single coronary artery. *Arch Intern Med (Chicago)* 117: 261, 1966.
6. Roberts JT, Loube SD: Congenital single coronary artery in man. *Amer Heart J* 34: 188, 1947.
7. Sanes S: Anomalous origin and course of the left coronary artery in a child. *Amer Heart J* 14: 219, 1937.
8. Maddox K, Isbister J: A case of single coronary artery, quadricuspid pulmonary valve and anomalous right subclavian artery: death from acute rheumatic carditis. *Med J Aust* 1: 50, 1940.
9. Smith JC: Review of single coronary artery with report of 2 cases. *Circulation* 1: 1168, 1950.
10. Ogden JA: *Congenital Variations of the Coronary Arteries*. Thesis, Yale University School of Medicine, 1968, p. 48.

Case 138 Aneurysm of the Nonpatent Ductus Arteriosus

M. Wayne Falcone, MD*, Joseph K. Perloff, MD, FACC†
and William C. Roberts, MD, FACC
Bethesda, Maryland

Clinical and necropsy findings are described in a 6 week old infant with aneurysm of the ductus arteriosus. It was obliterated at the pulmonary arterial end and patent at the aortic end. Observations in this case and in 60 previously described cases of ductal aneurysm disclosed that 46 of the aneurysms occurred in infants less than 2 months old, 4 in children, and 11 in adults. The aortic end of the ductal aneurysm is always patent. The pulmonary arterial end may or may not be patent. Since complications (rupture, embolism or infection) tend to develop in nearly half of the ductal aneurysms, operative resection appears indicated.

Persistent patency of the ductus arteriosus is a common congenital cardiovascular malformation. Aneurysmal dilatation is an occasional complication of patent ductus arteriosus in adults. Aneurysm of the ductus arteriosus in infancy—in contrast to simple patency—is rare. However, such was the case in an infant we recently studied. Clinical and necropsy observations in this patient with ductal aneurysm and in those previously reported by others are described in this communication.

REPORT OF PATIENT

A 52 day old white boy, the first-born of twins, delivered at a referring hospital, weighed 2.2 kg after a term gestation. At birth he showed flaccidity, cyanosis and regurgitation; Apgar scores were 2 and 8 at 1 and 5 minutes, respectively. Positive pressure respirator and intubation were required initially with spontaneous onset of respirations at 5 minutes. He had multiple congenital abnormalities including an elongated neck, cloudy cornea, low-set and posteriorly rotated ears, complete cleft palate, long thumbs, fetal hypospadius and undescended testes. No precordial murmur was ever heard. Chest roentgenogram (Figure 1) showed cardiomegaly. A large convex shadow at the left base was initially thought to be thymus.

On day 1, the hematocrit was 33 vol percent; leukocyte and platelet counts and serum electrolytes, including calcium and phosphorus, were normal. Chromosome pattern was 46 XY without any structural abnormality.

From the Departments of Medicine and Pediatrics, Georgetown University School of Medicine, Division of Cardiology, Georgetown University Hospital, Washington, D. C., and the Section of Pathology, National Heart and Lung Institute, National Institutes of Health, Bethesda, Md. Manuscript received January 8, 1971, accepted March 25, 1971.

Address for reprints: William C. Roberts, MD, Section of Pathology, National Heart and Lung Institute, National Institutes of Health, 9000 Rockville Pike, Bethesda, Md. 20014.

* Clinical fellow of the Washington Heart Association, Washington, D. C.

† Holder of Research Career Program Award HE 14,009 from the U. S. Public Health Service, Bethesda, Md.

DOI: 10.1201/9781003409342-17

Initially the infant was hypotonic, fed poorly and had respiratory difficulties. Barium swallow on day 12 ruled out tracheoesophageal fistula. The cardiac silhouette was smaller (Figure 1). The shadow in the angle between the aortic knob and pulmonary trunk was still interpreted as representing thymus.

The baby continued to lose weight and by day 22 he began to vomit almost all feedings, necessitating parenteral fluids to maintain electrolyte and caloric balance. The next day a mass was palpated in the right upper quadrant of the abdomen, and upper gastrointestinal series demonstrated pyloric stenosis (Figure 1). On the same day, he was transferred to Georgetown University Hospital, and pyloromyotomy under local anesthesia was performed immediately. Postoperatively, he had several apneic spells and continued to feed poorly; poor Moro and suck reflexes and generalized hypotonicity persisted. He died without an obvious precipitating cause.

At necropsy, a 1.5 by 2 by 1 cm ductal aneurysm containing thrombus was found (Figure 2). The pulmonary arterial end of the ductus was closed, and the aortic end was open. The wall of the aneurysm was composed primarily of smooth muscle and elastic fibrils; young connective tissue with focal calcific deposits was present at the junction of intraaneurysmal thrombus and ductal wall (Figure 3). The right atrium was dilated, and the valve over the fossa ovale was incompetent. No evidence of rupture, embolism or infection of the aneurysm was present.

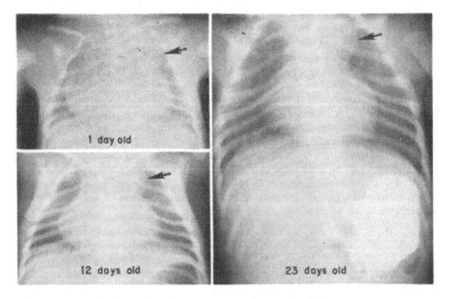

Figure 1 Chest roentgenograms. The arrows designate the ductal aneurysm. The cardiac size decreased from day 1 to day 23. Roentgenogram on the right demonstrates, in addition, pyloric stenosis with complete retention of contrast material 45 minutes after instillation of barium into the esophagus.

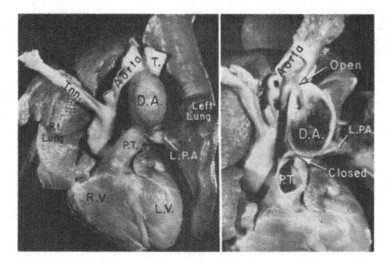

Figure 2 Unopened and opened views of the ductal aneurysm demonstrating its relation to surrounding structures. D.A. = ductal aneurysm; Inn. = innominate; L.P.A. = left main pulmonary artery; L.V. = left ventricle; P.T. = pulmonary trunk; R.V. = right ventricle; T. = trachea.

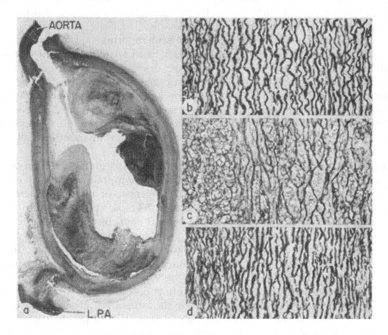

Figure 3 Photomicrographs of ductal aneurysm (**a**), and of portion of wall of aorta (**b**), ductal aneurysm (**c**) and left main pulmonary artery (L.P.A.) (**d**). The sites at which photomicrographs **b**, **c** and **d** were taken are shown by small blocks in **a**. The configuration of the elastic fibrils in the aorta (**b**) and left main pulmonary artery (**d**) are virtually identical. In contrast, fewer elastic fibrils are present in the wall of the ductal aneurysm (**c**), and the fibrils at this site have various spacial orientations. Movat stain, × 6 (**a**); elastic Van Gieson stains, each × 250 (**b** to **d**), all reduced by 43 percent.

Table 1: Aneurysm of the ductus arteriosus

I. Patent aortic and pulmonary arterial ends
    A. Fusiform* (with or without aneurysmal thrombus)
        1. Infected[4,13,19,20,23,26]
        2. Noninfected[3,6–8,22,24,25,27,31,39,40]
    B. Tubular dilatation[†16,18,28]
    C. Dissection[10,12,21,27]
II. Nonpatent pulmonary arterial end
    A. Fusiform* (with or without aneurysmal thrombus)
        1. Infected[33,34]
        2. Noninfected[5,14,27,29,35–37,42,43]
III. Postoperative[‡52,53]

* Both aortic and pulmonary arterial openings are small in comparison to the diameter of the aneurysm.
† Openings into aorta and pulmonary artery are of similar diameter to that of the aneurysm.
‡ After operative ligation of a patent ductus arteriosus.

DISCUSSION

Ductal aneurysm was described originally by Martin[1] in 1827 and by Billard[2] in 1828. Thore[3] in 1850 reported 8 cases of ductal aneurysm, and Hammerschlag[4] in 1925 reviewed the literature and excluded cases of aortic aneurysms involving the site of ductal insertion. Cruickshank and Marquis[5] in 1958 summarized the previous literature and added the tenth adult case.

At least 60 cases of ductal aneurysm have been reported.[1–43] The anatomic types are summarized in Table 1 and Figures 4 and 5. Exact anatomic classification is not possible in 19 cases[3, 8, 9, 11, 14, 15, 17, 27, 29, 32] because of insufficient information regarding the status of the pulmonary arterial end of the ductus. Six cases[44–49] previously considered ductal aneurysm were excluded because of inadequate anatomic detail. Observations in the remaining 42 cases are summarized in Table 2. Ductal aneurysm also may be classified by age— infantile, childhood and adult. Complications of the aneurysm in the 61 patients grouped by age are summarized in Table 3 and Figure 4.

Infantile ductal aneurysm: Nonpatent ductal aneurysm has been reported in 13 patients, including the infant described herein. The pulmonary arterial end was closed and the aortic end open in all 13. The pathogenesis of nonpatent ductal aneurysm is uncertain. Normally, the ductus arteriosus closes physiologically shortly after birth, but anatomic closure requires several days. By intimal proliferation[50] the ductus becomes obliterated first at the pulmonary arterial end, then the aortic end.[21, 51] The walls of the ductus undergo involutional changes by a decrease in elastica in comparison with the pulmonary trunk and aorta, and by increase of fibrous connective tissue, giving rise to the ligamentum arteriosum. If closure of the aortic end is delayed, the ductus in effect becomes an aortic diverticulum, subject to systemic pressure at a time when its walls are undergoing involution. This circumstance favors dilatation of the patent portion of the ductus with subsequent aneurysm formation. This mechanism is the most attractive explanation of nonpatent ductal aneurysm in the infants described, all of whom were less than 2 months old. Necrosis of the walls of the ductus was thought to have been etiologically important in several cases[23, 26, 27] but was not present in our patient. In those cases in which the histologic features were presented, decrease in elastic tissue in the wall of the aneurysm was observed.

Table 2: Spontaneous* aneurysm of the ductus arteriosus

Anatomic Classification	no.	Age Range	Complications			Assoc Mal
			Rupture	Embolism	Infection	
Patent ductal aneurysm						
Fusiform	19	2 days–51 yr	2	5	5	3[†]
Tubular dilatation	3	3 days–27 days	0	1	0	0
Dissection	7	12 hr–1 mo	3	0	0	1[‡]
Nonpatent ductal aneurysm						
Fusiform	13	13 days–66 yr	4	2	2	6[§]
Totals	42[¶]	12 hr–66 yr	9	8	7	10

* Excludes postoperative patients.
[†] Extrophie vesicale,[8] valvular incompetent patent foramen ovale,[31] aortic coarctation.[41]
[‡] Hydrocele.[27]
[§] Exomphalos,[27] double pelvis and ureter,[33] atresia of left pulmonary artery, stenosis of right pulmonary artery and aneurysm of pulmonary trunk,[36] right aortic arch,[39] coarctation of aorta.[42]
[¶] Autopsy in 39.
Assoc Mal = associated congenital malformations

Adult ductal aneurysm: The origin of nonpatent ductal aneurysms in adults is less certain. Documented persistence into adulthood of an infantile ductal aneurysm is lacking. However, the anatomic similarities between adult and infantile ductal aneurysms suggest that the adult ductal aneurysm may represent persistence of the infantile variety. Other mechanisms have been proposed to explain adult nonpatent ductal aneurysm including trauma to a persistently patent ductus,[38–40] infective arteritis in a patient with subsequent inflammatory closure of the pulmonary arterial end,[33] and delayed spontaneous closure with arrest at the stage of obliteration of the pulmonary arterial end.

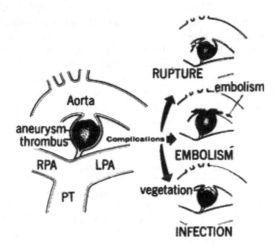

Figure 4 Diagram of aneurysm of the nonpatent ductus arteriosus and its complications. LPA = left main pulmonary artery; PT = pulmonary trunk; RPA = right main pulmonary artery.

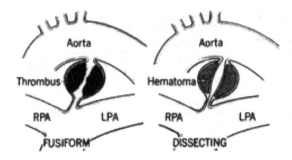

Figure 5 Diagram of aneurysm of the patent ductus arteriosus. In the fusiform aneurysm, the lumen contains thrombus which may or may not occlude blood flow. In the dissecting aneurysm a hematoma is present in the wall of the ductus but not in its lumen. Abbreviations as in Figure 4.

The latter mechanism, long considered the most likely one, was recently challenged by Bosman and Leoncini[42] as not being responsible by itself for aneurysm formation. These authors described a 66 year old man with a ductal aneurysm located just proximal to an aortic coarctation. They reasoned that in addition to obliteration of the pulmonary arterial end there must be some distal aortic obstruction causing increased systemic pressures in the patent portion of the ductus in order to initiate an aneurysm; 2 similar previously described patients were cited.[37, 41] Perhaps this additional lesion is necessary in the genesis of aneurysm in some adults with arrest at the stage of obliteration of the pulmonary arterial end; the ductus under these circumstances has been subject to systemic pressure for a considerable period of time and there would not appear to be any stimulus for the walls to undergo involution. In fact, in the majority of patients with isolated delayed spontaneous closure, the ductus appears as an inverted cone with the apex at the pulmonary arterial end and the base at the aortic end. Whether the pathogenesis of ductal aneurysm in childhood is the same as that operative in the infant or the adult remains uncertain.

Diagnosis: Correct antemortem diagnosis of ductal aneurysm has not been established in any infant. Because of the lack of related symptoms or physical signs, attention has not been drawn to the cardiovascular system in this age group. A soft tissue density at the upper border of the left cardiac silhouette may be mistaken for thymus, as it was in our patient (Figure 1), or hilar adenopathy, as in Scheef's patient.[20] A nonpatent ductal aneurysm was established by angiocardiography and successfully resected in 1 patient[35] in the childhood group. The diagnosis has been

Table 3: Spontaneous* aneurysm of the ductus arteriosus

Classification	no.	Age Range	Complications			Assoc Mal
			Rupture	Embolism	Infection	
Infantile[3,6–31]	46	12 hr–2 mo	5	6	5	5
Childhood[32–35]	4	20 mo–15 yr	3	1	1	1
Adult[4,5,36–43]	11	23 yr–66 yr	3	1	1	4
Totals	61†	12 hr–66 yr	11	8	7	10

* Excludes postoperative patients.
† Autopsy in 57.

made antemortem in only 1 adult patient.[43] The soft tissue density seen on chest roentgenogram was believed to represent aortic aneurysm in 2 patients,[5, 42] and tumor of the mediastinum in a third.[38] Graham[38] incised a ductal aneurysm, having considered it to be a solid mediastinal tumor, and emphasized the importance of the correct diagnosis. He pointed out that the differential diagnosis of a mediastinal mass at the level of the pulmonary trunk with displacement of the trachea rightward must include ductal aneurysm.

Complications: Complications of ductal aneurysm resemble those of aortic aneurysm: rupture, embolism and infection. Of the 13 nonpatent ductal aneurysms reported (Table 1), 4 ruptured, 2 embolized and 3 were infected. Death was directly attributable to 1 of these complications in 5 patients.[5, 30, 33, 34, 42] (The complication rate of the entire 61 patients was 43 percent, causing death in 19 patients [31 percent].)

Treatment: Tutassaura and Mustard[35] demonstrated the feasibility of total resection of a nonpatent ductal aneurysm, and there has been sufficient experience with postoperative ductal aneurysm[52, 53] to encourage resection, Because of the high incidence of complications operative excision appears indicated.

REFERENCES

1. Martin: Dilatation aneurysmal du canal arteriel. *Bull Soc Anat Paris* 22:17, 1827.
2. Billard CM: *Traité des Maladies des Enfans Nouveaux —Nés et à la Mamelle*, Paris, JB Bailliere, 1828, p. 567.
3. Thore: De l'anevrisme du canal arteriel. *Arch Gen Med (Paris)* 23:30–39, 1850 [8 cases]*.
4. Hammerschlag E: Ein Fall von wahrem Aneurysma des Ductus arteriosus Botalli. *Virchow Arch Path Anat* 258:1–8, 1925.
5. Cruickshank B, Marquis RM: Spontaneous aneurysm of the ductus arteriosus. *Amer J Med* 25:140–149, 1958.
6. Parise: Dilatation fusiforme-anevrisme du canal arteriel. *Bull Soc Anat Paris* 12:95–96, 1837.
7. Virchow R: *Gesammette Abhandlungen zur Wissen-chaftlichen Medicin*, Frankfurt-a-Main, Meidinger Sohn, 1856, p. 595.
8. Renaut MJ: Deux cas d'anevrisme du canal arteriel. *Bull Soc Anat Paris* 45:238–240, 1870 [2 cases]*.
9. Roeder H: Die Ruptur des Ductus arteriosus Botalli: eine monographische Studie zur Pathologie des Ductus. *Arch Kinderheilk* 30:157–216, 1900 [1 case]*.
10. Roeder H: Zwei Fälle von Ruptur des Ductus arteriosus Botalli. *Berl Klin Wschr* 38:72–78, 1901 [1 case]*.
11. Roeder H: Ein Fall eines solid thrombiesten Dilatationsaneurysma des Ductus arteriosus Botalli. *Virchow Arch Path Anat* 166:513–526, 1901 [1 case]*.
12. Bednar: Quoted in Ref 7.
13. Buhl: Quoted in Ref 49 [1 case]*.
14. Gerard G: De l'aneurysme du canal arteriel. Etude anatomique. *J Anat (Paris)* 39:1–10, 1903 [2 cases]*.
15. Gruner: Quoted in Ref 35.
16. Weller CV: Cardiac anomalies. Two rare cardiac malformations. *Bull Int Ass Med Mus* 5:122–125, 1915 [1 case]*
17. Schattman: Inaug-Dissertation, Breslau, 1919. Quoted in Ref 36.
18. Dry DM: Congenital aneurysmal dilatation of ductus Botalli. *Amer J Dis Child* 22:181–185, 1921.
19. Kaufmann E: *Lehbuch der speziellen Pathologischen Anatomie für Studierende und Ärzte*, Erster Band, Berlin and Leipzig, Walter de Gruyter, 1922, p. 71.

---

* Number of well documented cases of ductal aneurysm in this report. In the other cited references 1 case is described in each.

20. Scheef S: Über die Ruptur eines mykotischen Aneurysmas des Ductus Botalli und die röntgenologische Darstellung des erweiterten Duktus beim Säugling. *Arch Kinderheilk* 117:234–243, 1939.
21. Jager BV, Wollenmann OJ Jr: An anatomical study of the closure of the ductus arteriosus. *Amer J Path* 18:595–613, 1942 [4 cases]*.
22. Gross RE: Arterial embolism and thrombosis in infancy. *Amer J Dis Child* 70:61–73, 1945.
23. Pinninger JL: Aneurysm of the ductus arteriosus. *J Path Bact* 61:458–460, 1949.
24. Kneidel JH: A case of aneurysm of the ductus arteriosus, with post mortem roentgenologic study after instillation of barium paste. *Amer J Roentgen* 62:223–228, 1949.
25. Fell EH, Davis CB: Surgical problems associated with treatment of patent ductus arteriosus. *Arch Surg (Chicago)* 61:738–747, 1950 [1 case]*.
26. Lennox B, MacCarthy D: Aneurysm of the ductus arteriosus and umbilical haemorrhage in the new-born. *Arch Dis Child* 26:169–174, 1951.
27. Birrell JHW: Three aneurysms of the ductus arteriosus in the new-born. *Aust Ann Med* 3:37–43, 1954 [5 cases]*.
28. Lyon RA, Kaplan S: Patent ductus arteriosus in infancy. *Pediatrics* 13:357–362, 1954 [1 case]*.
29. Cuccurullo L: Contributo allo studio delle dilatazioni aneurismatche del dotto di Botallo. Presentazione di un caso e rassegna della litteratura. *Riv Anat Pat Oncol* 22:422–438, 1962.
30. Weisser E: Aneurysma des Ductus arteriosus Botalli und thrombotischer Verschluß der erkrankten Aorta abdominalis bei einem Säugling, eine anscheinend typische Kombination. *Frankfurt Z Path* 73:149–162, 1963.
31. Payan H, Blaustein A: Aneurysm of the ductus arteriosus. *Amer J Clin Path* 44:449–452, 1965.
32. Thorel C: Pathologie der Kreislauforgane. *Ergebn Allg Path* 9:594, 1903.
33. Hutchison R: A case of aneurysm of the ductus arteriosus. *Brit J Child Dis* 19:85–86, 1922.
34. Guggenheim A: Aneurysma des Ductus arteriosus Botalli mit Ruptur. *Frankfurt Z Path* 40:436–443, 1930.
35. Tutassaura H, Goldman B, Moes CAF, et al: Spontaneous aneurysm of the ductus arteriosus in childhood. *J Thorac Cardiovasc Surg* 57:180–184, 1969.
36. Hebb RG: Aneurysm of ductus arteriosus and atheroma of pulmonary artery. *Tr Path Soc London* 44:45–47, 1893.
37. Monckeburg JG: Die Missbildungen des Herzen. In, *Handbuch der speziellen pathologischen Anatomie und Histologie, Zweiter Band: Herz und Fefässe* (Henke F, Lubarsch O, ed). Berlin, Julius Springer, 1924, p. 163–165.
38. Graham EA: Aneurysm of the ductus arteriosus, with consideration of its importance to the thoracic surgeon. *Arch Surg* 41:324–333, 1940 [2 cases].
39. Mackler S, Graham EA: Aneurysm of the ductus Botalli as a surgical problem, with a review of the literature and report of an additional case diagnosed before operation. *J Thorac Surg* 12:719–727, 1943.
40. Dvorak L, Schmittovia M: Aneurysma arteriove duceje. Klinickoanatomicka studie. *Cas Lek Cesk* 92:1171–1174, 1953.
41. Otto L: Tödliche Ruptur eines Aneurysmas des Ductus arteriosus Botalli im Erwachsenenalter. *Thoraxchirurgie* 12:340–344, 1964.
42. Bosman C, Leoncini B: On pathogenesis of a case of ductus arteriosus aneurysm. *Acta Cardiol (Brux)* 22:279–288, 1967.

---

* Number of well documented cases of ductal aneurysm in this report. In the other cited references 1 case is described in each.

43. Cheng TO: Aneurysm of a nonpatent ductus arteriosus. An unusual cause of mediastinal mass. *Dis Chest* 55:497–500, 1969.
44. Baron: Quoted in Ref 2.
45. Westhoff: Inaug Dissertation, Gottingen, 1873. Quoted in Ref 18.
46. Voss M: Inaug Dissertation, Kiel, 1900. Quoted in Ref 18.
47. Buhl: Quoted in Ref 7 [2 cases].
48. Schmorl: Quoted in Ref 7.
49. Abbott ME: Congenital cardiac disease. In, *Modern Medicine*, third edition, vol. 4 (Osler W, McCrae T, ed), London, Oxford University Press, 1927, pp. 770–772.
50. Wilcox BR, Roberts WC, Carney EK: The effect of reduced atmospheric oxygen concentration on closure of the ductus arteriosus in the dog. *J Surg Res* 2:312–316, 1962.
51. Barclay AE, Barcroft J, Barron DH, et al: X-ray studies of closing of ductus arteriosus. *Brit J Radiol* 11:570–585, 1938.
52. Das JB, Chesterman JT: Aneurysms of the patent ductus arteriosus. *Thorax* 11:295–302, 1956.
53. Ross RS, Feder FP, Spencer FC: Aneurysms of the previously ligated patent ductus arteriosus. *Circulation* 23:350–357, 1961.

---

* Number of well documented cases of ductal aneurysm in this report. In the other cited references 1 case is described in each.

Case 145 Atresia of the Right Atrial Ostium of the Coronary Sinus Unassociated With Persistence of the Left Superior Vena Cava

A Clinicopathologic Study of Four Adult Patients

M. Wayne Falcone, MD,* and William C. Roberts, MD,
Bethesda, MD

Atresia of the ostium of the coronary sinus in the right atrium is rare, particularly so in the absence of a left superior vena cava.[1-8] We have studied at necropsy four adult patients with atresia of the right atrial ostium of the coronary sinus unassociated with left superior cava. This report describes physiologic and morphologic features of the anomalies in them.

PATIENTS STUDIED

Pertinent clinical and hemodynamic observations in the four patients are shown in Table 1. In each, atresia of the right atrial ostium of the coronary sinus was unsuspected clinically. Three patients (Nos. 1, 2, and 3) had other congenital cardiac malformations (Figures 1 to 6), and patient No. 4 clinically was considered to have primary myocardial disease (Figures 7 to 9). No patient had a persistent left superior vena cava. In patients Nos. 1, 2, and 3, a left atrial ostium of the coronary sinus was present, but in patient No. 4 no such opening was present, although a "dimple" was present in the left atrium where this ostium would be expected.

COMMENTS

Atresia of the right atrial ostium of the coronary sinus associated with persistence of the left superior vena cava (Figure 10) is of little functional significance.[8] With this combination coronary venous blood is delivered to the right atrium via retrograde flow in the left superior vena cava and then forward flow in the innominate artery and the right superior vena cava.

In atresia of the right atrial ostium of the coronary sinus and absent left superior vena cava, return of coronary venous blood is governed by communications between coronary veins and sinus and their related atria and ventricles.

From the Section of Pathology, National Heart and Lung Institute, National Institutes of Health, Bethesda, Md., and the Division of Cardiology, Department of Medicine, Georgetown University School of Medicine and Georgetown University Hospital, Washington, D. C.

Reprint requests to: William C. Roberts, M.D., Section of Pathology, National Heart and Lung Institute, National Institutes of Health, Bethesda, Md. 20014.

Received for publication July 20, 1971.

* Fellow, Cardiology Division, Department of Medicine, Georgetown University School of Medicine and Georgetown University Hospital, Washington, D. C. Supported as a clinical fellow of the Washington Heart Association, Washington, D. C.

DOI: 10.1201/9781003409342-18

Commonly, this communication is via the Thebesian vessels but occasionally it is by an ostium of the coronary sinus into the left atrium, as in three of our patients. The physiologic consequence of coronary venous return to the left atrium depends on the status of the atrial septum and on the distensibility characteristics of the receiving chambers. With an intact atrial septum and a left atrial ostium of the coronary sinus, systemic desaturation results.[7] In the presence of a fossa ovale type of atrial septal defect with left-to-right shunting, systemic desaturation still results because the left atrial ostium of the coronary sinus is below (caudal to) the defect and in closer proximity to the mitral valve orifice than to the septal defect. When the defect is located in the lowermost portion of the atrial septum (atrioventricular canal), the left atrial ostium is in close proximity to the defect and the flow of coronary venous blood is governed primarily by the distensibility characteristics of the receiving chambers, either right or left ventricle. With normal to moderately elevated right ventricular pressures, the right ventricle has greater distensibility and offers less resistance to inflow than does the left ventricle. Consequently, coronary sinus blood enters the right side of the heart and systemic arterial desaturation does not occur. If, however, hypertensive pulmonary vascular changes are present, the distensibility characteristics may change, with the left ventricle offering less resistance to inflow with both shunts (via the atrial septal defect and coronary sinus) becoming right-to-left.

With tricuspid atresia (patient No. 3), the presence of a left atrial ostium of the coronary sinus is of no physiologic consequence. All venous return is to the right atrium and all blood is delivered to the left atrium via the atrial septal defect. Thus, the coronary sinus return, be it to the right or left atrium, is delivered to the left side of the heart.

The physiologic consequences of absence of the right atrial ostium of the coronary sinus in patient No. 4 are unclear. Although an "ostium" was present in the left atrium it did not communicate with the coronary sinus. It would appear that in this patient the well-developed ostium and sinuslike structure attached to it became atretic before entering the coronary sinus. The Thebesian vessels were not dilated and the only egress of blood from the coronary sinus was via two small openings of the small cardiac vein into the right atrial appendage. The coronary sinus and posterior veins of the heart were greatly dilated, further suggesting venous obstruction. It is possible that the atresia of the left atrial coronary sinus was acquired later in life and that venous obstruction was somehow responsible for the myocardial disease. Although the long-term effects of coronary sinus obstruction are unknown, ligation of the coronary sinus in dogs causes immediate elevation of its pressure from average control values of 10/2 mm. Hg to pressures approaching or exceeding systolic aortic pressures.[9] Diastolic pressures range from 20 to 40 mm. Hg. Flow into the left coronary artery is reduced considerably while that into the right coronary artery is not affected. Normally,[10] 8 to 20 per cent of blood entering the right coronary artery is returned to the coronary sinus, and the remainder is returned directly to the right ventricle by the anterior cardiac veins. Approximately 75 per cent of the blood entering the left coronary artery is received in the coronary sinus, suggesting that coronary artery-coronary sinus communications are greater in the left coronary arterial system than in the right. Thus, hemodynamic consequence of coronary venous hypertension would be reflected to a much greater degree in the left coronary artery. Although increased coronary sinus pressure may cause increased flow in the Thebesian system with delivery of venous blood to left ventricle,[10] the long-range effects of chronically

Table 1: Data in 4 patients with atresia of right atrial ostium of coronary sinus and absent left superior vena cava

| Pt. No. | Age | Sex | SA* O₂ sat. (%) | Hemodynamics (pressures in mm. Hg) | | | | Major cardiac diagnoses |
				PA	SA	L→R shunt	R→L shunt	
1	31	F	81	90/30	125/70	1.7:1	0	VSD, ASD, MR, AR*
2	51	F	95	54/8		3.5:1	0	Partial A-V canal (ASD and MR)
3	27	M	88	—	112/66	0	+	Tricuspid atresia (large ASD, no VSD)
4	63	M						Idiopathic cardiomegaly

* *Abbreviations*: AR = aortic regurgitation; ASD = atrial septal defect; A-V = atrioventricular; MR = mitral regurgitation; PA = pulmonary artery; SA = systemic artery; sat. = saturation; VSD = ventricular septal defect.

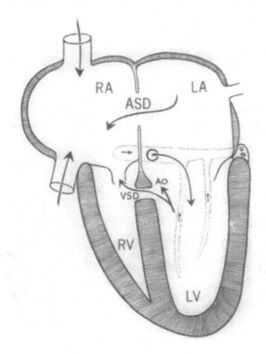

Figure 1 Patient No. 1 (A60–91). Diagram showing atresia of the right atrial (*RA*) ostium of the coronary sinus associated with a fossa ovale type of atrial septal defect (*ASD*), ventricular septal defect (VSD), and a left atrial (*LA*) ostium of the coronary sinus. Coronary venous blood is delivered to the left atrium, left ventricle (*LV*), and systemic arteries causing systemic desaturation in the absence of left-to-right shunting at atrial or ventricular levels. *RV* = right ventricle; *Ao* = aorta.

increased venous pressure and of decreased arterial flow on myocardial metabolism are unknown.

SUMMARY

Pertinent clinical and necropsy features are described in four patients with congenital atresia of the right atrial ostium of the coronary sinus unassociated with persistence of the left superior vena cava. Three patients had other congenital malformations and the fourth was suspected clinically of having primary myocardial disease. The latter patient not only had atresia of the right atrial ostium of the coronary sinus but communication between the coronary sinus and the left atrium, which occurred in the other three patients, was absent in the patient with "idiopathic" cardiomegaly. In the three patients with other congenital cardiac malformations, the anomaly of the coronary sinus did not cause any physiologic abnormality. Absence of a sizable communication between coronary sinus and atrium in the fourth patient led to varicosities of the coronary veins and sinus and possibly was the cause of the "idiopathic" cardiomegaly.

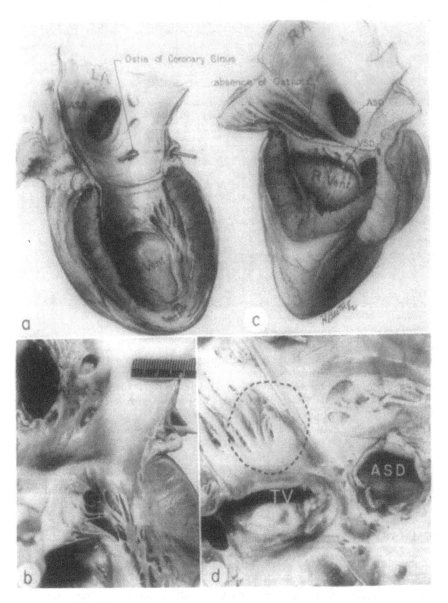

Figure 2 Patient No. 1. Drawings and photographs of opened left side (*a* and *b*) and right side (*c* and *d*) of the heart. *a*, Opened left atrium (*L.A.*), mitral valve, and left (*L.*) ventricle (*vent.*). A probe in the coronary sinus enters the left atrium. *A.S.D.* = fossa ovale type of atrial septal defect. *b*, Opened left atrium, mitral valve, and left ventricle. The tip of the stick in the coronary sinus is barely visible in the left atrial ostium of the coronary sinus. The atrial septal defect is apparent. *c*, Opened right atrium (*R.A.*), tricuspid valve, and right (*R.*) ventricle (*vent.*). The site of the absent ostium of the coronary sinus in the right atrium is designated. *VSD* = ventricular septal defect. *d*, Opened and flattened right atrium. The site of atresia of the ostium of the coronary sinus is indicated by the dashed circle. *TV* = tricuspid valve orifice.

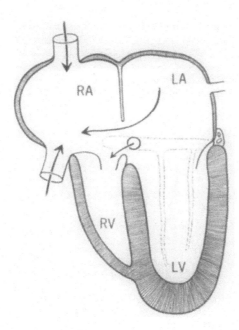

Figure 3 Patient No. 2 (A59–207). Diagram showing atresia of the right atrial ostium of the coronary sinus associated with an ostium primum type of atrial septal defect and a left atrial ostium of the coronary sinus. The left atrial ostium is in close proximity to the defect at the lowermost portion of the atrial septum. Coronary sinus blood enters the right ventricle due to the lower resistance and greater distensibility of this ventricle compared to the left one.

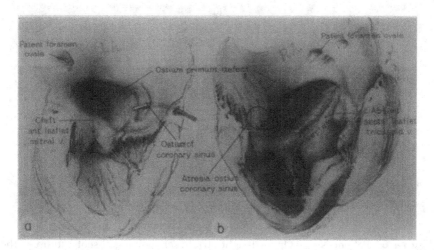

Figure 4 Patient No. 2. Drawing of opened left side (*a*) and right side (*b*) of the heart. *a*, Opened left atrium (*L.A.*), mitral valve (*v*) (showing a cleft in the anterior [*ant.*] leaflet), and left ventricle (*L.V.*). A probe in the coronary sinus extends into the left atrium in close proximity to the ostium primum type defect. *b*, Opened right atrium (*R.A.*), tricuspid valve (*v*), and right ventricle (*R.V.*). The site of atresia of the ostium of the coronary sinus is indicated by the circle.

141

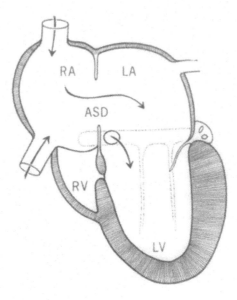

Figure 5 Patient No. 3 (A61–256). Diagram showing atresia of the right atrial ostium of the coronary sinus associated with tricuspid atresia, foramen ovale type of atrial septal defect (*ASD*), spontaneously closed ventricular septal defect, and a left atrial ostium of the coronary sinus.

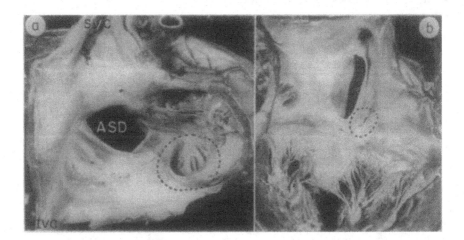

Figure 6 Patient No. 3. Opened right atrium (*a*) showing absent ostium of the coronary sinus (dashed circle), atresia of the tricuspid valve and a large atrial septal defect (*SVC* = superior vena cava; *IVC* = inferior vena cava), and opened left atrium, mitral valve, and left ventricle (*b*). The small ostium of the coronary sinus is indicated by the dashed circle in the left atrium (*b*).

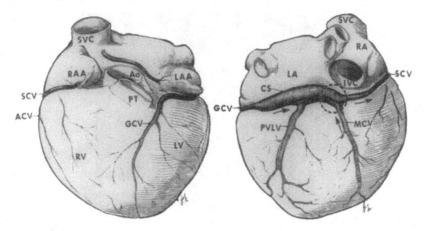

Figure 7 Patient No. 4 (GT No. 70A-353). Drawing depicting dilated coronary veins and coronary sinus. *a*, anterior view; *b*, posterior view. The veins, particularly the posterior vein of left ventricle (*PVLV*) and the middle cardiac vein (*MCV*), and the coronary sinus (*CS*) are greatly dilated. The small cardiac vein (*SCV*) drains into the left atrial appendage (*LAA*). The site of the atretic right atrial ostium of the coronary sinus is designated by the dashed circle in *b*. *GCV* = great cardiac vein; *ACV* = anterior cardiac vein; *SVC* = superior vena cava; *IVC* = inferior vena cava; *Ao* = aorta; *PT* = pulmonary trunk; and *RAA* = right atrial appendage. This 63-year-old man had overt congestive cardiac failure for 6 years before death and became functionally Class IV (New York Heart Association Classification). He never had chest pain, precordial murmur, or systemic hypertension. He ingested large quantities of alcohol chronically. Electrocardiogram showed a prolonged P-R interval and complete left bundle branch block.

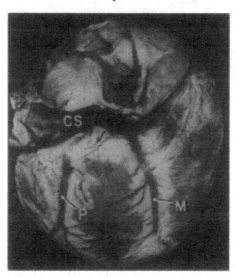

Figure 8 Patient No. 4. Posterior view of the heart showing the huge coronary sinus (*CS*) (now opened) and marked dilatation of the posterior (*P*) and middle (*M*) cardiac veins. The heart weighed 860 grams. The lumina of the coronary arteries were narrowed <25 per cent. No foci of fibrosis or necrosis were noted in the walls of either cardiac ventricle, both of which were quite dilated and hypertrophied. The 4 cardiac valves were normal.

143

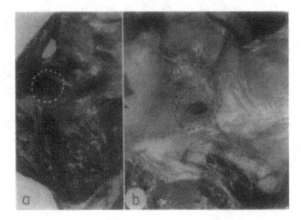

Figure 9 Patient No. 4. Opened right (*a*) and left sides (*b*) of the heart. *a*, The dashed circle designates the site of the absent right atrial ostium of the coronary sinus. *b*, The dashed circle designates the ostium of the coronary sinus in the left atrium.

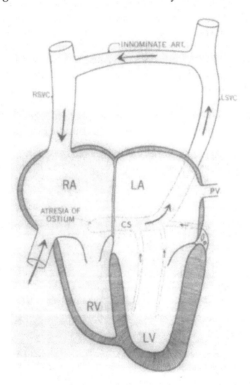

Figure 10 Diagram showing atresia of the right atrial ostium of the coronary sinus (*CS*) associated with persistence of the left superior vena cava (*LSVC*). Coronary venous blood is delivered to right atrium (*RA*) via retrograde flow in the *LSVC* and via forward flow in the innominate vein and right superior vena cava (*RSVC*). No patient described herein had a persistent left *SVC*, but this is the most common means of draining coronary sinus blood when the ostium in the right atrium is absent. *PV* = pulmonary vein.

REFERENCES

1. Meckel, J. F.: Über die Bildungsfehler des Herzens, *Arch. Physiol.* **6**:549, 1805.
2. Jeffray, J.: *Observations on the heart, and on peculiarities of the fetus*, Glasgow, John Smith and Son, Publisher, 1835, p. 1.
3. Bauer, K.: Ein Fall von Verdoppelung der oberen Hohlvene und ein Fall von ein Mündung des Sinus coronarius in den linken Vorhof, *Morphol. Arb.* **6**:221, 1896.
4. Ott, M.: Ein Fall von ein Mündung des Sinus coronarius in den linken Vorhof, *Arch. Entwick-lungsmechan Organ* **29**:33, 1910.
5. Bredt, H.: Formdeutung und Entstehung des missgebildeten menschlichen Herzens, *Virchows Arch.* **296**:114, 1935.
6. Fieldstein, L. E., and Pick, J.: Drainage of the coronary sinus into the left auricle, *Am. J. Clin. Pathol.* **12**:66, 1942.
7. MacMahon, H. E.: Communication of the coronary sinus with the left atrium, *Circulation* **28**:947, 1963.
8. Mantini, E., Grondin, C. M., Lillehei, C. W., and Edwards, J. E.: Congenital anomalies involving the coronary sinus, *Circulation* **33**:317, 1966.
9. Gregg, D. E., and Dewald, D.: The immediate effects of the occlusion of the coronary veins on the dynamics of the coronary circulation, *Am. J. Physiol.* **124**:444, 1938.
10. Gregg, D. E.: Some problems of the coronary circulation, *Verh. Dtsch. Ges. Kreislaufforsch.* **21**:22, 1955.

Case 215 Unruptured Sinus of Valsalva Aneurysm

Michael C. Fishbein, MD*, Robert Obma, MD[†]
and William C. Roberts, MD, FACC
Bethesda, Maryland
La Crosse, Wisconsin

An unruptured congenital sinus of Valsalva aneurysm (behind the right aortic valve cusp) is described as an incidental necropsy finding in an 82 year old man. Review of previous reports on aneurysms involving only one of the three aortic sinuses discloses that few cases have been described, and that these lesions are rarely diagnosed during life. It is probable, however, that unruptured aortic sinus aneurysm (involving only one sinus) is more common than previous reports indicate, but that, among patients with congenital sinus aneurysm, rupture is likely to occur.

One of the consequences of aging is dilatation of the aorta. The dilatation generally affects the ascending portion more than the descending portion, presumably because more elastic fibers are present in the proximal aorta. Included in the ascending aorta are the sinuses of Valsalva, that is, that portion of the aorta immediately behind the aortic valve cusps. Thus, with aging each of the three aortic sinuses dilates, and each sinus is affected more or less to a similar degree. This "senile-type dilatation" appears to be more pronounced in hypertensive than in normotensive persons, and tends to occur earlier in life in the hypertensive individual.

In addition to aging, there are at least three other causes of dilatation of all three aortic sinuses: (1) syphilis,[1, 2] (2) the Marfan and Marfan-like syndromes,[1, 2] and (3) ankylosing spondylitis.[3, 4] Although all three conditions may be associated with severe aortic regurgitation, each of the three sinuses may be dilated in the absence of aortic regurgitation. A congenital type of dilatation of all three aortic sinuses unassociated with other congenital anomalies of the heart or great vessels has been recorded,[5] but its occurrence, if indeed of congenital origin, must be unique.

In contrast to the common occurrence of dilatation of all three aortic sinuses, aneurysmal dilatation of only one or two of the three sinuses is unusual. The most common cause is probably infectious endocarditis with spread of the infective process into adjacent structures and formation of one or more ring abscesses.[6] Virtually always when this occurs one or more aortic valve cusps are severely damaged by the infective process so that severe aortic regurgitation results.

Aneurysmal dilatation of only one aortic sinus unassociated with infectious endocarditis is extremely rare. Generally, in this circumstance the localized aneurysmal dilatation is attributed to a congenital absence of media in the wall of the

From the Section of Pathology, National Heart and Lung Institute, National Institutes of Health, Bethesda, Md. and The Skemp-Grandview Clinic, La Crosse, Wisc. Manuscript accepted August 28, 1974.

Address for reprints: William C. Roberts, MD, Bldg. 10A, Rm. 3E30, National Institutes of Health, Bethesda, Md. 20014.

* Present address: Department of Pathology, Harbor General Hospital, Torrance, Calif. 90509.

[†] Present address: Skemp-Grandview Clinic, La Crosse, Wisc.

   DOI: 10.1201/9781003409342-19

aorta behind a sinus of Valsalva.[7] The sinus aneurysm may rupture, and several reports have described clinical consequences of the rupture and surgical procedures for correcting it.[8–12] Surprisingly, few patients with an *unruptured* sinus of Valsalva aneurysm have been described (Table 1). This report describes another patient with a large but unruptured sinus of Valsalva aneurysm, reviews previous reports of unruptured congenital aortic sinus aneurysms and poses certain questions, still unanswered, about this entity.

CASE REPORT

An 82 year old retired farmer, who was known to have systemic hypertension and cardiomegaly (on chest roentgenogram) since about age 65, had the onset of typical angina pectoris at age 70 years. At age 71 years he had an acute myocardial infarction. The frequency of angina pectoris decreased progressively thereafter and by age 73 years it had disappeared entirely; the blood pressure, however, remained elevated (180/105 mm Hg), exertional and nocturnal dyspnea appeared and the P-R interval widened to more than 0.20 second. By age 74 years, the blood pressure had decreased to 90/60 mm Hg and antihypertensive therapy with reserpine, given for 2 years, was discontinued. At age 76 years atrial fibrillation developed and digitalis therapy was begun. Chest roentgenograms revealed a larger heart than that previously recorded. At age 79 years, pedal edema appeared; the blood pressure was 110/60 mm Hg, and a grade 2/6 apical blowing systolic murmur and a third heart sound were audible. In retrospect this murmur was probably due to tricuspid regurgitation, caused by pulmonary hypertension secondary to an embolus. No precordial murmur had been heard previously on repeated examinations, and 2 weeks later no precordial murmur was present. The lung fields were clear but there was marked subcutaneous pitting edema of the legs and scrotum. Chest roentgenograms revealed an even larger heart than that recorded at age 76 years.

At age 80 years the patient had a cerebrovascular accident with residual right hemiparesis. The blood pressure was 130/90 mm Hg and the edema was still severe. In addition, a nodule that proved to be an adenocarcinoma was palpated in the prostate gland, and extensive distant metastases were found. He died suddenly several months later in a nursing home.

At necropsy, the formalin-fixed heart weighed 600 g. The sinus of Valsalva behind the right coronary (right anterior) aortic valve cusp was aneurysmally dilated (Figures 1 to 4). It protruded into the crista supraventricularis muscle of the right ventricular outflow tract. The right sinus was 2.5 cm deep and held 15 ml of fluid; the left coronary (left anterior) and posterior (noncoronary) sinuses were each 1.5 cm deep and each held only 5 ml of fluid. All four cardiac chambers were dilated. The atrial walls contained focal endocardial waxy deposits that proved to be amyloid. The left ventricular wall, which measured up to 1.9 cm in thickness, was firm and rubbery, and a transmural posterobasal scar was present. The lumen of the right coronary artery was more than 75 percent narrowed by atherosclerotic plaques.

Histologic sections revealed that the wall of the aortic sinus aneurysm consisted of endothelium covering a thin layer of connective tissue beneath which was myocardium (Figure 4). There was no aortic media within the aneurysmal wall. In addition to the posterobasal scar, the walls of all four cardiac chambers were infiltrated by small amounts of amyloid.

COMMENTS

Pathogenesis: The basic defect in patients with aneurysms involving only one or two of the three aortic valve sinuses is an absence of a portion or all of the media in

Table 1: Data in previously reported patients with an unruptured congenital sinus of valsalva aneurysm affecting only one or two aortic sinuses

Case no.	Year & Reference no.	Age (yr) & Sex	Clinical Problem	Associated Congenital Abnormalities	Cause of Death	Aortic Sinus Involved
1	1920[21]	23M	AR	Discrete subaortic stenosis	CHF	Right
2	1920[21]	23M	AR	Malformed AV	CHF	Right + posterior
3	1944[19]	49M	CHF, A-V block	Aortic stenosis	Arrhythmia	Posterior
4	1949[22]	29M	CHF, A-V block, RVOT obst.	0	CHF	Right + left
5	1953[23]	17F	Failure to thrive as child	0	Alive	Right
6	1957[13]	75M	?	0	?	Right
7	1963[24]	7F	CHF	Congenital PS, VSD	Operation	Left
8	1963[24]	38M	CHF	Acquired PS, VSD	Operation	Right + posterior
9	1963[25]	54F	Angina, AMI	Bicuspid AV	Compression of left coronary artery by aneurysm	Left
10	1969[12]	16M	AR	PDA	"Myocardial failure"	Right
11	1969[12]	14F	AR	0	Cerebral embolism	Right
12	1972[20]	62M	RVOT obst.	0	Alive	Right

AMI = acute myocardial infarction; AR = aortic regurgitation; AV = aortic valve; A-V = atrioventricular CHF = congestive heart failure; PDA = patent ductus arteriosus; PS = pulmonary stenosis; RVOT obst. = right ventricular outflow tract obstruction; VSD = ventricular septal defect.

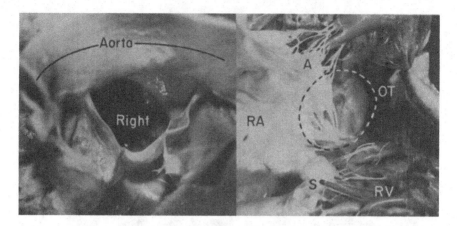

Figure 1 Aneurysm of right sinus of Valsalva viewed from aorta **(left)** and right ventricle **(right)**. The sinus aneurysm **(dashed circle, right)** bulges into the crista supraventricularis muscle. A and S = anterior and septal tricuspid valve leaflets, respectively; OT = right ventricular outflow tract; RA = right atrium; RV = right ventricle.

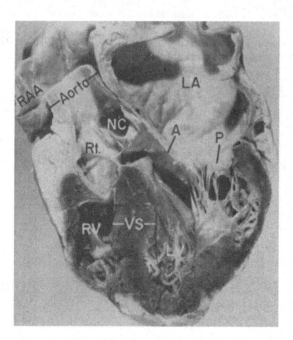

Figure 2 Coronal section of heart showing aneurysm of the right (Rt) sinus of Valsalva. If rupture had occurred, aorto-right ventricular communication would have resulted. A = anterior mitral leaflet; LA = left atrium; LV = left ventricle; NC = noncoronary sinus of Valsalva; P = posterior mitral leaflet; RAA = right atrial appendage; RV = right ventricle; VS = ventricular septum.

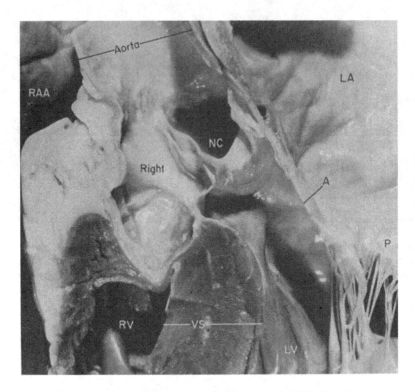

Figure 3 Close-up view of aneurysm of right sinus of Valsalva. The aortic wall behind the sinus aneurysm is very thin. Abbreviations as in Figure 2.

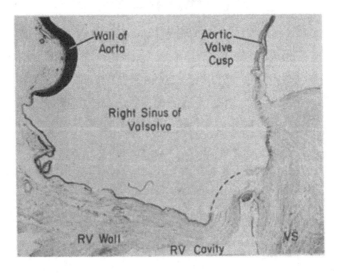

Figure 4 Photomicrograph of wall of sinus of Valsalva aneurysm. The aortic media is not present in the wall behind the sinus. Only thin connective tissue over supraventricularis muscle (RV wall) separates the sinus of Valsalva and right ventricular (RV) cavity. VS = ventricular septum. (Elastic-van Gieson stain × 4.5, reduced by 33 percent.)

the wall of the aorta behind the sinus[13] (Figure 5). Just because the media is deficient, however, does not assure the appearance of an aortic sinus aneurysm.[13, 14] Thus, when a single sinus aneurysm occurs the sinus wall is defective, but the sinus wall may be defective without the occurrence of an aneurysm. When a deficiency of aortic media occurs, the wall involved most commonly (about 70 percent of cases[8]) is that behind the right coronary (right anterior) cusp; occasionally (about 29 percent of cases[8]) it is the portion behind the noncoronary (posterior) cusp and virtually never (less than 1 percent of cases[15]) that portion behind the left coronary (left anterior) cusp. The explanation for these differences is uncertain.

Whether or not a sinus of Valsalva aneurysm is ever present from birth is uncertain; most likely the aneurysm is acquired, presumably the result of the aortic pressure. The higher the aortic pressure (for example, in patients with coarctation of the aortic isthmus) the more likely is an aortic sinus aneurysm to develop. The youngest child described with isolated sinus of Valsalva aneurysm was 4 years old.[16] Although the aneurysm itself may or may not be "congenital," the deficiency in aortic media behind the sinus must be congenital.

Incidence of rupture: Both the natural history and the frequency of media-deficient aortic sinus wall are uncertain.[17] The number of persons with a media-deficient aortic sinus wall in whom a sinus aneurysm developed is uncertain, as is the frequency of rupture of a developed sinus aneurysm. Among 78 cases of sinus of Valsalva aneurysm collected from previous publications by Kieffer and Winchell,[18] 59 (76 percent) had ruptured and 19 (24 percent) had not. In some of the cases included by these authors, however, the aneurysms involved all three sinuses and therefore were probably associated with the Marfan syndrome. Among seven hearts with aneurysm of one aortic sinus studied at necropsy by Edwards and Burchell,[7] four aneurysms had ruptured and three had not. Of five single (one of three sinuses involved) aortic sinus aneurysms studied at necropsy by us, four

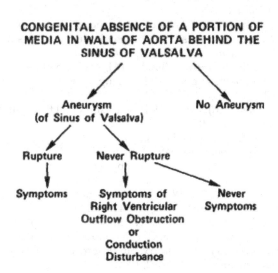

Figure 5 Diagram showing possible outcome in patients with congenital absence of a portion of media in aortic wall behind sinus of Valsalva. If no aneurysm occurs, the congenital defect will go unnoticed. If an aneurysm does occur it may or may not rupture. Rupture will virtually always produce clinical symptoms and signs of cardiac dysfunction. If rupture does not occur, symptoms will usually be present only if there is right ventricular outflow obstruction or conduction disturbances.

had ruptured and only one, that of the present case, was unruptured. These figures indicate that among reported cases of aortic sinus aneurysm, rupture is more common than nonrupture, but the data are probably considerably biased in favor of ruptured aneurysms. The nonruptured sinus aneurysm, for example, may be missed at necropsy (it was missed by the prosector in our case). The nonruptured aneurysm, with few exceptions,[19, 20] produces no evidence of cardiac dysfunction, and therefore at necropsy there may be no clinical sign or symptom to alert the pathologist to the presence of an aortic sinus aneurysm. Furthermore, incidental necropsy findings, which an unruptured aortic sinus aneurysm usually represents, are infrequently reported. Thus, it is likely that the frequency of unruptured aortic sinus aneurysm is considerably greater than has been reported.

Clinical features: An unruptured single aortic sinus aneurysm on rare occasion may produce evidence of cardiac dysfunction (Table 1). Kerber et al.[20] described clinical and operative findings in a 62 year old man who had evidence of right ventricular outflow obstruction as the result of an aortic sinus aneurysm's bulging into the crista supraventricularis. The aneurysm in our patient also bulged into the right ventricular outflow tract but not enough to cause outflow obstruction. Complete heart block has also been described in a patient with unruptured aortic sinus aneurysm.[19] The latter patient, however, also had calcific aortic stenosis, and thus it is not certain that the sinus aneurysm was responsible for the conduction defect.

REFERENCES

1. Roberts WC, Dangel JC, Bulkley BH: Non-rheumatic valvular cardiac disease: a clinicopathologic survey of 27 different conditions causing valvular dysfunction. *Cardiovasc Clin* 5:333–446, 1973.
2. Roberts WC: Left ventricular outflow tract obstruction and aortic regurgitation, chap 7. In, *The Heart* (Edwards JE, Lev M, Abell MR, ed). Baltimore, Williams & Wilkins, 1974, pp. 110–175.
3. Bulkley BH, Roberts WC: Ankylosing spondylitis and aortic regurgitation. Description of the characteristic cardiovascular lesion from study of eight necropsy patients. *Circulation* 48:1014–1027, 1973.
4. Roberts WC, Hollingsworth JF, Bulkley BH, et al: Combined mitral and aortic regurgitation in ankylosing spondylitis. Angiographic and anatomic features. *Am J Med* 56:237–243, 1974.
5. Pomerance A, Davies MJ: Congenital aneurysms of all three sinuses of Valsalva. *J Pathol Bact* 89:607–610, 1965.
6. Buchbinder NA, Roberts WC: Left-sided valvular active infective endocarditis. A study of forty-five necropsy patients. *Am J Med* 53:20–35, 1972.
7. Edwards JE, Burchell HB: Specimen exhibiting the essential lesion in aneurysm of the aortic sinus. *Proc Mayo Clin* 31:407–412, 1956.
8. Sawyers JL, Adams JE, Scott W: Surgical treatment for aneurysms of the aortic sinuses with aorticoatrial fistula. *Surgery* 41:26–42, 1957.
9. Morrow AG, Baker RR, Hanson HE, et al: Successful surgical repair of a ruptured aneurysm of the sinus of Valsalva. Circulation 16:533–538, 1957
10. McGoon DC, Edwards JE, Kirklin JW: Surgical treatment of ruptured aneurysm of aortic sinus. *Ann Surg* 147:387–392, 1958.
11. Spencer FC, Blake HA, Bahnson HT: Surgical repair of ruptured aneurysm of sinus of Valsalva in two patients. *Ann Surg* 152:963–968, 1960.
12. Taguchi K, Sasaki N, Matsuura Y, et al: Surgical correction of aneurysm of the sinus of Valsalva: a report of forty-five consecutive patients including eight with total replacement of the aortic valve. *Am J Cardiol* 23:180–191, 1969.

13. Edwards JE, Burchell HB: The pathological anatomy of deficiencies between the aortic root and the heart including aortic sinus aneurysms. *Thorax* 12:125–139, 1957.
14. Kwittken J, Christoponlos P, Dua NK, et al: Congenital and acquired aortic sinus aneurysm. A case report of each with histologic study. *Arch Intern Med* 115:684–691, 1965.
15. Sakakibara S, Konno S: Congenital aneurysm of the sinus of Valsalva. Anatomy and classification. *Am Heart J* 63:405–424, 1962.
16. Fowler REL, Bevel HH: Aneurysms of the sinus of Valsalva. *Pediatrics* 8:340–348, 1951.
17. Steinberg I, Finby N: Clinical manifestations of the unperforated aortic sinus aneurysm. *Circulation* 14:115–124, 1956.
18. Kieffer SA, Winchell P: Congenital aneurysms of the aortic sinuses with cardio-aortic fistula. *Dis Chest* 38:79–96, 1960.
19. Duras PF: Heart block with aneurysm of the aortic sinus. *Br Heart J* 6:61–65, 1944.
20. Kerber RE, Ridges JD, Kriss JP, et al: Unruptured aneurysm of the sinus of Valsalva producing right ventricular outflow obstruction. *Am J Med* 53:775–783, 1972.
21. Goehring C: Congenital aneurysm of the aortic sinus of Valsalva. *J Med Res* 42:49–60, 1920.
22. Raman TK, Menon TB: Aneurysms of the sinuses of Valsalva. *Indian Heart J* 1:1–14, 1949.
23. Falholt W, Thomsen G: Congenital aneurysm of the right sinus of Valsalva diagnosed by aortography. *Circulation* 8:549–553, 1953.
24. Gialloreto OP, Loiselle G: Aneurysm of aortic sinus of Valsalva associated with high ventricular septal defect. *Am J Cardiol* 11:537–546, 1963.
25. Eliot RB, Wolbrink A, Edwards JE: Congenital aneurysm of the left aortic sinus. A rare lesion and a rare cause of coronary insufficiency. *Circulation* 28:951–956, 1963.

Case 327 Complex Congenital Heart Disease

A Multiplicity of Therapeutic Options

Lewis P. Scott, MD, Roma S. Chandra, MD,** and
William C. Roberts, MD****
Washington, D.C., and Bethesda, MD

Dr. Roberts: In this report, a boy with cyanotic congenital cardiac disease will be presented and problems manifested in him will be discussed. Dr. Scott will describe his patient.

Dr. Scott: T. H. (CHNMC No. 299 3972), a 7-year-old black boy who died in December 1976, was noted to have cyanosis and a precordial murmur at 2 weeks of age. Shortly thereafter signs of congestive heart failure developed. At 3 months of age, cardiac catheterization (Table 1) provided a diagnosis of transposition of the great arteries with single ventricle. The pulmonary trunk was banded at this time with reduction of the systolic pressure in this artery from 85 to 45 mm. Hg (Figure 1). Despite this procedure, however, the child failed to thrive and cyanosis increased. Inadequate intracardiac mixing of blood was considered the reason and accordingly a Rashkind atrial septostomy was performed at 9 months of age (Figure 1). The transatrial pressure difference was reduced by this procedure from 9 to 3 mm. Hg.

Because of persistent growth failure and cyanosis, catheterization was repeated at 19 months of age (Table 1). Subsequently, growth continued to be slow, exercise tolerance poor, and polycythemia increased. Still another catheterization at 5 years of age disclosed severe reduction in systemic arterial saturation compared to previous studies (Table 1). Although the pulmonary trunk was not entered by the catheter, the pressure in the distal pulmonary artery, by clinical examination, was believed to be low. Accordingly, a left subclavian-to-pulmonary arterial anastomosis was performed (Figure 1). The distal portion of this left subclavian artery, however, thrombosed

---

From the Division of Pediatric Cardiology, Department of Child Health and Development and Department of Pathology, Children's Hospital National Medical Center, Washington, D.C., The Departments of Pediatrics and Pathology, George Washington University School of Medicine, Washington, D.C., and the Pathology Branch, National Heart, Lung, and Blood Institute, National Institutes of Health, Bethesda, Maryland.

Received for publication Nov. 15, 1977.

Reprint requests: William C. Roberts, M.D., Chief, Pathology Branch, NIH, National Heart, Lung and Blood Institute, Bethesda, Md. 20014.

* Chief, Department of Cardiology, Children's Hospital National Medical Center and Professor, Department of Child Health and Development, George Washington University School of Medicine, Washington, D.C.

** Chairman, Department of Anatomical Pathology, Children's Hospital, National Medical Center and Associate Professor of Pathology and of Child Health and Development, George Washington University School of Medicine, Washington, D.C.

*** Chief, Pathology Branch, National Heart, Lung, and Blood Institute, National Institutes of Health, Bethesda, Maryland and Clinical Professor of Pathology and Medicine (Cardiology), Georgetown University, Washington, D.C.

DOI: 10.1201/9781003409342-20

almost immediately and then a right subclavian-to-right pulmonary arterial anastomosis was done (Figure 1). This second shunt remained open as evidenced by the development of a continuous murmur over the precordium. Nevertheless, cyanosis persisted and polycythemia worsened. Multiple hospitalizations for phlebotomies followed. During the next several months, fever periodically appeared and a diastolic, basal precordial murmur suggesting aortic regurgitation developed. Blood cultures were always negative and the cause of the recurring fever was never determined.

The last hospitalization was at age 7 years for another cardiac catheterization. Its purpose was to again try to measure the pulmonary arterial pressure and resistance. The right subclavian artery was entered retrogradely from the femoral artery. The catheter was advanced into the right main pulmonary artery where pressures were elevated. With apparent occlusion of the right subclavian artery by the catheter, the child became severely hypoxic and heart beats ceased.

Dr. Roberts: Doctor Chandra, could you summarize the finding at necropsy?

Dr. Chandra: The findings at necropsy (A-111–76) are summarized in Figures 2 to 4. There was corrected or "L" transposition and common ventricle. The aorta arose anterior to the pulmonary trunk from a small, coarsely trabeculated subaortic chamber (right ventricular type). The anatomic left ventricle was on the right. Both atrioventricular valves entered the large ventricle which anatomically was left

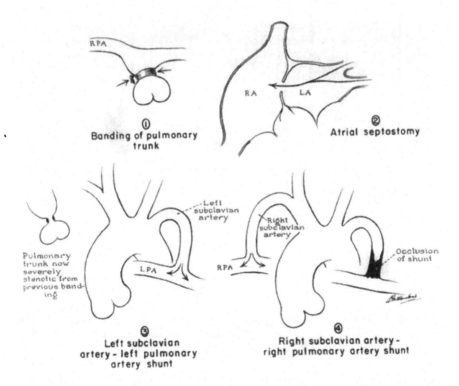

Figure 1 Diagram illustrating the operative procedures carried out in the child described. *RPA* and *LPA* = right and left main pulmonary arteries; *RA* = right atrium; *LA* = left atrium.

Table 1: Hemodynamic data in patient T. H.

Age at study (months)	3		10		19		60		84	
	P	**O**	**P**	**O**	**P**	**O**	**P**	**O**	**P**	**O**
Superior vena cava	–	–	–	–	3	70	5	33	–	–
Right atrial mean	6	47	3	50	3	70	5	33		–
"Right" ventricle	85/10	94	110	–	110/10	86	125/5	44	80/50	60
Pulmonary artery	–	–	–	–	–	–	–		–	–
Pulmonary vein	–	97	–	–	8	97	–	–		–
Left atrial mean	12	94	9		95	8	97	–	–		–
"Left" ventricle	85/9	93	–	–	–	–	–	–	–	–
Aorta	–	–	150/90	80	110/60	86	125/78	44	120/40	60
qP:qS					1.7:1		1:5.4			

Abbreviation: P = pressure in mm. Hg; O = oxygen saturation in per cent; qP:qS = pulmonic-to-systemic flow ratio.

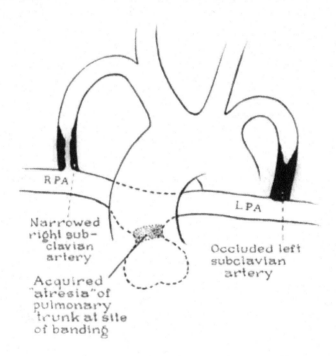

Figure 2 Diagram summarizing the operative procedures carried out on the pulmonary trunk and main right (*RPA*) and left (*LPA*) pulmonary arteries and their consequences.

ventricular in type. The coronary arteries were mirror-image of normal (Figure 4). On the ventricular aspects of each of the three cusps of the aortic valve, small bumps, composed mainly of fibrous tissue but also some calcific deposits, were present. The pulmonary trunk was totally occluded by fibrous tissue at the site of the banding.

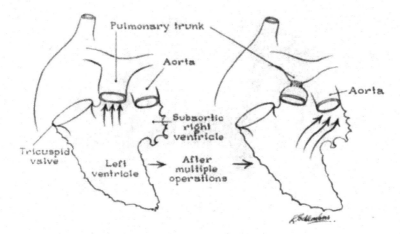

Figure 3 Diagram showing the change in intracardiac blood flow which occurred before any cardiac operation (*left*) and after complete occlusion of the pulmonary trunk by the banding procedure (*right*).

The distal portion of the left subclavian artery also was occluded by fibrous tissue (resulting from organization of thrombus) just proximal to its anastomosis to the left main pulmonary artery. The right subclavian artery was wide open. Histologic examination of sections from both lungs showed entirely normal pulmonary arteries and arterioles.

Dr. Roberts: This child's course and therapeutic interventions raise questions regarding management of patients with cyanotic congenital heart disease secondary to complex malformations. This boy's early course was characterized by evidence of *excessive* pulmonary blood flow and consequently the pulmonary trunk was banded. His course thereafter was characterized by evidence of *inadequate* pulmonary blood flow and consequently attempts (Blalock-Taussig anastomoses) were made to increase pulmonary blood flow. Dr. Scott, I am aware that the banding of the pulmonary trunk in this child was done before the child presented to you. If, however, we could "start again" in this child, *what would be the initial operative procedure you would recommend and why?*

Dr. Scott: Our major concern in a child presenting with pulmonary overflow associated with single ventricle and transposition is to control congestive heart failure and to prevent growth failure, the usual major presenting problems in this situation. Over the long run, of course, prevention of the development of pulmonary vascular disease is essential. Consequently, banding of the pulmonary trunk remains an excellent procedure to reduce congestive cardiac failure and prevent growth failure. In the presence of moderately elevated left atrial pressures, however, we would perform atrial septostomy at the time of the initial cardiac catheterization. There appears to be a relationship between the elevation of the left atrial pressure and the rapidity with which the pulmonary vascular disease develops.

Dr. Roberts: Dr. Scott, *why does pulmonary vascular disease develop so rapidly*, as a rule, in the child with single ventricle and transposed great arteries?

Dr. Scott: There are multiple factors. The high pressure and flow through the pulmonary arteries are certainly major contributors to the induction of these vascular changes. Just as important, however, are the left atrial pressure and the presence of hypoxemic blood in the bronchial circulation.

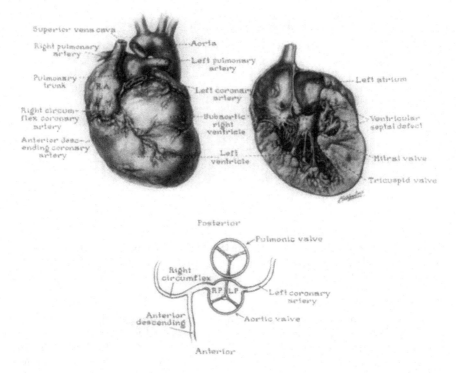

Figure 4 Drawings showing the various intrathoracic cardiovascular malformations observed in the patient described. The aorta arises anteriorly and from a small subaortic chamber. The large ventricle, located mainly on the right side, has the interior lining of an anatomic left ventricle. The coronary arteries are mirror-image of normal.

Dr. Roberts: The banding of the pulmonary trunk in this child diminished the pulmonary arterial systolic pressure measured at the time of operation from approximately 85 to 45 mm. Hg. Yet by the time necropsy was performed, nearly six years later, the pulmonary trunk was totally obstructed at the site of the band. Dr. Scott, do you have an *explanation for this acquired "atresia" of the pulmonary trunk at the site of banding*?

Dr. Scott: I have never observed a patient previously in whom banding of the pulmonary trunk progressed to total occlusion of its lumen. It is recognized that total obstruction to right ventricular outflow may occur in a patient with tetralogy of Fallot who has had a systemic-to-pulmonary arterial shunt created operatively.[1] What caused the especially severe fibrosis around the band in the present patient with eventual total occlusion of the pulmonary trunk is unclear.

Dr. Roberts: As I understand it, Dr. Scott, you did the last cardiac catheterization on this child to see if the pulmonary arterial pressure was elevated and indeed you did find that the pressure in this artery was quite elevated. Yet at necropsy, the pulmonary arteries in both lungs were devoid of changes suggestive of pulmonary hypertension. Indeed, many of the pulmonary arteries showed changes suggestive of pulmonary hypotension rather than hypertension. *What is your explanation for the finding of pulmonary hypertension in this child at the final catheterization?*

Dr. Scott: It is apparent from the necropsy findings that there was no pulmonary blood flow entering the lesser circuit from the right ventricular outflow tract. The only perfusion of the pulmonary circuit was through the right subclavian anastomosis and bronchial vessels. With the catheter in the right subclavian artery, pulmonary blood flow apparently was severely decreased. In all probability, near occlusion of the right subclavian artery by the catheter produced acute hypoxia, which caused severe spastic constriction of the smaller pulmonary arteries and arterioles resulting in severe elevation of the pulmonary arterial pressure.

Dr. Roberts: Dr. Scott, I believe you were quite concerned with the increasing polycythemia in this child during his last several years and consequently several therapeutic phlebotomies were performed. *What are your indications today for doing phlebotomy in individuals with cyanotic congenital heart disease?*

Dr. Scott: With rising hematocrit, the resulting increased viscosity in blood can induce intravascular thrombosis in both pulmonary and systemic vessels. When a child develops hematocrit values above 65 per cent, we usually recommend phlebotomy. By reducing viscosity, the tendency for intravascular thrombosis is reduced, and, in addition, the stroke work of the ventricle is reduced and consequently cardiac output improves.

Dr. Roberts: Dr. Scott, suppose that in this patient the banding procedure had been ideal, i.e., the pulmonary arterial pressure distal to the band was normal and that growth and development progressed well. Had that occurred, what would have been your subsequent plan for this child?

Dr. Scott: There are several options open to the cardiologist and cardiovascular surgeon today. None of these options, however, are truly optimal and I would not recommend any of them as long as the patient was relatively asymptomatic and grew normally. In the event that deterioration began, a total corrective operation wherein a ventricular septum would be created, assuming of course, that two well-developed atrioventricular valves existed, should be considered. At the same time, one would have to remove the band on the pulmonary trunk. A second option would be a modified Fontan operation: the tricuspid valve orifice would be closed and a conduit connected from the right atrial appendage to the distal pulmonary artery. To carry out such a procedure, pulmonary vascular resistance would have to be low and the function of the single ventricle would have to be excellent. Before performing the Fontan operation, the right pulmonary artery should be anastomosed to the superior vena cava. Had the Blalock-Taussig anastomoses already been performed, a third operative option would be to reanastomose or close off the anastomoses and perform a Waterston type shunt between ascending aorta and pulmonary artery.

Dr. Roberts: Dr. Scott, I understand that a basal diastolic blowing murmur was audible in this child during the last few months of life. What was your *explanation for this murmur?*

Dr. Scott: I initially thought that the diastolic murmur was produced by insufficiency of the pulmonic valve. As the aortic diastolic pressure began to fall, however, it was apparent that this murmur was due to runoff through the aortic valve. On several occasions, this patient had fever for rather protracted periods. Multiple blood cultures were obtained, but all were negative. Short-term courses of antibiotics for upper respiratory tract and ear infections probably allowed cure of the probable associated infective endocarditis, which caused the aortic regurgitation.

Dr. Roberts: At necropsy, there were lesions on each of the three aortic valve cusps which were consistent with healed infective endocarditis.[2] Occurrence of infective endocarditis in children is quite unusual. Those with endocarditis in childhood nearly always have underlying congenital heart disease, but, in contrast to this child, it is usually of the acyanotic variety.[3]

REFERENCES

1. Roberts, W. C., Friesinger, G. C., Cohen, L. S., Mason, D. T., and Ross, R. S.: Acquired pulmonic atresia. Total obstruction to right ventricular outflow after systemic to pulmonary arterial anastomoses for cyanotic congenital cardiac disease, *Am. J. Cardiol.* 24:335, 1969.
2. Roberts, W. C., and Buchbinder, N. A.: Healed left-sided infective endocarditis. A clinico-pathologic study of 59 patients, *Am. J. Cardiol.* 40:876, 1977.
3. Arnett, E. N., and Roberts, W. C.: Active infective endocarditis: A clinico-pathologic analysis of 137 necropsy patients, *Curr. Probl. Cardiol.* 1:1, 1976 (October).

Case 332 Calcific Pulmonic Stenosis in Adulthood*

Treatment by Valve Replacement (Porcine Xenograft) With Postoperative Hemodynamic Evaluation

Edgar A. Covarrubias, MD, Mazhar U. Sheikh, MD, Jeffrey M. Isner, MD, Mario Gomes, MD, F.C.C.P., Charles A. Hufnagel, MD, F.C.C.P. and William C. Roberts, MD, F.C.C.P.

Clinical and morphologic features are described in a 56-year-old man in whom severe, isolated pulmonic valve stenosis was treated by valve replacement with a porcine prosthesis. The calcific deposits were located on the ventricular aspect of the pulmonic valve, opposite the location (arterial aspect) of calcific deposits on stenotic aortic valves, and calcific deposits also were present in the tricuspid valve anulus.

Isolated pulmonic valve stenosis of severe degree in persons over 50 years of age is rare.[1-4] Calcific deposits in stenotic pulmonic valves also are rare,[2-4] and calcific deposits in the tricuspid valve anulus are even more rare.[5, 6] Treatment of isolated pulmonic valve stenosis by valve replacement has not been reported. Although each of the above occurrences is rare, all of them occurred together in our patient. In addition, the patient had postoperative hemodynamic evaluation after pulmonic valve replacement with a porcine xenograft.

CASE REPORT

A 56-year-old man was easily fatigued during his teens and was denied military service because of a "heart murmur." He was asymptomatic until age 46 years when exertional dyspnea occurred, and he was digitalized. At age 52, atrial fibrillation was noted, and cardioversion was done. During the next four years, the exertional dyspnea gradually progressed so that by age 56, he had considerable dyspnea when walking three flat blocks at a normal pace or climbing one flight of stairs.

Examination in November 1977 (age 56) disclosed a prominent "a" wave in the jugular veins, no precordial thrills, a decreased pulmonic component of the second heart sound at the base, a grade 3/6 harsh, systolic precordial murmur loudest over the upper left sternal border, and no organomegaly or subcutaneous edema. Electrocardiogram showed sinus rhythm and right bundle branch block. Chest roentgenogram (Figure 1) disclosed cardiomegaly and heavy calcific deposits in the pulmonic valve. The catheterization data are summarized in Table 1.

At operation on Feb 2, 1978, palpation via the right atrium disclosed calcific deposits in the tricuspid valve anular region. The pulmonary trunk was dilated, and a thrill was palpated. The pulmonic valve was dome-shaped with a central stenotic orifice and heavy calcific deposits on its ventricular aspect (Figure 2). The infundibulum

* From the Georgetown Cardiology Service, District of Columbia Hospital, and the Departments of Surgery, Medicine, and Pathology, Georgetown University Hospital, Washington, DC; and the Pathology Branch, National Heart, Lung, and Blood Institute, National Institutes of Health, Bethesda.
Reprint requests: Dr. Roberts, Chief, Pathology Branch, NHLBI, Bldg 10A, Room 3E30, 9000 Rockville Pike, Bethesda 20014

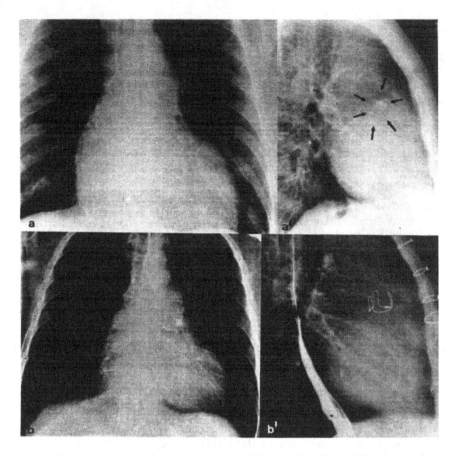

Figure 1 Three days before (*a* and *a'*) and 75 days after (*b* and *b'*) valve replacement. In preoperative lateral view, (a'), calcific deposits (*arrows*) are apparent. In postoperative roentgenograms (b and b'), wire of prosthetic cage is readily visible.

by palpation appeared narrowed, and therefore, several fragments of crista supraventricularis muscle were excised. The pulmonic valve was replaced with a 25-mm Hancock porcine xenograft via an incision in the pulmonary trunk. The postoperative course was smooth. The QRS complex on the ECG widened from 0.12 to 0.16 sec.

When evaluated nearly three months postoperatively, the patient stated that he had noted no change in his exercise tolerance. The precordial systolic ejection-type murmur was now of grade 2/6 intensity. Chest roentgenogram (Figure 1) showed a decrease in the size of the cardiac silhouette. Repeat catheterization disclosed a 36 mm Hg peak systolic pressure gradient at the level of the porcine valve and no subvalvular gradient.

DISCUSSION

Calcific deposits in stenotic pulmonic valves have been reported previously in at least 27 patients,[2–4] 15 (56 percent) with intact ventricular septa and 12 (44 percent) with associated ventricular septal defect. A prerequisite for calcium deposition in this valve is a severe degree of valvular stenosis, and with rare exception,[3] an age of

Table 1: Cardiac catheterization data

Date	RA	RV (s/d)	PT (s/d)	Pressures, mm Hg PAW mean	LV (s/d)	SA	CI liters/min/sq meter
12/15/77	a = 18 v = 14 Mean = 12	150/11	...	...	150/8	150/80	2.7
2/2/78*	...	106/16	17/5	...	...	...	...
2/2/78**	...	59/7	30/18	...	...	...	...
4/26/78	a = 14 v = 10	60/12	24/14	10	...	140/85	3.0
	Mean = 10						

CI = cardiac index; LV = left ventricle; PAW = pulmonary artery wedge; PT = pulmonary trunk; RA = right atrium; RV = right ventricle; SA = systemic artery; and s/d = systole/diastole.
*During operation, before cardiopulmonary bypass.
**During operation, after discontinuing bypass.

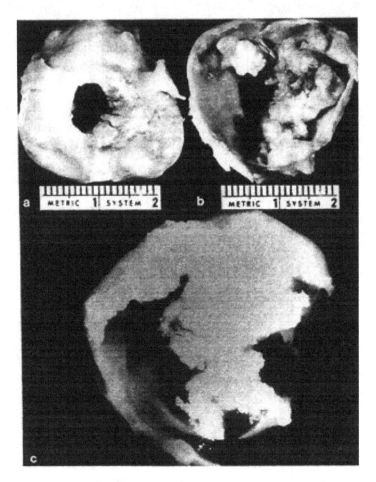

Figure 2 Operatively excised pulmonic valve. *a*, View from pulmonary arterial aspect; *b*, view from right ventricular aspect showing heavy calcific deposits on this undersurface; and *c*, roentgenogram again showing heavy calcific deposits.

greater than 30 years, usually greater than 40 years. Both of these requirements were fulfilled by our patient.

Calcific deposits on dome-shaped stenotic *pulmonic* valves appear to occur on the undersurface or ventricular aspect of the cusp, whereas calcific deposits on stenotic *aortic* valves are located entirely or predominantly on the arterial (aortic) aspect of the cusps. The following two reasons appear to account for these differences in location: (1) the low diastolic pressure in the pulmonary trunk as contrasted to the relatively high diastolic pressure in the aorta; and (2) the difference in configuration of the stenotic pulmonic valve compared to that of the stenotic aortic valve. Blood ejected from the right ventricle during systole initially contacts the concave surface of a stenotic dome-shaped pulmonic valve, whereas that ejected from the left ventricle contacts initially the convex surface of a stenotic aortic valve. Deposition of calcium on a convex surface appears to be more difficult than on a concave surface. Despite the location of the calcific deposits on the ventricular aspect of the pulmonic cusp and the high (150 mm Hg) right ventricular systolic pressure preoperatively, intravascular hemolysis was either absent or insignificant in our patient.

Calcific deposits in the mitral valve anulus are common, particularly in persons over 65 years of age, and they may occur at an earlier age at this site in patients with elevated left ventricular systolic pressures (systemic hypertension, aortic stenosis, hypertrophic cardiomyopathy).[5] In contrast, calcific deposits in the tricuspid valve anulus, as occurred in our patient, are rare.[6] The prerequisite for tricuspid valve anular calcification appears to be a right ventricular systolic pressure equal to or higher than the normal left ventricular systolic pressure and an age greater than 40 years. Because our patient's stenotic pulmonic valve was accommissural, it is likely that the valve in him was considerably stenotic from the time of birth and that his right ventricular systolic pressure was similar to his left ventricular systolic pressure for his entire 56 years before operation. A systolic closing pressure on the tricuspid valve five times that of normal for 56 years appears to be an adequate explanation for the tricuspid valve anular calcification.

Our patient is the first, to our knowledge, to undergo pulmonic valve replacement with a porcine xenograft for isolated pulmonic valve stenosis. Although this procedure reduced the right ventricular systolic pressure from 150 to 60 mm Hg, and the right ventricular outflow peak systolic pressure gradient from approximately 125 to 36 mm Hg, the right ventricular diastolic pressure remained unchanged and elevated (12 mm Hg). Because of the heavy calcific deposits in the pulmonic valve, partial valvulotomy would not have been feasible, and valve replacement appears to have been a better option than total valvulectomy despite the 36 mm Hg systolic pressure gradient across the prosthesis three months postoperatively. This degree of right ventricular outflow obstruction, however, should not in itself be responsible for symptoms of cardiac dysfunction. Possibly, there is considerable right ventricular fibrosis as a consequence of the severe elevation of the right ventricular systolic pressure for nearly six decades.

REFERENCES

1. Tinker J, Howitt G, Markman P, et al: The natural history of isolated pulmonary stenosis. *Br Heart J* 27:151–160, 1965.
2. Dinsmore RE, Sanders CA, Harthorne JW, et al: Calcification of the congenitally stenotic pulmonary valve. *N Engl J Med* 275:99–100, 1966.
3. Roberts WC, Mason DT, Morrow AG, et al: Calcific pulmonic stenosis. *Circulation* 37:973–978, 1968.
4. Rodriguez GR, Bennett KR, Lehan PH: Calcification of the pulmonary valve. *Chest* 59:160–164, 1971.
5. Roberts WC, Perloff JK: Mitral valvular disease: A clinicopathologic survey of the conditions causing the mitral valve to function abnormally. *Ann Intern Med* 77:939–975, 1972.
6. Arnold JR, Ghahramani AR, Hernandez FA, et al: Calcification of annulus of tricuspid valve (observation in two patients with congenital pulmonary stenosis). *Chest* 60:229–232, 1971.

Case 387 Congenital Heart Disease with Trisomy 13

Use of the Echocardiogram in Delineating the Location of a Left-to-Right Shunt

Henry S. Cabin, MD, Lucille A. Lester, MD, and William C. Roberts, MD
Bethesda, MD

DR. ROBERTS: Herein we will discuss a child with congenital heart disease and trisomy 13. Dr. Cabin will present the patient's clinical and morphologic findings.

DR. CABIN: J. M. (CC No. 13-31-03) was a 4.5-month-old girl who died on July 10, 1979. She weighed 2.4 kilograms at birth after a 37 week gestation. A precordial murmur was noted during the first 2 weeks of life and she was acyanotic. At age 15 days, she was transferred to the Clinical Center of the National Institutes of Health because of feeding difficulties and intermittent signs of congestive heart failure. Her blood pressure was 70/40 mm. Hg, her heart rate was 172 beats/minute, and the respiratory rate was 80 breaths/minute. Her head was small (microcephaly); both eyes were small (microphthalmia), and a fissure was present in the left iris (coloboma). She had a cleft upper lip and palate, a preauricular skin tag, transpalmar (Simian) creases, partial fusion (frog-like) of her toes (syndactylism), and a rudimentary extra digit (polydactyly) on her left hand and left foot. The right ventricular impulse was palpable, S_2 was single and loud, and a Grade 3/6 systolic ejection type murmur was heard along the upper sternal border. The lungs were clear. The chest radiograph (Figure 1) disclosed cardiomegaly and evidences of increased pulmonary blood flow. The electrocardiogram (Figure 1) disclosed biventricular hypertrophy and the echocardiogram (Figure 1) disclosed no abnormalities. Despite furosemide, digoxin, and supplemental oxygen, the congestive heart failure worsened. The feeding problem was found to be the result of partial antral obstruction. She died quietly.

At autopsy (A79-831), the heart weighed 34 gms. (expected weight for her age = 29 gms.). The right atrium was clearly dilated; the walls of the right atrium, right ventricle, and left ventricle were thickened. The left atrium was normal in size. The four cardiac valves were normal. A large *ventricular septal defect (VSD)*, located posterior and inferior to the crista supraventricularis, a large ostium secundum type *atrial septal defect (ASD)*, and a *patent ductus arteriosus (PDA)* were present (Figure 2).

DR. ROBERTS: The child presented had several abnormalities associated with trisomy 13. Dr. Cabin, will you describe the usual findings in patients with trisomy 13 and contrast them to those in patients with trisomy 18 and 21?

DR. CABIN: The abnormalities frequently found in patients with trisomy 13 are listed in Table 1, along with an indication of which abnormalities also are seen in

From the Pathology Branch, National Heart, Lung, and Blood Institute, and the Pediatric Metabolism Branch, National Institute of Arthritis, Metabolism and Digestive Diseases, National Institutes of Health, Bethesda, Md.

Received for publication Nov. 2, 1979.

Reprint requests: William C. Roberts, M.D., Chief, Pathology Branch, National Institutes of Health, National Heart, Lung, and Blood Institute, Bethesda, Md. 20014.

DOI: 10.1201/9781003409342-22

Table 1: Major clinical and necropsy findings in trisomy 13 and the presence or absence of these findings in trisomy 18 and 21

	Trisomy 13	Trisomy 18	Trisomy 21
Incidence	1/5,000	1/4,000	1/700
Increased maternal age*	+	+	+
Survival beyond 1 year	Rare	Rare	Rare
Male:Female	1:1	1:4	1:1
Mental retardation*	+	+	+
Feeding difficulty*	+	+	0
Deafness*	+	+	0
Congenital heart disease*	+	+	+
Microcephaly*	+	0	0
Microphthalmia*	+	0	0
Cleft lip and palate*	+	0	0
Malformed ears*	+	+	+
Coloboma of the iris*	+	0	0
Simian crease*	+	+	+
Polydactyly*	+	0	0
Syndactyly*	+	+	0
Rocker-bottom feet	+	+	0
Long hyperconvex fingernails	+	+	+
Undescended testes	+	+	+
Double renal pelvis	+	0	0
Absent olfactory bulbs*	+	0	0
Biseptate uterus*	+	0	0

* Indicates that this abnormality was present in our patient.

trisomy 18 and 21. Our patient had several of the listed abnormalities (those with asterisks) and, consequently, the diagnosis of trisomy 13 in her was obvious and also it was confirmed by chromosome study. Diagnostic features of trisomy 18 include: small lower jaw, short palpebral fissure, clenched hands, short sternum, narrow pelvis, short stature, and mental deficiency. Characteristic findings in infants with trisomy 21 include: flat facies, protruded tongue, slanted palpebral fissures, hypotonia, short hands, and mental deficiency. In all three trisomy syndromes congenital heart disease is common. Of 388 patients reported by Warkany and associates,[1] congenital heart disease occurred in 27 (84%) of 32 necropsy patients with trisomy 13, in 83 (99%) of 84 patients with trisomy 18, and in 141 (52%) of 272 patients with trisomy 21. The most commonly found malformations in trisomy 13 were VSD, PDA, and ASD, and two or three of these three defects occurred more frequently than a single defect. These three defects also were common in patients with trisomy 18 and 21. The most common type of atrial septal defect in trisomy 21 is one located in the lowermost portion of the atrial septum (ostium primum or endocardial cushion type) and in trisomy 13 and 18, the defect most commonly is in the mid-portion of the atrial septum (secundum type).

The occurrence in our patient of signs of congestive heart failure, acyanosis, and enlarged right-sided cardiac chambers with evidences of increased pulmonary blood flow strongly suggested the presence of a left-to-right shunt at the atrial, ventricular, or great-artery level, or combinations of these three. The presence of trisomy 13 strongly suggested the presence of two or more of these defects.

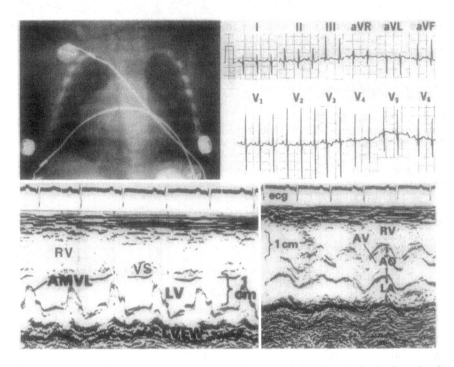

Figure 1 Posteroanterior chest radiograph *(upper left)* 2.5 months before death showing considerable prominence of the right-sided chambers. The pulmonary vascular markings are prominent. Electrocardiogram *(ECG) (upper right)*, obtained 3 months before death, shows sinus tachycardia and biventricular hypertrophy. The echocardiogram *(lower)*, obtained 3 months before death, shows the right ventricle *(RV)*, left ventricle *(LV)*, and left atrium *(LA)* to be of normal size. The aorta *(Ao)* is at the upper limit of normal. The ventricular septum *(VS)* moves normally. *AMVL* = anterior mitral valve leaflet; *AV* = aortic valve.

DR. ROBERTS: The echocardiogram has proved useful in delineating the level of a left-to-right shunt. Dr. Lester has recently analyzed the usefulness of echocardiography for characterization and quantitation of a left-to-right shunt in patients with ventricular septal defect.[2] Dr. Lester, can you summarize the echocardiographic findings in patient J. M., and, from your previously collected data, how useful is the echocardiogram in predicting the level of the shunt in patients with left-to-right shunts?

DR. LESTER: An echocardiogram was performed at 15 days of life (Figure 1). The left and right ventricles and left atrium were normal in size. The ventricular septum did not move paradoxically. The aorta was mildly enlarged and the left atrial to aortic ratio was normal (1.0 [normal range = 0.8 to 1.21]). These findings are of considerable help in sorting out the level of a left-to-right shunt. Both VSD and PDA result in dilated left atria and left ventricles,[3-5] because of volume overload of the left-sided chambers from the left-to-right shunt. The right ventricle may enlarge to some extent; the right atrium does not dilate. An ASD causes right atrial and right ventricular volume overload without left-sided enlargement. This right-sided

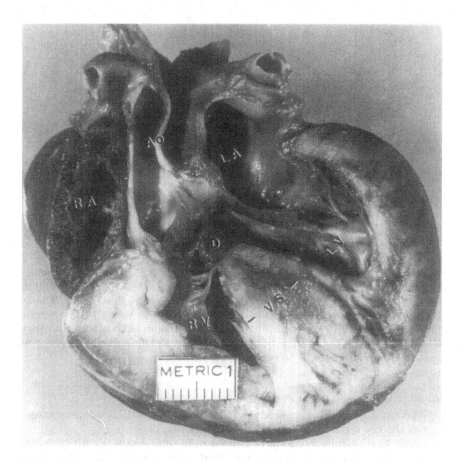

Figure 2 Longitudinal section of the heart. The walls of both the right *(RV)* and left *(LV)* ventricles are hypertrophied, a defect *(D)* is present in the most cephalad portion of the ventricular septum *(VS)*, the right atrium *(RA)* is large, and the aorta *(Ao)* and left atrium *(LA)* are of normal size. (Photo by M.M.M. Moore.)

overload may result in paradoxical movement of the ventricular septum during ventricular systole.[6-8] Thus, M-mode echocardiograms in infants with VSD (Figure 3) or PDA show increased left ventricular and left atrial dimensions with increased left atrial to aortic root ratios. ASD produces an increased right ventricular dimension; the left ventricular and left atrial dimension are normal or smaller than normal and the left atrial to aortic root ratios are normal (Figure 3).

In our infant, all three chambers seen by the M-mode echocardiogram were normal in size, and, therefore, the presence of ASD, VSD, or PDA as an isolated defect was most unlikely. The combination, however, of an ASD with a PDA and/or a VSD could result in a normal-sized left atrium, particularly if the atrial shunt were large. The left or right ventricle could be normal or increased in size depending upon the relative magnitude of each shunt. Thus, the M-mode echocardiogram in combination with the other findings in our patient suggested the diagnosis of ASD in combination with VSD and/or PDA.

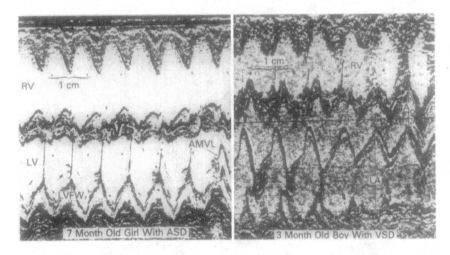

Figure 3 Echocardiograms from two patients. *Left*, A 7-month-old girl with a secundum type atrial septal defect *(ASD)*. The right ventricle *(RV)* is dilated and the ventricular septum *(VS)* moves paradoxically during ventricular systole. The left ventricle *(LV)* is of normal size. *LVFW* = left ventricular free wall; *AMVL* = anterior mitral valve leaflet. *Right*, Echocardiogram from a 3-month-old boy with a ventricular septal defect *(VSD)*. The left atrium *(LA)* is dilated and the aorta *(Ao)* is of normal size; consequently, the LA to Ao ratio is increased.

REFERENCES

1. Warkany, J., Passarge, E., and Smith, L. B.: Congenital malformations in autosomal trisomy syndromes, Am. J. Dis. Child. **112**:502; 1966.
2. Lester, L. A., Vitullo, D., Sodt, P., Hutcheon, N., and Arcilla, R.: An evaluation of the left atrial/aortic root ratio in children with ventricular septal defect, Circulation **60**:364, 1979.
3. Mathew, R., Thilenius, O. G., and Arciila, R.: Comparative response of right and left ventricles to volume overload, Am. J. Cardiol. **38**:209, 1976.
4. Lewis, A. B., and Takahashi, M.: Echocardiographic assessment of left-to-right shunt volume in children with ventricular septal defect, Circulation **54**:78, 1976.
5. Silverman, N. H., Lewis, A. B., Heymann, M. A., and Rudolph, A. M.: Echocardiographic assessment of ductus arteriosus shunt in premature infants, Circulation, **50**:821, 1974.
6. Diamond, M. A., Dillon, J. C., Haine, C. L., Chang, S., and Feigenbaum, H.: Echocardiographic feature of atrial septal defect, Circulation **43**:129, 1971.
7. Meyer, R. A., Schwartz, D. C., Benzing, G., III, and Kaplan, S.: Ventricular septum in right ventricular volume overload. An echocardiographic study, Am. J. Cardiol. **30**:349, 1972.
8. Radtke, W. E., Tajik, A. J., Gau, G. T., Schattenberg, T. T., Giuliani, E. R., and Tancredi, R. G.: Atrial septal defect: Echocardiographic observations. Studies in 120 patients, Ann. Intern. Med. **84**:246, 1976.

Case 399   Pulmonic Valve Stenosis, Atrial Septal Defect and Left-to-Right Interatrial Shunting with Intact Ventricular Septum

A Distinct Hemodynamic-Morphologic Syndrome

Ernest N. Arnett, MD, Seena C. Aisner, MD, Kenneth B. Lewis, MD, Paul Tecklenberg, MD, Robert K. Brawley, MD, and William C. Roberts, MD, F.C.C.P.

Herein we will discuss observations in two patients, each of whom had pulmonic-valve stenosis with secundum type atrial septal defect and large left-to-right shunts at the atrial level.

DESCRIPTION OF PATIENTS

Patient 1, a 69-year-old woman who died on Nov 29, 1978, was known to have had a precordial murmur for many years. She was asymptomatic, however, until eight days before death, when she suddenly had diplopia while washing dishes. She sat down, her right leg began shaking, and a generalized tonic-clonic seizure followed. Not long thereafter she was brought to the hospital in a comatose state, and examination disclosed unequal pupils and bilateral extensor plantar responses. The blood pressure was 190/100 mm Hg, and temperature 40.7 °C. A grade 4/6 holosystolic ejection type murmur was heard over the upper left sternal border. There was no cyanosis or clubbing. The ECG (Figure 1) disclosed atrial fibrillation and complete right bundle branch block, and chest roentgenogram (Figure 2) showed considerable cardiomegaly and prominent pulmonary arteries. She remained deeply comatose until death eight days later. The findings at necropsy are summarized in Figure 3.

Patient 2, a 55-year-old woman, was known to have had a precordial murmur since childhood. She was asymptomatic until age 48 years, when exertional dyspnea and fatigue were noted. At 52 years of age, cardiac catheterization was performed, and a 54 mm Hg peak systolic pressure gradient was recorded between right ventricle and pulmonary trunk. During the subsequent three years, exertional dyspnea and fatigue worsened, and she was again hospitalized. The blood pressure was 160/90 mm Hg and there was no cyanosis or clubbing. The jugular venous pressure was normal. A prominent systolic thrill was present at the upper left sternal border. A harsh grade 6/6 holosystolic ejection murmur and a grade 1/6 diastolic blowing murmur were heard over the left upper sternal border. The ECG (Figure 4) showed sinus rhythm and complete right bundle branch block. Chest roentgenogram (Figure 5) showed a normal sized heart but enlarged main pulmonary arteries.

Because of worsening symptoms, cardiac catheterization was performed again in May 1979 (Table 1). Oxygen saturation analysis disclosed a 1.8:1 left-to-right shunt at the atrial level, and indicator-dilution curves disclosed a minute right-to-left shunt.

From the Medicine and Pathology Departments, Franklin Square Hospital, The Department of Surgery, The Johns Hopkins Hospital, Baltimore, and the Pathology Branch, NHLBI, NIH, Bethesda, Md.

Reprint requests: Dr. Roberts, Building 10A, Room 3E30, National Institutes of Health, Bethesda 20205

DOI: 10.1201/9781003409342-23

171

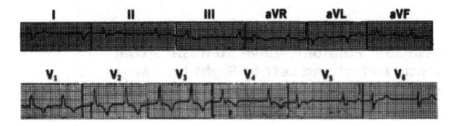

Figure 1 Patient 1. ECG showing atrial fibrillation and complete right bundle branch block.

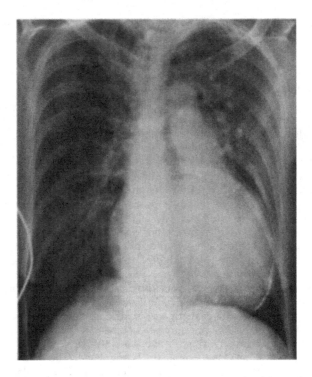

Figure 2 Patient 1. Chest roentgenogram showing considerable cardiomegaly and prominent main pulmonary arteries.

At operation (June 1979), the dome-shaped stenotic pulmonic valve was incised, and the large (4.5 × 3.0-cm) secundum type atrial septal defect was closed with a patch. The early postoperative course was uneventful, and since the early postoperative period she has been asymptomatic.

COMMENTS

Each of the two women described had pulmonic-valve stenosis (PS) and atrial septal defect (ASD) with large left-to-right shunts at the atrial level. Neither had ever had cyanosis, even with strenuous exertion. One lived 69 years without symptoms

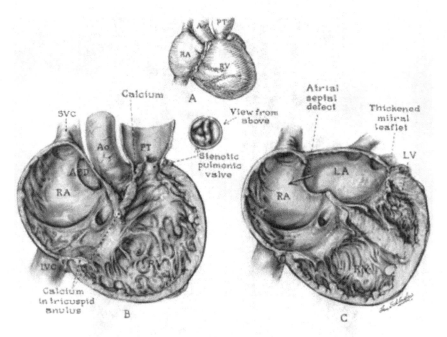

Figure 3   Patient 1. Drawing showing the major cardiac findings at necropsy. Right atrial (RA) and right ventricular (RV) cavities severely dilated; left atrial (LA) and left ventricular (LV) cavities normal in size. From anterior aspect (A), left ventricle was not visible, and only appendage of left atrium was visible. Secundum type atrial septal defect (ASD) was approximately 2.7 cm in largest diameter. Orifice of pulmonic valve was eccentric, stenotic, and valvular cusps, severely thickened by fibrous tissue and calcific deposits. Pulmonic trunk (PT) dilated. Calcific deposits also present in the tricuspid-valve annulus. IVC and SVC = inferior and superior vena cava, respectively; Ao = ascending aorta.

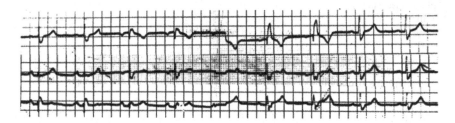

Figure 4   Patient 2. ECG showing sinus rhythm and complete right bundle branch block.

of cardiac dysfunction, and the second was asymptomatic until the age of 48 years. At necropsy or operation, both had stenotic pulmonic valves and large secundum type ASD.

Each of our two patients demonstrated typical morphologic features produced by the combination of PS and ASD with left-to-right shunting, but both are unique because of their age. Recently, Roberts and associates[1] reviewed hemodynamic and

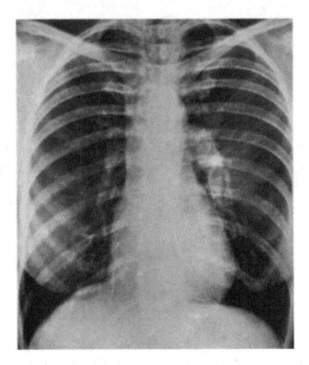

Figure 5 Patient 2. Chest roentgenograms, posteroanterior view (*left*) and lateral view (*right*) showing considerable enlargement of major pulmonary arteries.

Table 1: Hemodynamic findings in patient 2

	Pressure, mm Hg	Oxygen Saturation, %
Pulmonary artery (s/d)	20/5	92.2
Right ventricle (s/d)		
Outflow	70/1	. . .
Inflow	77/1	78.7
Right atrium		
Mean: A:V	0:5:1	76.2
Superior vena cava	. . .	68.6
Inferior vena cava	. . .	74.0
Left atrium		
Mean: A:V	0:5:1	96.6
Left ventricle (s/d)	120/1	. . .
Aorta (s/d)	120/56	94.4
Pulmonic valve area (index)	1.2 cm^2 (0.8 cm^2/M^2)	
Left-to-right shunt	1.8 liters/minute	

operative findings in 30 patients with PS and ASD: in 19 (63 percent), the shunt at the atrial level was exclusively, or nearly so, right-to-left, and in the other 11 (37 percent), the shunt was entirely, or nearly so, left-to-right. The ages at operation of the 19 patients with right-to-left shunts ranged from 3 to 43 years (mean, 19 years), and the ages of the 11 patients with left-to-right shunts ranged from 4 to 28 years (mean, 14 years). Of the 30 patients, 21 (70 percent) were female, including seven of the 11 with entirely left-to-right shunts. The explanation for the differing direction of the shunting at the atrial level in the 30 patients was the size of the defect in the atrial septum and the degree of obstruction to right ventricular outflow. The patients with right-to-left interatrial shunting had small (average diameter, 1.1 ± 0.1-cm) sized defects in the atrial septum (patent foramen ovale) and severe pulmonic valve stenosis (average peak systolic pressure gradient, 120 ± 11 mm Hg). In contrast, the patients with left-to-right shunts had mild to moderate pulmonic valve stenosis (average peak systolic pressure gradient, 60 ± 5 mm Hg) and relatively large (average diameter, 2.8 ± –.1 cm) defects in the atrial septum (true atrial septal defect). Both of our patients had secundum atrial septal defects larger than 2.5 cm in diameter, and both had moderate pulmonic valve stenosis (54 mm Hg peak systolic pressure gradient in patient 2). Surprisingly, the patients described earlier by Roberts and associates[1] with right-to-left interatrial shunts had no significant differences in right vs left atrial pressures. The patients with left-to-right interatrial shunts, however, had left atrial pressures (7 ± 0.5 vs 5 ± 0.5 mm Hg, $P <.05$), significantly greater than right atrial pressures. No significant differences in ventricular end-diastolic pressures were observed.

Although numerous reports have emphasized the frequency of right-to-left interatrial shunting in patients with valvular PS with intact ventricular septa, few have focused on patients with exclusive or nearly exclusive left-to-right shunting at the atrial level. The first to do so seems to have been Abrahams and Wood in 1951.[2] Among their 52 patients with "isolated" pulmonic stenosis, 15 had defects in the atrial septum, producing exclusive right-to-left shunting in eight and left-to-right shunting in seven. Each of the latter seven had only mild PS, whereas each of the former eight had evidence of severe PS. Although not confirmed anatomically, these authors reasoned that the patients with severe PS had venoarterial interatrial shunting via a patent foramen ovale, and that the patients with arteriovenous interatrial shunting had a true atrial septal defect. This reasoning was confirmed anatomically by the recent report by Roberts and associates[1] and by the morphologic and hemodynamic findings in the two patients just described.

REFERENCES

1 Roberts WC, Shemin RJ, Kent KM. Frequency and direction of interatrial shunting in valvular pulmonic stenosis with intact ventricular septum and without left ventricular inflow or outflow obstruction. *Am Heart J* 1980; 99:142–48.
2 Abrahams DG, Wood P. Pulmonary stenosis with normal aortic root. *Br Heart J* 1971; 13:519–24.

Case 406 Prolapsing Atrioventricular Valve in Partial Atrioventricular Defect

Bruce F. Waller, MD, Mazhar U. Sheikh, MD,
and William C. Roberts, MD
Bethesda, Md. and Washington, D.C.

Prolapse of the posterior mitral leaflet is now recognized to occur fairly frequently in patients with secundum-type atrial septal defect.[1-5] In contrast, prolapse of an atrioventricular (AV) valve in patients with primum-type atrial septal defect (AV defect or canal) has not been reported to our knowledge. Such an occurrence, however, was observed in a woman with partial AV defect and clinical and morphologic cardiac findings are described in this report.

A 56-year-old mongoloid black woman, who died on September 28, 1978, had been in her usual state of health until 8 days before death. In October, 1977 (9 months before death), she was seen at a cardiology clinic because of a precordial murmur. The cardiac silhouette on chest radiograph was of normal size, but the major pulmonary arteries were mildly dilated. She remained asymptomatic until September 20, 1978, when she became dyspneic and febrile. When hospitalized, she was lethargic and the systemic blood pressure was 100/70 mm Hg. The intensity of the second cardiac sound (S_2) was slightly increased (Figure 1); a grade 3/6 holosystolic murmur, loudest over the cardiac apical impulse and in the left axilla (Figure 1), was heard. A simultaneously recorded phonocardiogram and echocardiogram (Figure 1) disclosed "holosystolic" prolapse of a mitral leaflet. Pulmonary parenchymal infiltrates were present on chest radiogram. An electrocardiogram (Figure 2) showed a heart rate of 105 beats/min, a QRS axis of –75 degrees, QRS complexes typical of incomplete bundle branch block. Despite antibiotic therapy, her condition worsened, and she died after aspirating gastric contents.

At necropsy, the heart weighed 340 gm. Partial AV defect with ballooning of the AV leaflets was present (Figure 3). A large defect was present in the lowermost portion of the atrial septum (Figure 4). The right ventricle was mildly dilated. Thromboembolic material was present in the intrapulmonary pulmonary arteries and infarcts were present in the lower lobes of the lungs. Histologically, both the media and intima of the pulmonary arteries were normal.

No previous report, to our knowledge, has described prolapse or floppiness of one or more AV valve leaflets in AV defect (canal). Long survival in our patient appears to have been made possible because of the lack of development of evidence of pulmonary arterial hypertension or overt evidence of chronic congestive heart failure. The prolapsing AV valvular leaflet may have played a role in reducing the left-to-right shunt and therefore contributed to rather than detracted from prolonged survival.

From the Pathology Branch, National Heart, Lung, and Blood Institute, National Institutes of Health, Bethesda, and District of Columbia General Hospital, Washington, D.C.

Reprint requests: William C. Roberts, M.D., Building 10A, Room 3E-30, National Institutes of Health, Bethesda, MD 20205.

   DOI: 10.1201/9781003409342-24

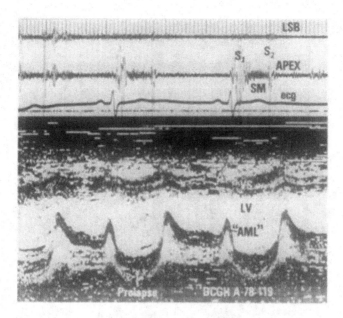

Figure 1   Phonocardiogram and echocardiogram obtained 8 days before death. A pansystolic murmur (*SM*) was recorded during "holosystolic" prolapse of a mitral leaflet (*"AML"*). *ecg* = electrocardiogram, *LV* = left ventricular cavity, *LSB* = left sternal border, *VS* = ventricular septum.

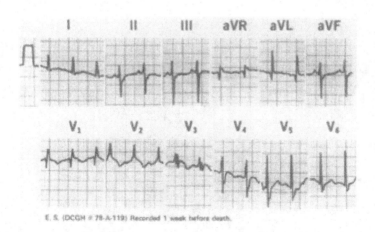

Figure 2   Electrocardiogram recorded 1 week before death.

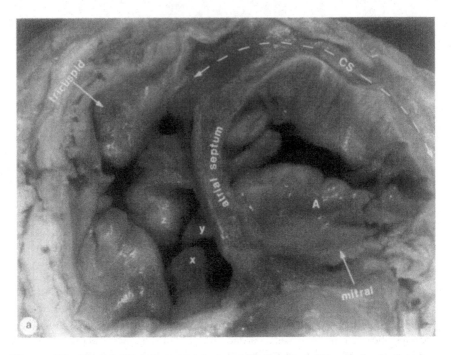

Figure 3A Partial AV defect. Atrial view of ballooning AV valvular leaflets (*x, y, z*). *A* = anterior leaflet, *CS* = ostium of the coronary sinus.

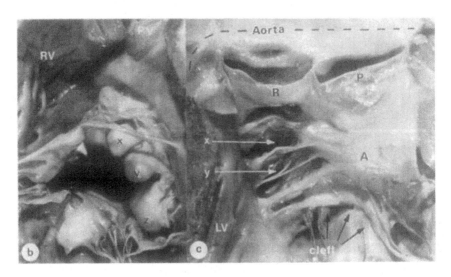

Figure 3B and **C. b,** View of prolapsed leaflets (*x, y, z*) from right ventricle (*RV*). c, outflow tract of left ventricle (*LV*) showing cleft anterior (*A*) and prolapsed portions (*x, y*) of the AV valve. *R* = right and *P* = posterior aortic cusps.

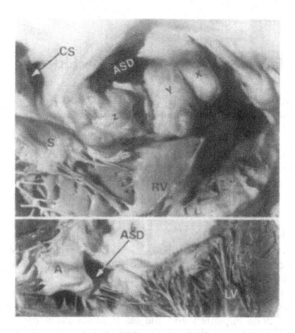

Figure 4 Right (*RV*) and left (*LV*) ventricular views of anterior (*A*), septal (*S*), and ballooning portions of the AV valve. An ostium primum atrial septal defect (*ASD*) is seen. *CS* = ostium of the coronary sinus.

REFERENCES

1. McDonald A, Harris A, Jetterson K, Marshall J, McDonald L: Association of prolapse of posterior cusp of mitral valve and atrial septal defect. *Br Heart J* **33**:383, 1971.
2. Pocock WA, Barlow JB: An association between billowing posterior mitral leaflet syndrome and congenital heart disease, particularly atrial septal defect. *Am Heart J* **81**:720, 1971.
3. Jeresaty RM: Atrial septal defect and myxomatous mitral-valve prolapse. *N Engl J Med* **290**:1088, 1974.
4. Leachman RD, Cokkinos DV, Cooley DA: Association of ostium secundum atrial septal defects with mitral valve prolapse. *Am J Cardiol* **38**:167, 1976.
5. Rippe JM, Sloss LJ, Angoff G, Alpert JS: Mitral valve prolapse in adults with congenital heart disease. *Am Heart J* **97**:561, 1979.

Case 435 Ebstein's Anomaly in the Elderly

Henry Scott Cabin, MD, Thomas P. Wood, MD, J. Orson Smith, MD, and William C. Roberts, MD, F.C.C.P.

Although the average survival with Ebstein's anomaly, when isolated, (except for a defect in the atrial septum) is about 25 years, at least seven patients surviving for 70 years or longer have been reported.[1-6] Herein we describe an elderly patient with Ebstein's anomaly and analyze factors allowing such survival.

CASE REPORT

A 72-year-old man who died on October 2, 1979 had paroxysmal supraventricular tachycardia since infancy without associated symptoms of cardiac dysfunction. He was asymptomatic until February, 1975 when at age 68 he had several episodes of near-syncope. The electrocardiogram showed a prolonged PR interval and right bundle branch block, and a pericardial friction rub was heard. In July, 1975, chest pain and palpitations appeared and the electrocardiogram disclosed atrial flutter with 2:1 atrioventricular block. After cardioversion, Holter monitor disclosed episodes of ventricular tachycardia unassociated with symptoms of cardiac dysfunction and he was treated with procainamide. In July, 1979, atrial flutter again appeared and he was again cardioverted to sinus rhythm and then begun on quinidine sulfate. He again did well until seven days before death when severe dyspnea and substernal chest pain with minimal exertion occurred, which was relieved by nitroglycerin. Examination three days later disclosed large V waves in the jugular venous pulse. The first and second heart sounds split widely. Midsystolic clicks, a third heart sound, and a soft systolic murmur (at the lower left sternal border) were heard. Pitting edema in the legs was present. The chest radiograph (Figure 1), electrocardiogram (Figure 2) and echocardiogram were all compatible with Ebstein's anomaly.[7-10] The final four days were characterized by recurrent episodes of chest pain, dyspnea and finally electromechanical dissociation.

At necropsy, the parietal and visceral pericardia were everywhere adherent to one another by fibrous adhesions. The heart weighed 560 grams. The amount of downward displacement into the right ventricle of the basal attachments of the septal and posterior tricuspid valve leaflets was severe (Figure 3). The interior circumference of the right atrioventricular junction, *ie*, the site where the tricuspid valve leaflets should have had their basal attachments, was 16 cm (normal ≤ 11 cm). The mitral valve anulus measured 11 cm in circumference. The lumina of the left anterior descending and right coronary arteries were narrowed 76–95 percent, and the left circumflex coronary artery from 51–75 percent in cross-sectional area by atherosclerotic plaques (Figure 4). A transmural scar was present in the

From the Pathology Branch, National Heart, Lung and Blood Institute, National Institutes of Health, Bethesda, Maryland and from the Departments of Pathology and Medicine, Tallahassee Memorial Regional Medical Center, Tallahassee, Florida.

Reprint requests: Dr. Roberts, National Institutes of Health, Bldg 10A, Room 3E30, Bethesda 20205

DOI: 10.1201/9781003409342-25

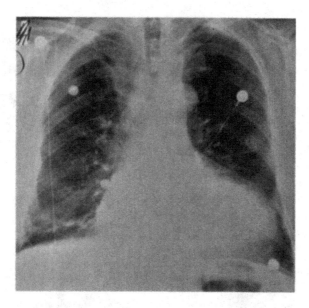

Figure 1 Posteroanterior chest radiograph one day before death showing a very large cardiac silhouette.

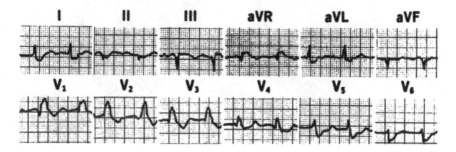

Figure 2 Electrocardiogram four days before death showing complete right bundle branch block, left axis deviation and a supraventricular rhythm.

anterobasal wall of left ventricle. A valvular competent patent foramen ovale was present.

COMMENTS

Of 121 previously reported necropsy patients with Ebstein's anomaly in whom the ages at death and the status of the atrial septa were described,[1-5, 11-16] 28 (23 percent) died during the first year of life and 84 (69 percent) by age 20 (Figure 5). The mean age of the 93 patients surviving past the first year of life was 26 years. To determine anatomic factors that might affect prognosis, we examined the relationship, if any, of survival to presence of an atrial septal defect or patent foramen ovale (Figure 5) or

181

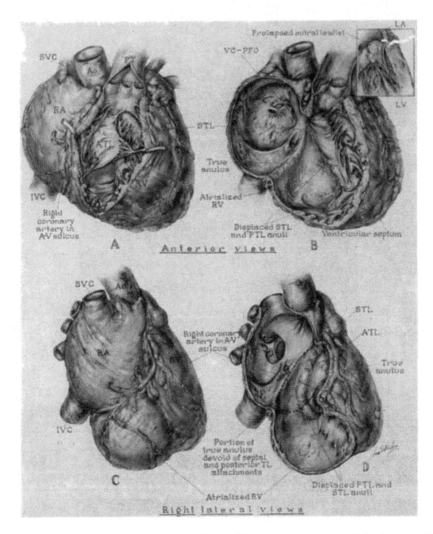

Figure 3 Drawing of the heart. *A*, View of the anterior surface of the heart with the anterior wall of the right ventricle (RV) opened to show the elongated anterior tricuspid valve leaflet (ATL) attached at the true anulus. Ao = aorta; AV = atrioventricular; IVC = inferior vena cava; PT = pulmonary trunk; RA = right atrium, STL = septal tricuspid leaflet; SVC = superior vena cava. *B*, View of the heart with the anterior walls of the RA and RV removed to show the posterior and septal portions of the true anulus devoid of leaflet attachments with the basal portions of the STL and posterior tricuspid leaflet (PTL) attached to the body of the RV. Caudal to the true anulus and cephalad to the attachments of the STL and PTL is the atrialized portion of RV. Shown in the *inset is* a portion of the left ventricle (LV) and left atrium (LA). The posterior leaflet of the mitral valve prolapsed mildly into the LA. VC-PFO = valvular competent patent foramen ovale. *C*, View of the right lateral surface of the heart showing the dilated RA and the posteriorly protruding atrialized portion of RV. *D*, View of the heart with the right lateral wall removed showing the basal attachment of the ATL to the true anulus (*dashed line*), but that of the PTL and STL displaced caudally into the body of RV.

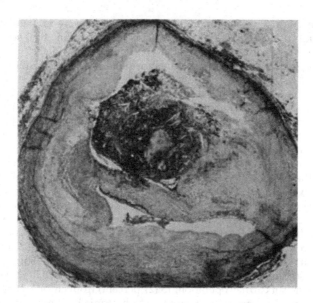

Figure 4 Left anterior descending coronary artery at its site of maximal narrowing. Hemorrhage into the lipid portion of the plaque has occurred (Movat stain × 22).

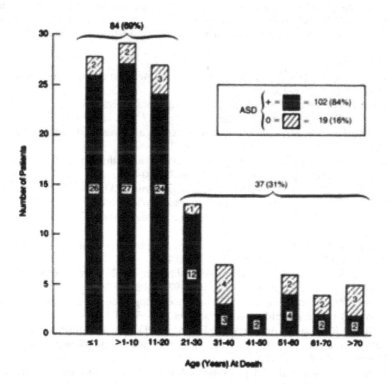

Figure 5 Length of life and frequency of true atrial septal defect or patent foramen ovale (ASD) in 121 previously reported necropsy patients with Ebstein's anomaly of the tricuspid valve.

183

other congenital cardiovascular anomalies in these 121 necropsy patients. Of the 28 patients dying in the first year of life, 26 (93 percent) had an atrial septal defect or patent foramen ovale; five (18 percent), a ventricular septal defect (in combination with atrial septal defect or patent foramen ovale in four), and six (21 percent), pulmonic valve atresia or stenosis. Of the 93 patients surviving the first year of life, 76 (82 percent) had an atrial septal defect or patent foramen ovale, and 17 (18 percent) did not; three (3 percent) had a ventricular septal defect (in combination with atrial septal defect or patent foramen ovale in two), and four (4 percent) had pulmonic valve atresia or stenosis. The mean age at death of those surviving the first year of life with an atrial septal defect or patent foramen ovale was 20 years, whereas it was 41 years in those with an intact atrial septum (P<.001). Thus, although there are exceptions, the presence of an atrial septal defect or patent foramen ovale overall appears to adversely affect survival.

Death in our patient, as well as chest pain during the final week of life, was secondary to coronary arterial narrowing by atherosclerotic plaques rather than to the congenitally abnormal tricuspid valve. To our knowledge, our patient is the first reported with Ebstein's anomaly in whom death was attributed to atherosclerotic coronary heart disease. Of 63 reported necropsy patients who survived past one month of age and in whom the cause of death was determined, 16 (25 percent) died as a consequence of cardiac operation; 13 (21 percent) from chronic congestive heart failure; 12 (19 percent), presumably from an arrhythmia because death was sudden; six (10 percent) from paradoxic embolus or brain abscess, five (8 percent), from complications of cardiac catheterization, and 11 (17 percent) from noncardiac causes.

Thus, prolonged symptom-free survival with an anatomically severe form of Ebstein's anomaly is possible. The presence of an atrial septal defect or valvular incompetent patent foramen ovale generally adversely affects survival.

REFERENCES

1. Adams JCL, Hudson R. A case of Ebstein's anomaly surviving to the age of 79. *Br Heart J* 1956; 18:129–132.
2. Vacca JB, Bussmann DW, Mudd JG. Ebstein's anomaly: complete review of 108 cases. *Am J Cardiol* 1958; 2:210–226.
3. Harris RHD. Ebstein's anomaly: discovered in a 75-year-old subject in the dissecting laboratory. *Can Med Assoc J* 1960; 83:653–655.
4. Makous N, Vander Veer JB. Ebstein's anomaly and life expectancy: report of a survival to over age 79. *Am J Cardiol* 1966; 18:100–104.
5. Lev M, Liberthson RR, Joseph RH, Seten CE, Kunske RD, Eckner FAO, Miller RA. The pathologic anatomy of Ebstein's disease. *Arch Path* 1970; 90:334–343.
6. Seward JB, Tajik AJ, Feist DJ, Smith HC. Ebstein's anomaly in an 85-year-old man. *Mayo Clin Proc* 1979; 54:193–196.
7. Kumar AE, Fyler DC, Miettinen OS, Nadas AS. Ebstein's anomaly: clinical profile and natural history. *Am J Cardiol* 1971; 28:84–85.
8. Bialostozky D, Horwitz S, Espino-Vela J. Ebstein's malformation of the tricuspid valve: a review of 65 cases. *Am J Cardiol* 1972; 29:826–836.
9. Farooki ZQ, Henry JG, Green EW. Echocardiographic spectrum of Ebstein's anomaly of the tricuspid valve. *Circulation* 1976; 53:63–68.
10. Giuliani ER, Fuster V, Brandenburg RO, Mair DD. Ebstein's anomaly: the clinical features and natural history of Ebstein's anomaly of the tricuspid valve. *Mayo Clin Proc* 1979; 54:163–173.
11. Livesay WR. Clinical and physiologic studies in Ebstein's malformation. *Am Heart J* 1959; 57:701–711.
12. Oldenburg FA, Nichol AD. Ebstein's anomaly in the adult. *Ann Intern Med* 1960; 52:710–717.

13. Genton E, Blount SG Jr. The spectrum of Ebstein's anomaly. *Am Heart J* 1967; 73:395–425.
14. Sekelj P, Benfey BG. Historical landmarks: Ebstein's anomaly of the tricuspid valve. *Am Heart J* 1974; 88:108–114.
15. Hansen JF, Leth A, Dorph S, Wennevold A. The prognosis in Ebstein's disease of the heart: long-term follow-up of 22 patients. *Acta Med Scand* 1977; 201:331–335.
16. Anderson KR, Lie JT. Pathologic anatomy of Ebstein's anomaly of the heart revisited. *Am J Cardiol* 1978; 41:739–745.

Case 460 Total Anomalous Pulmonary Venous Connection

Survival for 62 Years Without Surgical Intervention

Bruce M. McManus, MD, PhD, Josef Luetzeler, MD, and
William C. Roberts, MD
Bethesda and Silver Spring, MD

Most patients with total anomalous pulmonary venous connection (TAPVC), irrespective of the drainage site, live for less than 6 months.[1, 2] Of reported nonoperated necropsy patients with TAPVC with drainage of a common pulmonary vein into the left innominate vein via a left vertical vein ("Snowman" type), none had survived as long as 10 years[1] (Figure 1). The oldest reported patient with TAPVC of any type with necropsy verification was 39 years of age.[1] Recently, we studied at necropsy a 62-year-old man with unoperated TAPVC with drainage of a retroatrial common vein into the left innominate vein. He was cyanotic shortly after birth, acyanotic from about age 20 to 40 years, and cyanotic again during approximately his last 20 years. He was dyspneic on moderate exertion during his last 20 years. He had an acute febrile illness at age 48 years characterized by cough and excessive dyspnea. At that time chest roentgenogram disclosed cardiomegaly and a cavity in the left upper lobe. The pulmonic second sound was increased in intensity. After antibiotic therapy the signs suggestive of infection vanished. Because of cyanosis and cardiomegaly he underwent cardiac catheterization 6 months later. Pressures (mm Hg) and oxygen saturations (%) respectively were femoral artery (130/90, 78), left ventricle (110/3, 78), right ventricle (94/5, 78), left atrium (5, 76), right atrium (6, 78); oxygen saturations (%) superior vena cava (90), low left innominate vein (92), left subclavian vein (77), left brachial vein (59); and cardiac output 5.6 L/min. The ECG at that time and 2 days before death are shown in Figure 2. He never had overt congestive cardiac failure or a precordial murmur. He died from complications of a perforated duodenal ulcer. The findings in the heart and lungs at necropsy are delineated in Figures 3 to 6.

Besides lack of excessive pulmonary vascular resistance, survival in TAPVC appears to be dependent primarily on three factors: (1) the size of the defect in the atrial septum; 2) the length of the anomalous pulmonary veins(s), and (3) the degree of obstruction to flow in the anomalous pulmonary vein(s). Our patient appeared to have survived so long because of nearly ideal characteristics of each of these three factors. The atrial septum was virtually absent and therefore there was no interference to flow to the left side of the heart. The anomalous pulmonary vein was relatively short and free of any degree of obstruction. The cause of the total thrombotic occlusion of the left main pulmonary artery in our patient was not determined. It is clear, however, that this artery was totally occluded for at least 13 years and maybe considerably longer. Its occlusion in the presence of the left-to-right shunt (via the TAPVC) may have further elevated the pulmonary arterial pressures.[3–7]

From the Pathology Branch, National Heart, Lung and Blood Institute, National Institutes of Health; and the Department of Pathology, Holy Cross Hospital of Silver Spring.

Received for publication Sept, 28, 1981; accepted Oct. 6, 1981.

DOI: 10.1201/9781003409342-26

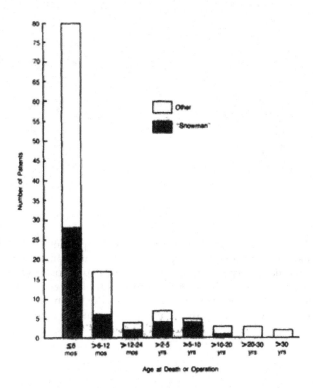

Figure 1 Age at death or operation in 121 previously reported patients with isolated TAPVC.[1, 2] Of those patients with the supracardiac "Snowman" type of TAPVC, 76% (34 of 45) had died or been operated upon by age 1 year, compared with 83% (63 of 76) of those with other types of TAPVC. Only five patients lived longer than 20 years of age and none of them had the "Snowman" type of pulmonary venous anomaly.

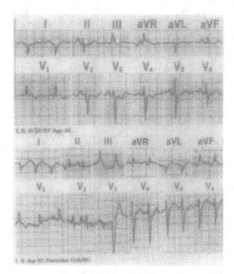

Figure 2 Electrocardiograms at age 48 years, when the diagnosis of TAPVC was made initially, and at age 62 years, 2 days before death. On both occasions, sinus rhythm, right axis deviation, right atrial abnormality, and right ventricular hypertrophy are present.

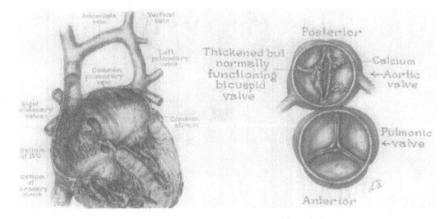

Figure 3 Drawing of four-chamber view of the patient's heart illustrating the common atrium and anomalous pulmonary venous connection. Despite the presence of calcific deposits, the congenitally bicuspid aortic valve appears to have functioned normally. The anterior commissure of the aortic valve was not in apposition with the posterior commissure of the pulmonic valve as is normally the case. The pulmonic valve is normal, as was the right ventricular outflow tract.

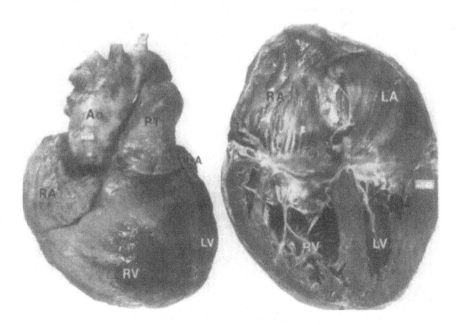

Figure 4 Exterior (*left*) and interior (*right*) of heart. *Ao* = aorta; *LA* = left atrium; *LV* = left ventricle; *PT* = pulmonary trunk; *RA* = right atrium; *RV* = right ventricle. (Photographs by M.M.M. Moore)

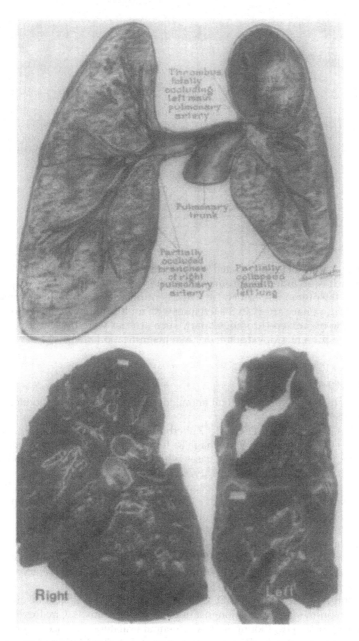

Figure 5 The right and left lungs demonstrating marked collapse and fibrosis of the left lung and cavitation of the left upper lobe which contained *Aspergillus* species. The left main pulmonary artery was completely occluded by thrombus. Extensive thrombus also was present in the proximal branches of the right pulmonary artery (*arrows*). The distal pulmonary arteries in the right lung are dilated.

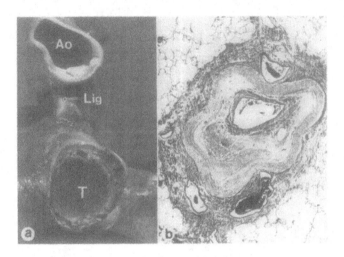

Figure 6 *a*, View of the transected aorta (*Ao*) at its isthmus and left main pulmonary artery which is occluded by thrombus (*T*). Extensive calcific deposits are present in the wall of the pulmonary artery. *Lig* = ligamentum arteriosum. *b*, Photomicrograph of a small pulmonary artery in the left lung with multiluminal channels presumably representing organized thrombus. Many such arteries were present. No plexiform lesions were present. (Movat stain; original magnification ×18.)

REFERENCES

1. Burroughs JT, Edwards JE: Total anomalous pulmonary venous connection. Am Heart J **59**:913, 1960.
2. Delisle G, Ando M, Calder AL, Zuberbuhler JR, Rochenmacher S, Alday LE, Mangini O, Van Praagh S, Van Praagh R: Total anomalous pulmonary venous connection: Report of 93 autopsied cases with emphasis on diagnostic and surgical considerations. Am Heart J **91**:99, 1976.
3. Harrison RW, Buehler WB, Thompson RG, Long ET, Carlson R, Charbon B, Adams WE: Cardiopulmonary reserve five to fifteen years following 50 percent or more reduction of lung volume. Surg Forum **8**:209, 1956.
4. Harrison RW, Adams WE, Beuhler WB, Long ET: Effects of acute and chronic reduction of lung volumes on cardiopulmonary reserve. Arch Surg **75**:546, 1957.
5. Harrison RW, Adams WE, Long ET, Burrows B, Reimann A: The clinical significance of cor pulmonale in the reduction of cardiopulmonary reserve following extensive pulmonary resection. J Thorac Surg **36**:352, 1958.
6. Rudolph AM, Neuhauser EBD, Golinko RJ, Auld PAM: Effects of pneumonectomy on pulmonary circulation in adult and young animals. Circ Res **9**:856, 1961.
7. Pool PE, Vogel JHK, Blount SG Jr: Congenital unilateral absence of a pulmonary artery. The importance of pulmonary hypertension. Am J Cardiol **10**:706, 1962.

Case 479 Fetal Rubella 27 Years Later

Bruce F. Waller, MD, F.C.C.P., Frederick A. Smith, MD, Donald M. Kerwin, MD, and William C. Roberts, MD, F.C.C.P.

Rubella infection in the first trimester of pregnancy is now well recognized to produce abnormalities in one or more body organs, including the cardiovascular system, but few detailed descriptions of the morphologic alterations affecting this system are available. Since 1963 at least six reports[1-6] have appeared describing cardiovascular findings at autopsy in 45 patients born from women having had rubella during early pregnancy: their ages in 37 were < one year; in four, one to five years; in three, six to ten years, and the oldest was 17 years of age. The present report was prompted by study at autopsy of an even older patient with typical features of the "congenital rubella syndrome."

A 27-year-old, severely mentally retarded woman who was born on Sept 14, 1952, and died on March 12, 1980, had been asymptomatic all her life until 18 hours before death, when evidence of acute pneumonia developed, which proved fatal. At birth she had been full-term but weighed only 2.2 kg. A precordial murmur was first noted at age three months. Her jaw protruded (prognathia), her teeth were malformed, her palate was arched, and her left foot turned inward (valgus) when walking. A grade 4/6 precordial systolic ejection-type murmur, with a thrill, was present, loudest along the upper left sternal border. In the axillae and back, the murmur had both systolic and diastolic components. An ECG showed right ventricular hypertrophy, and a chest roentgenogram disclosed a dilated pulmonary trunk. Catheterization (Table 1) disclosed multiple, severe (peak systolic pressure gradient, 90 mm Hg) peripheral pulmonary stenoses. She did well until the day of death, when she began coughing, became rapidly dyspneic, febrile, hypotensive, hypoxic, and died. The blood hematocrit was 55 percent; leukocyte count, 17,000/cu mm, and urinary protein level, 3 + /4 +.

Injection of contrast material into the major extrapulmonary pulmonary arteries at autopsy disclosed many discrete stenoses of the intrapulmonary pulmonary arteries (Figure 1). The pulmonary arteries proximal to the stenoses had severely thickened walls and the thickening resulted entirely from thickening of the media (Figure 2). The right ventricular wall was severely hypertrophied, and its cavity was not dilated (Figure 3). The wall of the entire aorta also was severely thickened, and again the thickening resulted entirely from thickening of the media (Figures 4 and 5). The wall of the left ventricle also was hypertrophied and its cavity was not dilated (Figure 3). The heart weighed 340 g. Histologically, the myocardium was normal except for hypertrophy of the myocardial fibers. Each kidney weighed about 100 g, and histologically, hemosiderin deposits were present in the cytoplasm of many renal tubular cells, indicating that intravascular hemolysis had occurred during life. The liver (1,200 g) and

From the Pathology Branch, National Heart, Lung and Blood Institute, National Institutes of Health, Bethesda, Md, and the Department of Pathology, Georgetown University Medical Center, Washington, D.C.

Reprint requests: Dr. Roberts, Bldg 10A, Room 3E30, National Institutes of Health, Bethesda 20205

spleen (90 g) were normal and free from iron deposits. The rubella-neutralizing antibody titer on a postmortem blood specimen was 1:32 (normal, ≤1:8).

The patient described had fetal rubella with abnormalities of the cardiovascular and pulmonary systems and was asymptomatic until acute pneumonia proved fatal. She had severe peripheral pulmonary arterial stenoses resulting in severe proximal pulmonary arterial hypertension. The walls of the major pulmonary arteries proximal to the narrowings were severely thickened, and the walls of these arteries distal to the narrowings were thin. Of the eight previously reported patients with the congenital rubella syndrome who died after one year of age, only one had peripheral pulmonary arterial stenosis.[1] The thickening of the pulmonary artery walls in our patient was due entirely to thickening of the media by elastic fibers, smooth muscle cells and collagen. Only two of the eight previously reported patients surviving longer than one year had had thickened walls of the major pulmonary arteries, which has been attributed to thickening of the intima.

Table 1: Cardiac catheterization data at age 18 years*

Pressures, mm Hg
Left: P→M→PT→RV = 25/-→ 89/45→115/45→114/13
Right: P→M→PT→RV = 24/-→108/38→114/45→114/13
Ascending aorta→Abdominal aorta→Femoral artery = 147/90→140/89→145/75

* Abbreviations: M = recording from a portion of pulmonary artery somewhere between an intrapulmonary artery and the pulmonary trunk; PT = pulmonary trunk; and RV = right ventricle.

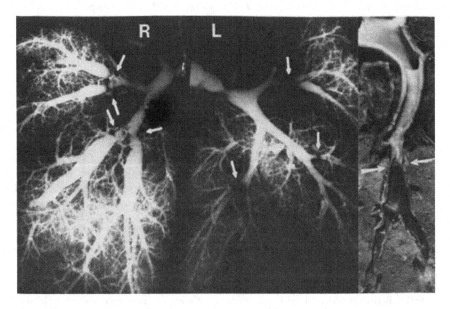

Figure 1 Postmortem roentgenogram (*left*) after injection of contrast material into right (R) and left (L) major extrapulmonary pulmonary arteries, disclosing multiple discrete stenoses of the intrapulmonary arteries (*arrows*). Opened pulmonary artery (*right*) showing marked thickening of walls proximal to stenosis (*between arrows*) and thinned walls distally.

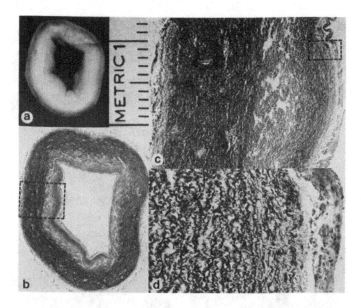

Figure 2 Thickened wall of portion of left main pulmonary artery proximal to intrapulmonary pulmonary arterial stenosis. *A,* Cross-section of gross specimen. *B,* Photomicrograph of section shown in A. *C,* Photomicrograph of boxed area in B showing increased wall thickness resulting primarily from proliferation of elastic tissue in media. *D,* Photomicrograph of boxed area in C showing irregular and fragmented elastic fibers. Movat stains, original magnifications, × 8.5 (B), × 38 (C), × 220 (D).

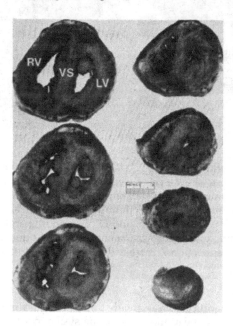

Figure 3 Transverse slices of cardiac ventricles showing severe thickening of right (RV) and mild thickening of left (LV) ventricular walls. Neither cavity was dilated. VS = ventricular septum.

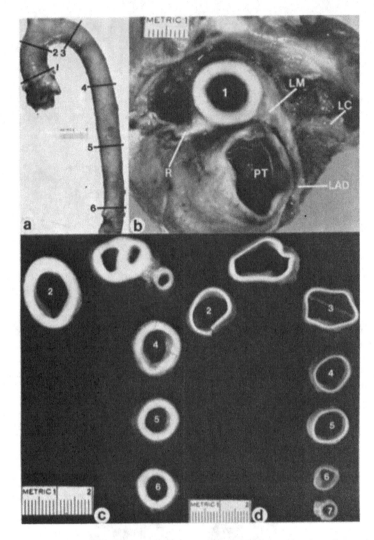

Figure 4 Thickened aorta in study patient (*B* and *C*) compared with similar portions of aorta from control subject (*D*), a 27-year-old woman who died of leukemia, and with normal aorta to show level of sections (*A*). *B*, Ascending aorta at level 1; wall severely thickened compared with wall of pulmonic trunk (*PT*). LAD = left anterior descending coronary artery; LC = left circumflex coronary artery; R = right coronary artery. Similar portions (levels 2, 4, 5, and 6) of ascending and thoracic aorta from study patient (*C*) and control subject (*D*) show diffusely thickened walls of aorta in study patient. Cross-section 7 is from distal abdominal aorta. (Photographs by Margaret M. M. Moore).

The wall of the entire aorta also was greatly thickened by a similar medial proliferation and appears to have been the cause of the systemic arterial hypertension. Of three previously reported autopsy patients with fetal rubella and systemic hypertension,[2, 6] each had severely thickened renal arteries, but the renal arteries in our patient were normal.

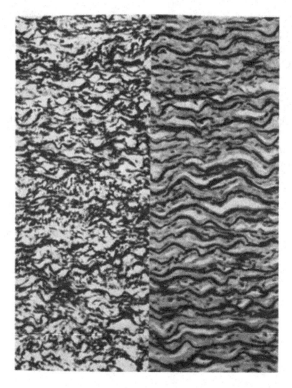

Figure 5 Photomicrographs of wall of ascending aorta (level 1, Figure 5) from study patient (*left*) and control subject (*right*) showing disorganized and fragmented elastic fibers in study patient. Movat stains, original magnifications, × 220.

Clinical manifestations of cardiovascular rubella may be absent early in life. Of eight previously reported autopsy patients with fetal rubella who had survived over one year of life,[1-6] clinical information was available for only two. The 17-year-old boy with fetal rubella and peripheral stenosis described by Franch and Gay[1] was similar to our patient in that he was asymptomatic until shortly before death. The seven-year-old boy described by Fortuin and associates[6] also had no symptoms of systemic vascular disease until shortly before death. The cause of the vascular changes later in life may not be appreciated if other nonvascular manifestations of the rubella syndrome are absent. Fetal rubella infection should be considered, however, as a cause of occlusive pulmonary or systemic vascular disease in young persons.

A surprising finding in our patient at autopsy was renal hemosiderosis, which indicates that intravascular hemolysis had occurred. Its cause is unclear, but it seems reasonable to consider the possibility that trauma to the erythrocytes being ejected through the multiple peripheral pulmonic stenosis under near systemic pressures was responsible. It has been demonstrated previously that ejection of blood through one severely stenotic, native, calcified aortic valve or through a prosthetic valve produces intravascular hemolysis.[7, 8] Possibly, ejection through many noncalcified but severely stenotic pulmonary stenoses under similar pressure also may produce some degree of intravascular hemolysis.

REFERENCES

1. Franch RH, Gay BB Jr. Congenital stenosis of the pulmonary artery branches: a classification, with postmortem findings in two cases. Am J Med 1963; 35:512–529.
2. Esterly JR, Oppenheimer EH. Vascular lesions in infants with congenital rubella. Circulation 1967; 36:544–554.
3. Singer DB, Rudolph AJ, Rosenberg HS, Rawls WE, Boniuk M. Pathology of the congenital rubella syndrome. J Pediatr 1967; 71:665–675.
4. Esterly JR, Oppenheimer EH. Pathological lesions due to congenital rubella. Arch Pathol 1969; 87:380–388.
5. Tang JS, Kauffman SL, Lynfield J. Hypoplasia of the pulmonary arteries in infants with congenital rubella. Am J Cardiol 1971; 27:491–496.
6. Fortuin NJ, Morrow AG, Roberts WC. Late vascular manifestations of the rubella syndrome. Am J Med 1971; 51:134–140.
7. Roberts WC. Renal hemosiderosis (blue kidney) in patients with valvular heart disease. Am J Pathol 1966; 48:409–419.
8. Roberts WC, Morrow AG. Renal hemosiderosis in patients with prosthetic aortic valves. Circulation 1966; 33:390–398.

Case 482 Separate Aortic Ostium of the Left Anterior Descending and Left Circumflex Coronary Arteries From the Left Aortic Sinus of Valsalva (Absent Left Main Coronary Artery)

Barry S. Dicicco, MD, Bruce M. McManus, MD, PhD, Bruce F. Waller, MD, and William C. Roberts, MD
Bethesda, MD

Ordinarily, of course, only one coronary artery arises from the left sinus of Valsalva and that is the left main (LM) coronary artery. On rare occasion, the LM coronary artery is absent and both left anterior descending (LAD) and left circumflex (LC) coronary arteries arise independently, each from a separate ostium in the left sinus of Valsalva (Figures 1 to 3). Schlesinger et al.[1] found a separate ostium for both LAD and LC coronary arteries in the left aortic sinus in 2 (0.2%) of 1000 consecutive necropsies, and Zumbo et al.[2] observed coronary arterial anomalies in 33 of 2089 necropsied patients, 21 (1%) of whom had a separate aortic ostium of the LAD and LC coronary arteries. During the past 3 years, we have studied at necropsy four patients (three men) aged 61 to 74 years (mean 67) in whom the LAD and LC arose separately in the left aortic sinus; three died from consequences of coronary atherosclerosis and one from a noncardiac cause.

We call attention to this anomaly because its nonrecognition at angiography or operation could potentially lead to serious consequences. If at coronary angiography contrast material is injected into only one or the other of the two arteries arising from the left aortic sinus, the noninjected artery might mistakenly be interpreted as being totally occluded at its origin from the LM coronary artery. If either the LAD or LC coronary arteries are not visualized by selective injection of contrast material, injection into the sinuses of Valsalva may prevent confusing an anomalously arising coronary artery with a totally occluded coronary artery. If either ostium is not perfused at the time of cardiopulmonary bypass, a portion of left ventricular myocardium might not be adequately oxygenated, as observed in a patient described by Ogden.[3] A theoretical advantage of a separate ostium of both the LAD and LC coronary arteries from the left aortic sinus is the inability to have complications resulting from narrowing of the LM coronary artery. Two of our four patients with separate origin of the LAD and LC coronary arteries, however, had severe (> 75% cross-sectional area) narrowing of both LAD and LC coronary arteries proximal to any major branches and therefore had so-called "LM equivalent" narrowing (Figure 2). This coronary anomaly does not appear to accelerate atherosclerosis in either of the separately arising coronary arteries.[2]

From the Pathology Branch, National Heart, Lung and Blood Institute, National Institutes of Health.

Received for publication March 11, 1982; accepted March 19, 1982.

Reprint requests: William C. Roberts, M.D., Pathology Branch, NHLBI-NIH, Bldg. 10A, Room 3E-30, Bethesda, MD 20205.

DOI: 10.1201/9781003409342-28

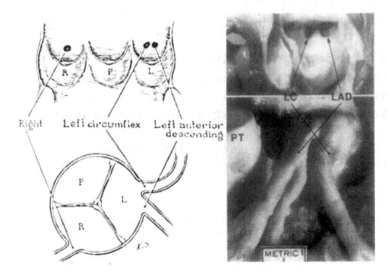

Figure 1 Drawing (*left*) of aorta showing origin of each of the left circumflex (*LC*) and left anterior descending (*LAD*) coronary arteries from a separate ostium in the left sinus of Valsalva. *Right upper*, Interior of left sinus showing each ostium (SH No. A81–49). *Lower right*, Exterior view showing both LC and LAD coronary arteries arising separately. *PT* = pulmonary trunk. (Photo by M.M.M. Moore.)

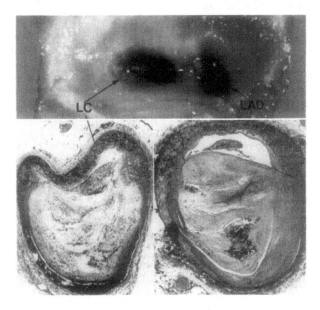

Figure 2 *Upper*, Portion of aorta behind left sinus showing a separate ostium for each of the left circumflex (*LC*) and left anterior descending (LAD) coronary arteries in 63-year-old woman (GT No. 81A-209). (Photo by M.M.M. Moore.) *Lower left*, Cross-section of LAD coronary artery in its first 5 mm segment. *Lower right*, Cross-section of LC coronary artery in its first 5 mm segment. Both the LAD and LC are considerably narrowed proximally (left main equivalent). (Movat stains; each original magnification ×14.)

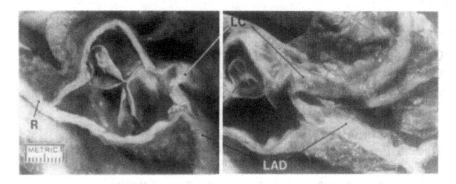

Figure 3 Aortic valve from above showing separate origins of the right (*R*), left anterior descending (*LAD*), and left circumflex (*LC*) coronary arteries from the aorta in a 74-year-old man (GT No. 79A-74). (Photo by M.M.M. Moore.)

REFERENCES

1. Schlesinger MJ, Zoll PM, Wessler S: The conus artery: A third coronary artery. Am Heart J **38**:823, 1949.
2. Zumbo O, Fani K, Jarmdyeh J, Daoud AS: Coronary atherosclerosis and myocardial infarction in hearts with anomalous coronary arteries. Laboratory Investigation **14**:571, 1965.
3. Ogden JA: Anomalous aortic origin: Circumflex, anterior descending or main left coronary arteries. Arch Pathol **88**:323, 1969.

Case 490 Origin of the Left Main from the Right Coronary Artery or from the Right Aortic Sinus with Intramyocardial Tunneling to the Left Side of the Heart via the Ventricular Septum

The Case Against Clinical Significance of Myocardial Bridge or Coronary Tunnel

William C. Roberts, MD, Barry S. Dicicco, MD, Bruce F. Waller, MD, Joan C. Kishel, MD, Bruce M. McManus, MD, PhD, Stuart L. Dawson, MD, John C. Hunsaker, III, MD, and James L. Luke, MD
Bethesda, MD, and Washington, D.C.

Recently we studied the hearts of two patients who died from consequences of knife or bullet wounds. Although during life neither ever had clinical evidence of cardiac dysfunction, at necropsy both had origin of the left main (LM) coronary artery from either the right (R) coronary artery or directly from the right anterior sinus of Valsalva with intramyocardial coursing within the ventricular septum to the left side of the heart. The course within the septum was 5.0 cm in the 34-year-old man (Figure 1) and 4.5 cm in the 48-year-old man (Figure 2). In each patient, the LM exited from the ventricular septum anteriorly and immediately branched into the left anterior descending (LAD) and left circumflex (LC) coronary arteries which thereafter followed their usual courses. The walls of the tunneled LM in each patient were thinner than that of the R, LAD, or LC coronary arteries. The course of the R coronary artery was normal. The myocardium was normal. The major coronary arteries in both patients were free of atherosclerotic plaques.

Review of previous published reports on patients with origin of the LM from the R coronary artery or from the right anterior aortic sinus disclosed at least 11 necropsy patients (aged 28 to 87 years [mean = 55]; eight males and three females) in whom the LM arose either from the R coronary artery or directly from the right anterior aortic sinus and thereafter coursed within the ventricular septum to emerge in the epicardium above the anterior portion of septum.[1-7] Of these 11 previously reported necrospy patients, five died from noncardiac conditions and never had evidence of cardiac dysfunction during life; three died from coronary atherosclerotic heart disease[5, 6, 4]; one died from valvular heart disease[1]; and one died from amyloid heart disease.[7] In the remaining patient (case No. 9 of Cheitlin et al.[4]), a 36-year-old man with repeated episodes of ventricular tachycardia and finally fatal cardiac arrest, it is likely that the coronary anomaly in some way was responsible for the ventricular arrhythmia and sudden death. Although it is of course hazardous to attribute functional importance to a coronary anomaly when only 1 of 11 reported patients appears to have had a

From the Pathology Branch, National Heart, Lung and Blood institute, National Institutes of Health; and the Medical Examiner's Office, Washington, D.C.

Received for publication Apr. 15, 1982; accepted Apr. 19, 1982.

Reprint requests: William C. Roberts, M.D., Pathology Branch, NIH-NHLBI, Bldg. 10A, Room 3E-30, Bethesda, MD 20205.

DOI: 10.1201/9781003409342-29

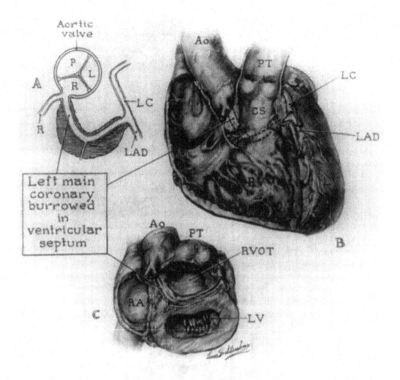

Figure 1 Drawing of the heart in our 34-year-old man (DCMEO No. 81-09-750). The left main (LM) coronary artery coursed within the ventricular septum beneath the right ventricular outflow tract before branching above the septum into the left anterior descending (*LAD*) and left circumflex (*LC*) coronary arteries. *Ao* = aorta; *CS* = crista supraventricularis; *LV* = left ventricle; *RA* = right atrium; *PT* = pulmonary trunk; *RV* = right ventricle.

fatal or nonfatal cardiac problem not explainable by another cardiac condition, the anomaly in this one patient suggests that this coronary anomaly may occasionally be of clinical importance. We found no reports of this anomaly being diagnosed by coronary angiography during life.[8] In three additional reported necropsy patients (aged 4, 39, and 60 years; two males), the LAD arose from the R coronary artery or right sinus of Valsalva and thereafter coursed similarly in the ventricular septum; the LC arose from the R coronary artery and coursed behind the aorta before reaching the left atrioventricular sulcus.[9-11] None of these three patients ever had evidence of cardiac dysfunction.

Although angina pectoris[12] and sudden death[13] have been attributed to tunneling of one (LAD) of the four major coronary arteries, the absence of evidences of myocardial ischemia both clinically and at necropsy in our two patients and in 10 of 11 previously reported patients suggests that tunneling is an unlikely cause of myocardial ischemia. In each of our two patients the tunneled LM was over 4 cm in length. When only the LAD is tunneled, the tunneled segment is usually less than 3 cm in length and, of course, only one artery is affected in this circumstance rather than two which is the situation when the LM is tunneled. Tunneling of a

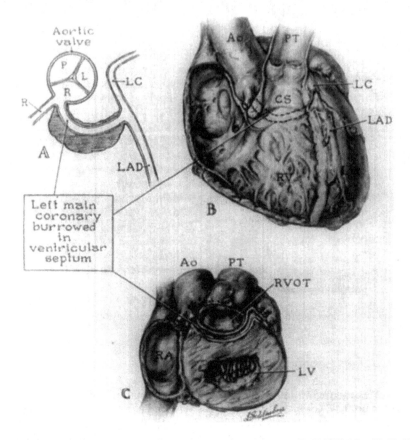

Figure 2 Drawing of the heart in our 48-year-old man (DCMEO No. 82-03-291). Abbreviations as in Figure 1.

major coronary artery within myocardium protects the intramyocardial segment from atherosclerotic plaques.

REFERENCES

1. Gallavardin L, Ravault P: Anomalie d'origine de la coronaire anterieure. Lyon Med **136**:270, 1925.
2. Kintner AR: Anomalous origin and course of the left coronary artery. Arch Pathol **12**:586, 1931.
3. Born E: Uber Missbildungen der Kranzarterien und ihre Beziehungen zu Zirkulationsstorungen und plotzlichem Tod. Virchows Arch Pathol Anat **290**:688, 1933.
4. Cheitlin MD, De Castro CM, McAllister HA: Sudden death as a complication of anomalous left coronary origin from the anterior sinus of Valsalva. A not-so-minor congenital anomaly. Circulation **50**:780, 1974.
5. Roberts JT, Loube SD: Congenital single coronary artery in man. Report of nine new cases, one having thrombosis with right ventricular and atrial (auricular) infarction. Am Heart J **34**:188, 1947.

6. Allen GL, Snider TH: Myocardial infarction with a single coronary artery. Report of a case. Arch Intern Med **117**:261, 1966.
7. Snow PJD: A case of single coronary artery with stereographic demonstration of the arterial distribution. Br Heart J **15**:261, 1953.
8. Moodie DS, Gill C, Loop FD, Sheldon WC: Anomalous left main coronary artery originating from the right sinus of Valsalva. Pathophysiology, angiographic definition, and surgical approaches. J Thorac Cardiovasc Surg **80**:198, 1980.
9. Bochdalek J: Anomaler Verlauf der Kranzartenen des Herzens. Virchows Arch Pathol Anat **41**:260, 1967.
10. Sanes S: Anomalous origin and course of the left coronary artery in a child. So-called congenital absence of the left coronary artery. Am Heart J **14**:219, 1937.
11. White NK, Edwards JE: Anomalies of the coronary arteries. Report of four cases. Arch Pathol **45**:766, 1948.
12. Rossi L, Dander B, Nidasio GP, Arbustini E, Paris B, Vassanelli C, Buonanno C, Poppi A: Myocardial bridges and ischemic heart disease. Eur Heart J **1**:239, 1980.
13. Morales AR, Romanelli R, Boucek RJ: The mural left anterior descending coronary artery, strenuous exercise and sudden death. Circulation **62**:230, 1980.

Case 508 Crisscrossed Atrioventricular Valves and Prolonged Survival

William C. Roberts, MD, Thomas L. Spray, MD,
Richard J. Shemin, MD and Barry J. Maron, MD

Normally, of course, the atrioventricular (AV) cardiac valves have a right-to-left relationship with one another (Figure 1). The right-sided AV valve connects the right-sided atrium to the right-sided ventricle, and the left-sided AV valve connects the left-sided atrium to the left-sided ventricle. In rare cases, however, the AV valves are not parallel to one another but are crisscrossed, so that the right-sided atrium connects to the left-sided ventricle and the left-sided atrium connects to the right-sided ventricle (Figure 1). When this occurs, the AV valves have an anteroposterior relation. Since 1974, a number of patients with crisscrossed AV valves have been reported on, and most died early in life from either inadequate or excessive pulmonary blood flow, the latter by way of an associated large ventricular septal defect. This report was prompted by studying a man who lived 55 years with crisscrossed AV valves associated with double outlet right ventricle and pulmonic valve stenosis.

Although cyanosis and a precordial murmur were present at birth and throughout life, the patient was asymptomatic except on extreme exertion until age 46 years when syncope occurred; cardiac catheterization was performed, and operation refused. At age 54 years (10 months before death), 2,500 ml of blood was removed because of a hematocrit level of about 65%. Two months later, diplopia, a sixth nerve palsy, and intermittent Mobitz II heart block with a left bundle branch block pattern appeared, and cardiac catheterization was repeated. The pressures (in mm Hg) were as follows: pulmonary artery, 15/7; right ventricular outflow, 60/10, and inflow, 135/7; right, atrial mean, 5; pulmonary artery wedge mean, 7; left ventricle, 125/10; and aorta, 125/71. Examination 4 months before death disclosed a grade 3/6 precordial systolic murmur with thrill, most prominent at the left sternal border. The electrocardiogram, chest roentgenograms, and M-mode echocardiogram are shown in Figures 2 to 4. The right subclavian artery was anastomosed to the right pulmonary artery 70 days before death. Immediately after operation, intractable congestive heart failure developed and 6 days later the Blalock-Taussig shunt was closed; his condition improved briefly, but gradually evidence of poor perfusion of the kidneys, heart, and brain developed and the patient died.

The findings at necropsy are summarized in Figures 1, 5, and 6. The mitral valve, located posterior to the tricuspid valve, connected the right-sided anatomic right atrium to the left-sided anatomic left ventricle, and the tricuspid valve, located anterior to the mitral valve, connected the left-sided anatomic left atrium to the right-sided anatomic right ventricle. The only outlet for blood from the left ventricle was a ventricular septal defect. Both aorta and pulmonary trunk arose from the right ventricle. The pulmonic value was severely stenotic and heavily calcified (Figure 6), and a portion of its sinus wall protruded anteriorly (Figure 1).

From the Pathology, Surgery, and Cardiology Branches, National Heart, Lung, and Blood Institute, National Institutes of Health, Bethesda, Maryland. Manuscript received and accepted July 2, 1982.

Address for reprints; William C. Roberts, MD, Building 10A, Room 3E-30, National Institutes of Health, Bethesda, Maryland 20205.

DOI: 10.1201/9781003409342-30

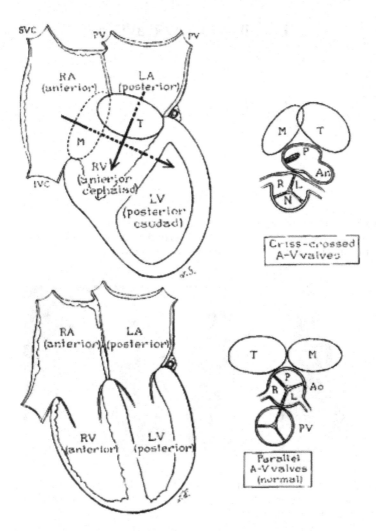

Figure 1   Diagram showing basic arrangement of the patient's crisscrossed heart (**top**) compared with the normal heart (**bottom**). The valves shown **on the right** are as they appeared after removing the aorta (Ao), pulmonary trunk, and walls of the right atrium (RA) and left atrium (LA). The ventricular septum in the crisscrossed heart is relatively perpendicular to the atrial septum, and this feature allows the crisscrossed valve arrangement. Blood traversing the tricuspid (T) valve from the posteriorly located LA flows anteriorly to the anteriorly located right ventricle (RV) and blood traversing the mitral (M) valve flows posteriorly to the posteriorly located left ventricle (LV). The pulmonic valve (P) (**top only**) is unicuspid and unicommissural, and an aneurysm (An) of its sinus protrudes anteriorly. L = left; N = noncoronary cusp or sinus; P = posterior sinuses of Valsalva of the aortic valve; R = right.

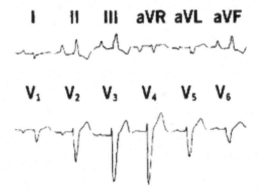

Figure 2 Electrocardiogram showing intermittent second-degree heart block, left bundle branch block, a P-R interval of 0.21 second, and lack of development of a significant r wave in the precordial leads. V leads ½ standard.

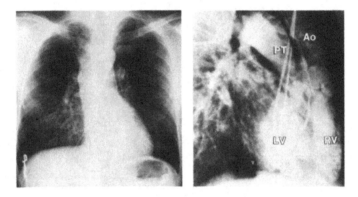

Figure 3 Posteroanterior radiograph (**left**) and lateral angiogram (**right**). The aorta (Ao) arises anterior to the stenotic pulmonic valve. LV = left ventricle; PT = pulmonary trunk; RV = right ventricle.

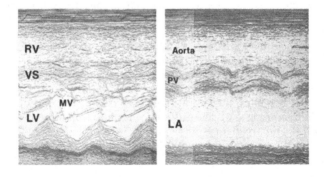

Figure 4 M-mode echocardiogram interpreted retrospectively showing (**left**) the mitral valve (MV) to occupy most of the left ventricular cavity (LV), and (**right**) the calcified pulmonic valve (PV) located anterior to the dilated left atrium (LA) and posterior to the aorta. RV = right ventricular cavity; VS = ventricular septum.

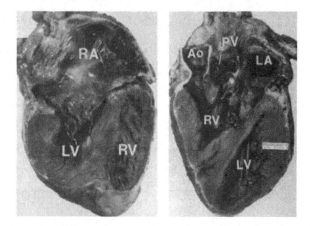

Figure 5 Anteroposterior cut of the heart showing (**left**) the right atrium (RA) draining into the left ventricle (LV) and (**right**) the left atrium (LA) draining directly into the right ventricle (RV). Both the aorta (Ao) and the pulmonary trunk arise from the right ventricle. The tricuspid valve is displaced toward the right ventricle, and its leaflets partly obstruct the ventricular septal defect. The conus is inverted. PV = stenotic pulmonic valve.

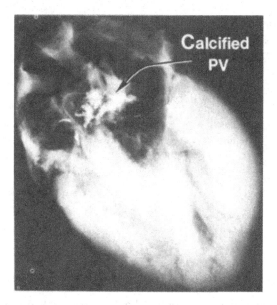

Figure 6 Radiograph of heart specimen disclosing heavy calcific deposits in the stenotic pulmonic valve (PV).

This case is by far the oldest reported thus far with crisscrossed AV valves. Of the other 9 necropsy cases reported,[1-6] 4 ([1][Case 13],[2,5][Case 2],[6][Case 7]) died during the first 2 months of life, 1 at 4 years,[3] 2 at 8 years ([1][Case 12],[4]), 1 at 23 years ([6][Case 5]) and 1 at 25 years ([5][Case 1]). Both of the 2 reported patients living longer than 20 years and our patient had obstruction to pulmonary blood flow, a near necessity for prolonged survival with transposition of the great arteries and ventricular septal defect or double-outlet right ventricle.

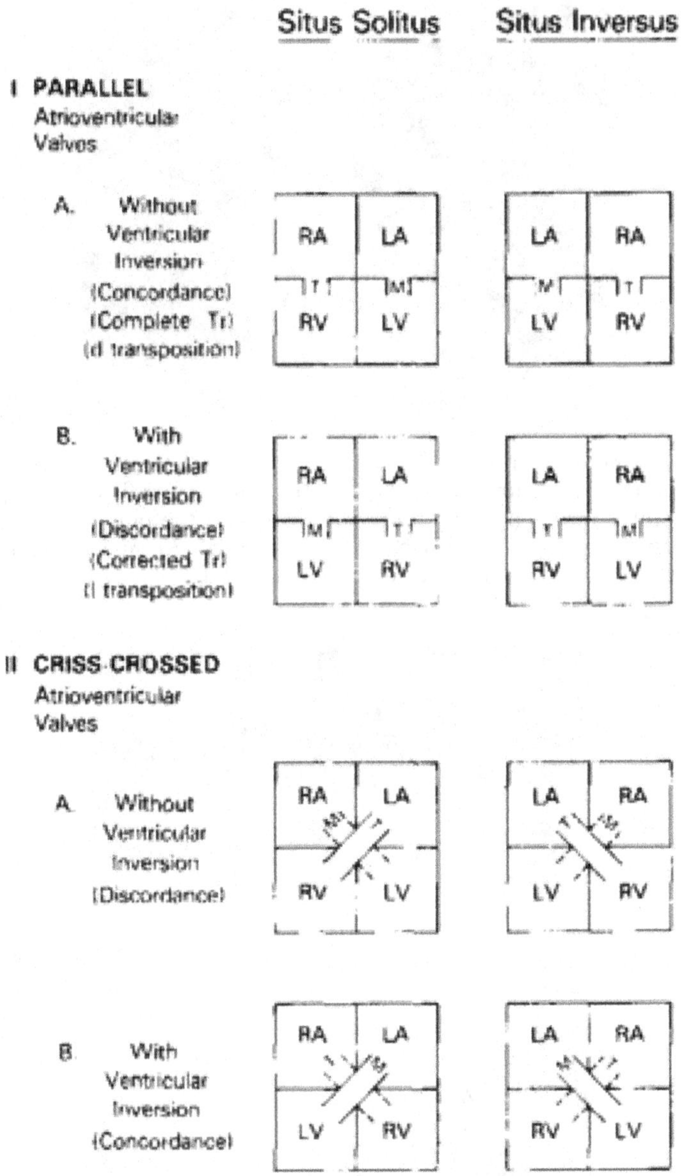

Figure 7 Transposition (Tr) of aorta and pulmonary trunk. A proposed classification of transposition complexes including both parallel and crisscrossed AV valves. Abbreviations as before.

Nearly all patients with crisscrossed AV valves have malformed or transposed great arteries, the most common being complete transposition and double-outlet, right ventricle. Because most present classifications of the transposition complexes assume that the relation of the AV valves to one another is parallel, it is important to delineate this relationship as parallel or crisscrossed because this factor affects intracardiac blood flow and operative therapy[7] (Figure 7).

REFERENCES

1. **Lev M, Rowlatt UF.** The pathologic anatomy of mixed levocardia. A review of thirteen cases of atrial or ventricular inversion with or without corrected transposition. Am J Cardiol 1961;8:216–263.

2. **Anderson RH, Shinebourne EA, Gerlis LM.** Criss-cross atrioventricular relationships producing paradoxical atrioventricular concordance or discordance. Their significance to nomenclature of congenital heart disease. Circulation 1974;50:176–180.

3. **Symons JC, Shinebourne EA, Joseph MC, Lincoln C, Ho Y, Anderson RH.** Criss-cross heart with congenitally corrected transposition: Report of a case with d-transposed aorta and ventricular preexcitation. Eur J Cardiol 1977;5(6):493–505.

4. **Anderson KR, Lie JT, Sieg K, Hagler DJ, Ritter DG. Davis GD.** A criss-cross heart. Detailed anatomic description and discussion of morphogenesis. Mayo Clin Proc 1977;52:569–575.

5. **Coto EO, Wilkinson JL, Dickinson DF, Rufilantchas J, Marquez J.** Gross distortion of atrioventricular and ventriculoarterial relations associated with left juxtaposition of atrial appendages. Bizarre form of atrioventricular criss-cross. Br Heart J 1979;41:486–492.

6. **Van Praagh S, LaCorte M, Fellows KE, Bossina K, Busch HJ, Keck EW, Weinberg PM, Van Praagh R.** Superoinferior ventricles: Anatomic and angiocardiographic findings in ten postmortem cases. In: Van Praagh R, Takao A, eds. Etiology and Morphogenesis of Congenital Heart Disease. Mount Kisco. NY: Futura, 1980:317–378.

7. **Danielson GK, Tabry IF, Ritter DG, Fulton RE.** Surgical repair of criss-cross heart with straddling atrioventricular valve. J Thorac Cardiovasc Surg 1979;77:847–851.

Case 534 Massive Right Ventricular Outflow Tract Aneurysm After Ventriculotomy for Subvalvular Pulmonic Stenosis Associated With Peripheral Pulmonary Arterial Stenoses

Jeffrey E. Saffitz, MD, PhD*, Charles L. McIntosh, MD, PhD and William C. Roberts, MD

Aneurysms that develop at sites of cardiac ventriculotomy incisions are recognized but infrequent consequences of such procedures.[1] Their development appears to be dependent on 2 major factors: (1) the peak systolic pressure within the ventricle after the incision, and (2) the length of the incision. The incidence of postventriculotomy aneurysm is far greater in the left ventricle than in the right because of the differences in peak pressures in each chamber. Herein, we describe a patient with *both* subvalvular pulmonic stenosis and peripheral pulmonary arterial stenoses in whom a massive right ventricular (RV) outflow tract aneurysm developed after operative relief of the subvalvular obstruction.

A 30-year-old woman (CC #05-28-81) had a precordial murmur at birth and cyanosis and clubbing of the digits by age 7 years. Results of 4 cardiac catheterization studies, summarized in Table 1, confirmed the presence of subpulmonic obstruction, peripheral pulmonary arterial stenoses, and a right-to-left shunt through a patent foramen ovale. Syncope occurred at age 12 years, and by age 15 had become frequent and severe. The subpulmonic stenosis was operatively relieved at age 15 years by excision of portions of crista supraventricularis myocardium. A Teflon® fabric patch was used to enlarge the RV outflow tract. The patent foramen ovale was sutured closed.

Six months after operation, a pulsatile mass was present at the upper left sternal border of the heart (Figure 1). During the next 13 years, the patient had no physical limitations and received no medications (functionally class 1). She died suddenly at age 30 years after a febrile illness with hemoptysis.

Table 1: Hemodynamic data

Pressures (mm Hg)	Age (yr)			
	8	15	Intra-Operative	(6 mo PO) 16
Pulmonary artery (s/d)	100/	75/5	115/20	120/60
Right ventricle (s/d)	175/	180/7	120/20	120/16
RV inflow-outflow peak systolic gradient	75	105	5	0
Systemic artery (s/d)	. . .	110/60	120/60	120/70

PO = postoperative; s/d = peak systole/end-diastole.

From the Pathology and Surgery Branches, National Heart, Lung, and Blood Institute, National Institutes of Health, Bethesda, Maryland. Manuscript received and accepted January 4, 1983.

* On leave from the Department of Pathology, Washington University, St. Louis, Missouri.

DOI: 10.1201/9781003409342-31

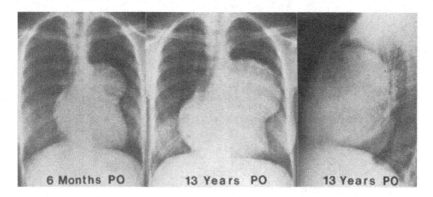

Figure 1 Radiographs of the chest 6 months and 13 years after operation, illustrating the development of the RV outflow tract aneurysm. A thin rim of calcium lines the wall of the aneurysm. PO = postoperative.

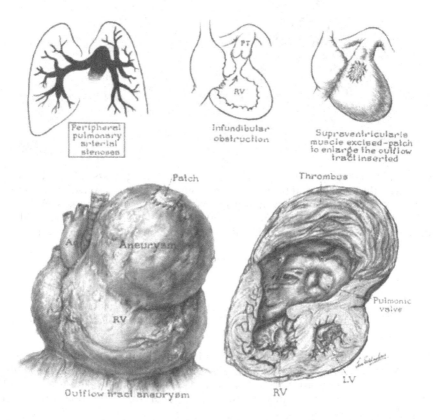

Figure 2 Diagrams illustrating various components of peripheral pulmonary arterial stenoses and RV infundibular obstruction, and the consequences of the right ventriculotomy. Ao = aorta; LV = left ventricle; PT = pulmonary trunk; RV = right ventricle.

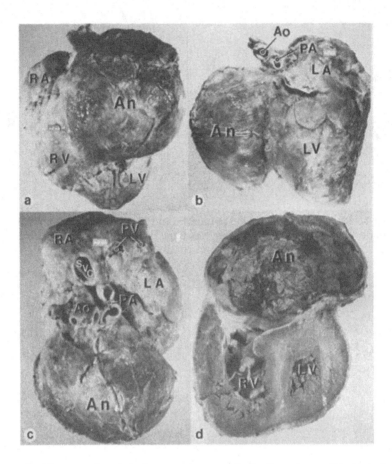

Figure 3 Photographs of the heart at necropsy including views of the anterior (a), left lateral (b), basal (c), and transverse cut (d) surfaces. The transverse cut illustrates the massive size of the aneurysm (thrombus removed) and the marked RV hypertropy. An = aneurysm; Ao = aorta; LA = left atrium; LV = left ventricle; PA = pulmonary artery; PV = pulmonary veins; RA = right atrium; SVC = superior vena cava. (Photographs by M. M. M. Moore.)

At necropsy, the heart with the aneurysm weighed 830 g (Figures 2 and 3). The RV outflow incisional aneurysm was partially filled with laminated thrombus and lined by focally calcified fibrous tissue. The aneurysm partially compressed the pulmonary trunk, left atrium, and left anterior descending coronary artery.

RV aneurysms of the magnitude described in this patient, to our knowledge, have not been described previously after right ventriculotomy. In this case, inoperable peripheral pulmonary arterial stenoses caused persistent, severe elevation of the RV systolic pressure, which in turn caused massive aneurysmal dilatation of the surgically incised RV outflow tract.

REFERENCE

1. **Kerr WF, Wilcken DEL, Steiner RE.** Incisional aneurysms of the left ventricle. Br Heart J 1961;23:88–102.

Case 598 Eisenmenger Ventricular Septal Defect with Prolonged Survival

Carole A. Warnes, MB, BS, MRCP, James E. Boger, MD and William C. Roberts, MD

Most patients with a large ventricular septal defect (VSD) are dead by age 40 years. In this report we describe a man with a large VSD who lived 63 years without ever having a cardiac operation.

V.M., a 63-year-old man at death, was told when he was 7 years old that he had a "heart murmur." During childhood he had occasional dizzy spells. At age 18 years, he was rejected from the Armed Services and later failed several insurance examinations because of the murmur. He worked as a professional gambler, married and had 3 children. At age 38 years (1958), dyspnea with hemoptysis appeared. Examination disclosed central cyanosis, a short systolic and a long, loud diastolic precordial murmur, loudest in the third left intercostal space. The blood hemoglobin was 22 g/dl and the hematocrit was 62%. An electrocardiogram showed right ventricular strain. The first of 3 cardiac catheterizations was performed at this time (Table 1). By age 41 years (1961), he was more dyspneic and cyanotic, and had chronic lethargy, and a second cardiac catheterization was performed (Table 1). A radiograph showed cardiac enlargement with large pulmonary arteries (Figure 1). By age 51 years, the diastolic murmur of pulmonary regurgitation was loud (grade 4/6). In addition, a grade 1/6 murmur of tricuspid regurgitation was heard. A third cardiac catheterization was performed (Table I). Although not physically active, he continued to support himself and his family through gambling. In the last 2 months of life signs of severe tricuspid regurgitation developed, and his condition deteriorated rapidly. He died in October 1983.

At necropsy, the heart weighed 525 g (Figure 2). A 2.5-cm subaortic VSD was present (Figures 2 and 3). The tricuspid anulus measured 13.5 cm and the mitral anulus was 10 cm in circumference. The configuration of the elastic fibrils in the pulmonary trunk and ascending aorta were identical, a finding indicating that the systolic pressure in the pulmonary artery was at systemic level from the time of birth[1] (Figure 4). The elastic and muscular pulmonary arteries were all dilated and virtually free of intimal thickening. Additionally, the media in some of these arteries were thicker than normal, but in most they appeared thinner than normal. The pulmonary arterioles, in contrast, were considerably narrowed by intimal fibrous tissue. Many plexiform lesions were present in the lungs (Figure 5), a finding indicating that the pulmonary hypertension was irreversible.

The average age at death in unoperated patients with an isolated, large (≥2 cm) VSD is about 35 years.[2] Thus, survival in our patient to 63 years with a 2.5-cm VSD is extraordinary. Indeed, we found detailed descriptions at necropsy in only 5 patients with isolated, large (≥1.5 cm) VSDs who survived more than 40 years without operation.[3-5] Their ages ranged from 44 to 60 years (mean 51). Only 1 had cardiac catheterization. The systemic arterial pressure was provided in only 1 patient and it was elevated (indirect = 180/120 mm Hg), as it was in our patient (indirect 170/120 mm Hg).

From the Pathology Branch, National Heart, Lung, and Blood Institute, National Institutes of Health, Bethesda, Maryland, and the University of Arkansas Medical Center, Little Rock, Arkansas. Manuscript received and accepted April 2, 1984.

DOI: 10.1201/9781003409342-32

Table 1: Hemodynamic data

Chamber or Artery	Age 38 Years Pressure (mm Hg)	Age 38 Years Oxygen Saturation (%)	Age 41 Years Pressure (mm Hg)	Age 41 Years Oxygen Saturation (%)	Age 51 Years Pressure (mm Hg)	Age 51 Years Oxygen Saturation (%)
SA (s/d)	117/75	88	176/115	81	150/90	81
LV (s/d)	...	...	...	...	150/10	...
PA (s/d)	100/47	71	142/71	70	150/70	70
RV outflow (s/d)	104/6	71	142/0	68	150/5	68
RV inflow	...	65	...	56	...	56
RA mean	2	67	0	50	a = 15, v = 5	50

LV = left ventricle; PA = pulmonary artery; RA = right atrium; RV = right ventricle; SA = systemic artery; and s/d = peak systole/end-diastole.

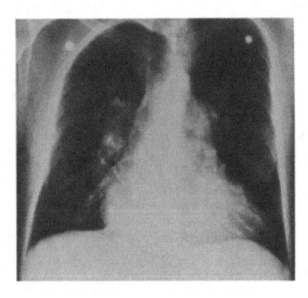

Figure 1 Chest radiograph at age 41 years showing a large heart and pulmonary arteries.

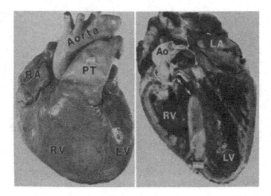

Figure 2 The heart at necropsy (**left**) and after an anteroposterior cut (**right**) showing dilated and hypertrophied right (RV) and left (LV) ventricles. The large ventricular septal defect is indicated by the **arrows**. Ao = aorta; LA = left atrium; PT = pulmonary trunk; RA = right atrium.

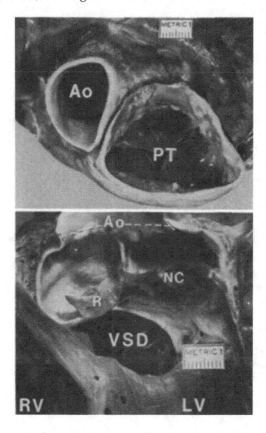

Figure 3 Top, ascending aorta (Ao) and pulmonary trunk (PT) from above. Atherosclerotic plaque is present in the pulmonary trunk. **Bottom**, close-up of the ventricular septal defect (VSD) and aortic valve (Ao). Three dilated intramural coronary arteries are seen in the ventricular septum. LV = left ventricle; NC and R = non-coronary and R = right coronary cusps; RV = right ventricle.

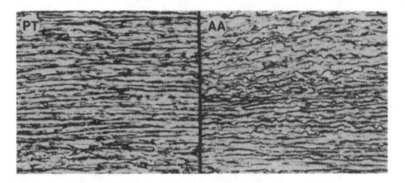

Figure 4 Transverse sections of pulmonary trunk (PT) and ascending aorta (AA) showing a near identical configuration of elastic fibrils in the media. Elastic van Gieson stain; magnification × 130.

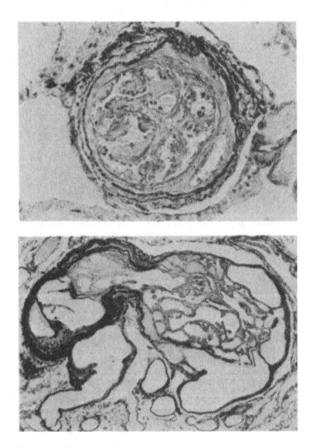

Figure 5 Pulmonary plexiform lesions (**top** and **bottom**). Elastic van Gieson stains; magnification (**top**) ×330, (**bottom**) ×80; both panels reduced 31%.

REFERENCES

1. **Heath D, DuShane JW, Wood EH, Edwards JE.** The structure of the pulmonary trunk at different ages and in cases of pulmonary hypertension and pulmonary stenosis. J Path Bacteriol 1959;77:443–456.
2. **Bloomfield DK.** The natural history of ventricular septal defect in patients surviving infancy. Circulation 1964;29:914–955.
3. **Selzer A, Laqueur GL.** The Eisenmenger complex and its relation to the uncomplicated defect of the ventricular septum. Arch Intern Med 1951;87:218–241.
4. **Stewart HL, Crawford BL.** Interventricular septal defect, dextroposition of the aorta and dilatation of the pulmonary artery. Am J Pathol 1933;9:637–648.
5. **Young D, Mark H.** Fate of the patient with the Eisenmenger syndrome. Am J Cardiol 1971;28:658–669.

Case 599 Eisenmenger Ductus Arteriosus with Prolonged Survival

Bruce M. McManus, MD, PhD, Peter F. Hahn, MD, PhD, John A. Smith, MD, PhD, William C. Roberts, MD and James H. Jackson, MD

Determinants of the outcome of nonsurgically treated patients with ductus arteriosus (DA) are not clearly understood. Generally, the smaller the DA, the smaller the left-to-right shunt, the lower the pulmonary artery (PA) pressure and PA resistance, and the longer the survival. However, not all patients with these favorable characteristics do well, and conversely, not all patients with a long-standing large DA and a large left-to-right shunt do poorly.[1] The latter was the case in the patient described herein.

A 44-year-old man, who was found to have a precordial murmur when 7 years old, had exertional dyspnea and palpitations at age 17 years and the first of 3 cardiac catheterizations were performed (Table 1). Increasing palpitations and lightheadedness led to a second cardiac catheterization at age 24 years. Aortogram disclosed a large DA with left-to-right shunting and large PAs. A machinery murmur typical of DA was heard from ages 28 to 44 years. At age 38, atrial flutter appeared but sinus rhythm was restored by cardioversion. The blood hematocrit was 48% at age 16, 64% at age 37 and 70% at age 41. From age 37 until 45 days before death at age 44 his symptoms were stable. Then exercise tolerance rapidly diminished and arrhythmias appeared: paroxysmal atrial tachycardia, then atrial flutter with 2 to 3:1 block, and then ventricular tachycardia. The precordial murmur was now that of mitral regurgitation. His toes were clubbed but not his fingers. The hematocrit was 58%. Thereafter, he had signs of worsening cardiac output, pneumonia with abscess formation, and right hemiparesis with dysphasia. Three days before death, the PA pressure was 90/25 mm Hg and the systemic arterial pressure was 120/70 mm Hg.

At necropsy, the DA was 2 cm long, 2.5 cm in maximal diameter and free of calcific deposits (Figure 1). Thrombus was present in all 3 major PAs and it occluded the PA to the left upper lobe, the site of a 6-cm abscess. Numerous atherosclerotic plaques were present in the major PAs. The configuration of the elastic fibrils in the pulmonary trunk and ascending aorta were virtually identical (Figure 2). The muscular PAs and arterioles were severely narrowed and occasional plexiform lesions were present (Figure 3). The heart weighed 840 g.

Our patient lived his entire life with elevated PA pressures, as reflected by the "fetal" pattern of elastic laminae in the pulmonary trunk,[2] and during his last 27 years, by measured near-systemic PA pressures. The course of our patient was typical of Eisenmenger's syndrome in adults.[3, 4] Congestive heart failure, tachyarrhythmias and PA thromboses ensued. The DA murmur was not heard during the final days of life.

Most patients today with DA have operative closure of the DA during childhood and few nonsurgically treated adult patients with DA are seen. Oldham et al[5]

From the Departments of Pathology and Medicine, Brigham and Women's Hospital, Boston, Massachusetts, and the Pathology Branch, National Heart, Lung, and Blood Institute, National Institutes of Health, Bethesda, Maryland. Manuscript received and accepted April 2, 1984.

DOI: 10.1201/9781003409342-33

Table 1: Hemodynamic data (pressures in mm Hg)

Site	Age 17 Years	Age 24 Years	Age 44 Years
Pulmonary artery (s/d)	—	103/68	90/25
Right ventricle (s/d)	102/9	103/0	120/20
Right atrium (mean)	12	0	—
Left ventricle (s/d)	—	120/0	—
Aorta (s/d)	112/61	120/65	120/70

s/d = systolic/diastolic.

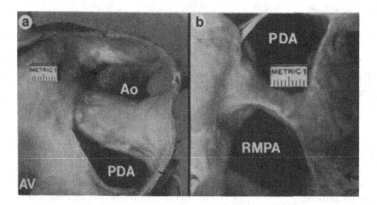

Figure 1 **a**, aortic (Ao) and **b**, pulmonary arterial ends of the patent ductus arteriosus (PDA) at necropsy. AV = aortic valve; RMPA = right main pulmonary artery.

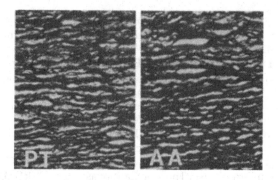

Figure 2 Photomicrographs of histologic sections of pulmonary trunk (PT) and proximal ascending aorta (AA). The configuration of the elastic fibers in the media are virtually identical. Elastic van Gieson stains; magnification each × 125, reduced 17%.

described 14 adults with "giant" (15 to 24 mm in diameter, comparable to our patient) DA and all 7 who had catheterization had severe PA hypertension. We found reports of 23 nonsurgically treated patients older than age 40 years with DA studied at necropsy.[6–22] They ranged in age from 44 to 90 years (mean 61 ± 13); 15 (65%) were women and 8 (35%) were men. The diameter of the DA (available in 13 patients)

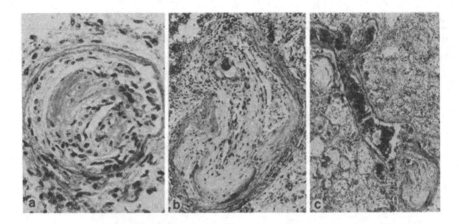

Figure 3 Pulmonary arteries with severe intimal fibrous thickening, plexiform lesion and dilatation lesions. Hematoxylin-eosin stains; magnification × 75 (**a**), × 225 (**b**), × 50 (**c**); reduced 29%.

ranged from 1 to 15 mm (mean 8). Three (13%)[16, 19, 21] had atrial fibrillation. The systemic arterial pulse pressure (available in 15 patients) ranged from 40 to 136 mm Hg (mean 82 ± 30). A ductal type precordial murmur was described in 14 (70%) of 20 patients. Fourteen patients died from the consequences of the DA: 6 from chronic congestive heart failure,[9, 12, 13, 16, 19, 22] 4 from infective endarteritis or endocarditis,[6, 11, 12, 14] and 1 each from PA rupture,[15] aortic rupture,[7] embolus[10] or PA thrombosis.[17] Calcific deposits were described in the wall of the DA in 7 patients,[8–10, 12, 15, 18, 23] in the mitral valve leaflets and anulus in 5,[8, 9, 14, 19, 20] and in the aortic valve cusps in 2.[16,22]

REFERENCES

1. **Marquis RM, Miller HC, McCormack RJM, Matthew MB, Kitchin AH.** Persistence of ductus arteriosus with left to right shunt in the older patient. Br Heart J 1982;48:469–484.

2. **Heath D, DuShane JW, Wood EH, Edwards JE.** The structure of the pulmonary trunk at different ages and in cases of pulmonary hypertension and pulmonary stenosis. J Path Bact 1959;77:443–456.

3. **Wood P.** The Eisenmenger syndrome: or pulmonary hypertension with reversed central shunt. Br Med J 1958;2:701–761.

4. **Rudolf AM.** High pulmonary vascular resistance after birth. 1. Pathophysiologic considerations and etiologic classification. Clin Pediatr 1980;19:586–590.

5. **Oldham HN, Perryman-Collins N, Pierce GE, Sabiston DC, Blalock A.** Giant patent ductus arteriosus. J Thoracic Cardiovasc Surg 1964;47:331–336.

6. **Reid J.** Four cases of aneurysm of the arch of the aorta and a case of diaphragmatic hernia. Edin Med and Surg J 1840;53:95–112.

7. **Hubeny MJ.** Roentgen diagnosis of patent ductus arteriosus; with report of a case complicated by presence of saccular aneurysm. AJR 1920;7:23–26.

8. **White PD.** Patent ductus arteriosus in a woman in her sixty-sixth year. JAMA 1928;91:1107–1108.

9. **Brody JG, Randall A.** Patent ductus arteriosus—case report of a woman sixty-five years, eleven and one-half months of age. Ohio State Med J 1935;31:599–602.

10. **Jager BV.** Noninfectious thrombosis of a patent ductus arteriosus. Am Heart J 1940;20:236–243.

11. **Gibb WT Jr.** Acute bacterial endarteritis of a patent ductus arteriosus. NY State J Med 1941;41:1861–1863.
12. **Keys A, Shapiro MJ.** Patency of the ductus in adults. Am Heart J 1943;25:158–186.
13. **Shapiro MJ, Keys A.** The prognosis of untreated patent ductus arteriosus and the results of surgical intervention—a clinical series of 50 cases and an analysis of 139 operations. Am J Med Sci 1943;206:174–183.
14. **Welch KJ, Kinney TD.** The effect of patent ductus arteriosus and of interventricular septal defects on the development of pulmonary vascular lesions. Am J Pathol 1948;24:729–761.
15. **Lindert MCF, Correll HL.** Rupture of pulmonary aneurysm accompanying patent ductus arteriosus. JAMA 1950;143:888–891.
16. **Fishman L, Silverthorne MC.** Persistent patent ductus arteriosus in the aged: including the report of the oldest case on record with diagnosis confirmed post mortem. Am Heart J 1951;41:762–769.
17. **Whitaker W, Heath D, Brown JW.** Patent ductus arteriosus with pulmonary hypertension. Br Heart J 1955;17:121–137.
18. **Bain CWC.** Longevity in patent ductus arteriosus. Br Heart J 1957:19:574–576.
19. **Fishman L.** Patent ductus arteriosus in a patient surviving to seventy-four years. Am J Cardiol 1960;6:685–688.
20. **Alken JE, Bifulco E, Sullivan JJ.** Patent ductus arteriosus in the aged. JAMA 1961;177(5):330–331.
21. **Caine DB, Raftery EB.** Patent ductus arteriosus in an elderly man. Br Heart J 1966;78:716–717.
22. **White PD, Mazurkle SJ, Boschetti AE.** Patency of the ductus arteriosus at 90. N Engl J Med 1969;280:146–147.

Case 604 Atrioventricular Septal Defect (Primum Atrial Septal Defect) with Prolonged Survival (Despite Severe Mitral Regurgitation and Pulmonary Hypertension) and Associated Cardiac Calcification (Mitral Anulus, Coronary Artery and Pulmonary Trunk)

Carole A. Warnes, MB, BS, MRCP, Gerald I. Shugoll, MD,
Robert B. Wallace, MD and William C. Roberts, MD

Atrioventricular (AV) septal defect (formerly called AV canal or endocardial cushion defect or primum atrial septal defect [ASD] with cleft mitral valve) may be either complete (single AV valve) or partial (2 well formed AV valves). Patients with complete AV septal defect rarely survive for more than a few years without operation. However, patients with partial AV septal defect often survive for many years, but not as long as patients with secundum ASD. Prolonged survival with partial AV septal defect (primum ASD), however, is unusual, particularly in the presence of severe mitral regurgitation and pulmonary hypertension, but such was the case in the patient described herein.

S.C., a 59-year-old woman, was found to have a precordial murmur in childhood. Episodic palpitations began at age 20 years and an episode of atrial fibrillation was documented when she was 37 years old. Although easily fatigued, she performed housework until her early 50s, when palpitations associated with dyspnea became more frequent and pedal edema developed. At age 59 years, orthopnea and angina pectoris appeared. The blood pressure was 110/70 mm Hg. A right ventricular lift was palpated, P_2 was loud and the interval between A_2 and P_2 was wider than normal and did not vary with respiration. A grade 3/6 systolic murmur was present at the apex and it radiated into the left axilla. A grade 2/6 systolic murmur along the lower left sternal border increased in intensity with inspiration. The electrocardiogram showed sinus rhythm with prolonged PR interval (0.24 s), right bundle branch block and left-axis deviation. The Holter monitor tracing showed both supraventricular and ventricular ectopic complexes with episodes of bigeminy and a 4-beat run of ventricular tachycardia. Chest radiography showed cardiomegaly with pulmonary congestion. The findings on cardiac catheterization are summarized in Table 1. Left ventriculography demonstrated a normally contracting left ventricle, a narrowed outflow tract with the characteristic "gooseneck" deformity, no ventricular septal defect, severe (grade 3+/4+) mitral regurgitation, and thickened, deformed, relatively immobile mitral leaflets. Calcium was visible in the mitral anular region. Pulmonary venogram demonstrated an ostium primum ASD. The pulmonary to systemic flow ratio was 1.7 and the net left-to-right shunt was 2.5 liters/min. The pulmonary resistance was 7 Wood units/m^2 and the systemic resistance was 28 Wood units/m^2. Coronary arteriography and, later, necropsy demonstrated a 50 to 75% diameter reduction in the midportion of the left anterior descending coronary artery. The ostium of the right coronary artery was located in the left coronary sinus (confirmed at necropsy).

From the Pathology Branch, National Heart, Lung, and Blood Institute, National Institutes of Health, Bethesda, Maryland, and Georgetown University Medical Center, Washington, D.C. Manuscript received May 8, 1984, accepted May 16, 1984.

  DOI: 10.1201/9781003409342-34

Table 1: Hemodynamic data

Chamber	Pressure (mm Hg) s/d	Oxygen Saturation (%)
IVC	...	69
SVC	...	53
RA mean	22	70
RV (s/d)	95/15	77
PA (s/d)	95/30	77
LA mean	20	85
LV (s/d)	120/20	83
Aorta (s/d)	120/65	83

IVC = inferior vena cava; LA = left atrium; LV = left ventricle; PA = pulmonary artery; RA = right atrium; RV = right ventricle; s/d = peak systole/end-diastole; SVC = superior vena cava.

On January 26, 1984, the deformed mitral valve was replaced with a 3M Starr-Edwards prosthesis, the primum ASD was closed with a pericardial patch, a de Vega tricuspid valve anuloplasty was performed, and a saphenous vein was inserted between the aorta and left anterior descending coronary artery (done first). Although atrial fibrillation developed, the early postoperative course was uneventful. She went home on February 4, 1984. Two days later she had an acute episode of dyspnea, and she died about 12 hours later.

At necropsy, the heart weighed 650g. The defect (4 cm in maximal diameter) in the lower most portion of the atrial septum had been closed securely, 1 of the 4 stents of the prosthesis in the mitral position contacted the left ventricular wall, and the aortocoronary conduit was patent (Figures 1 and 2). Heavy calcific deposits were present in the mitral anulus, pulmonary trunk and left anterior descending coronary artery (Figure 3). No clear anatomic cause of death was discernible at necropsy.

Few reported patients with partial AV septal defect have survived for more than 50 years. One man with this defect, confirmed at necropsy, lived 69 years.[1] Hynes et al[2] reported 52 such patients aged 20 years or older, 18 of whom were 45 years or older and 6 of whom were 60 years or older. Pulmonary hypertension was rare; the highest mean pulmonary artery pressure was 55 mm Hg. Somerville[3] reported 14 patients aged 30 years or older with primum ASD, 2 of whom had pulmonary hypertension (pulmonary vascular resistance ≥3 Wood units). Severe mitral regurgitation also was unusual in the patients of Hynes et al: Of 33 patients who underwent left ventricular angiography, mitral regurgitation was found in 4 (12%). In Somerville's 14 patients, severe mitral regurgitation was present in 2. Martin et al[4] described 7 adults, aged 34 to 48 years, with primum ASD; 1 had an elevated pulmonary artery pressure (86/33 mm Hg), and mitral regurgitation was minimal in all 7. Goodman et al[5] reported 12 patients aged 15 to 53 years (mean 30) with primum ASD: 1 had a pulmonary artery systolic pressure >50 mm Hg, and 2 had severe mitral regurgitation.

Although recognized as frequent in patients with mitral valve prolapse, which in turn is recognized as frequent in older patients with secundum type ASD, mitral anular calcium is infrequent in patients with secundum ASD,[6] (presumably because survival longer than 65 years is relatively uncommon) and it has never been reported in a patient with primum ASD. The occurrence of significant coronary atherosclerosis, also present in our patient, has not been described previously in a patient with primum ASD, and obviously, aortocoronary bypass grafting, as performed on our patient, has not been reported previously in such a case. Moreover, the occurrence of a calcified mass in the pulmonary trunk has not been reported previously in a

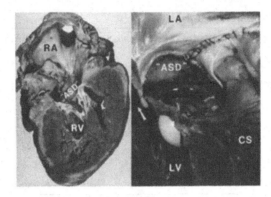

Figure 1 Opened right side of the heart (**left**) exposing the operatively closed atrial septal defect ("ASD"). The right atrium (RA) is dilated and the wall of right ventricle (RV) is markedly thickened. **Right**, opened left atrium (LA) showing the operatively closed ASD with a portion of the prosthetic ring attached to the most caudal margin of the ASD. The **arrow** points toward the aortic valve. CS = coronary sinus; LV = left ventricle.

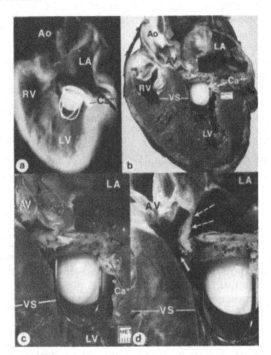

Figure 2 Left side of the heart. **a**, radiograph. Calcium (Ca^{++}) is present in the mitral anular region. **b**, long-axis view showing relative sizes of the right ventricle (RV), left ventricle (LV), left atrium (LA) and the relative thicknesses of the ventricular walls. The aortocoronary artery conduit is visible. **c**, close-up of the prosthesis. **d**, close-up of left ventricular outflow tract. The anterior mitral leaflet (**broken arrows**) is displaced anteriorly toward the ventricular septum (VS), and this displacement appears to have diminished the area of left ventricular outflow (**solid arrow**). Ao = ascending aorta; AV = aortic valve.

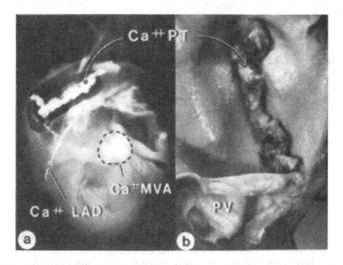

Figure 3 **a,** calcific deposit (Ca⁺⁺) in pulmonary trunk (PT), probably originally a thrombus, and in the mitral valve anulus (MVA) and left anterior descending coronary artery (LAD). **b,** close-up of the calcific deposit in the pulmonary trunk located just above the pulmonic valve (PV).

patient with primum ASD. Thus, the patient described herein is unusual on 7 counts (prolonged survival, severe mitral regurgitation, severe pulmonary hypertension, mitral anular calcium, pulmonary truncal calcium, coronary arterial calcium and severe coronary atherosclerosis necessitating aortocoronary bypass grafting).

REFERENCES

1. **Heath D.** Long survival in partial persistent common atrioventricular canal. Br J Dis Chest 1968;62:207–210.
2. **Hynes JK, Tajik AJ, Seward JB, Fuster V, Ritter DG, Brandenburg RO, Puga FJ, Danielson GK, McGoon DC.** Partial atrioventricular canal defect in adults. Circulation 1982;66:284–287.
3. **Somerville J.** Ostium primum defect: Factors causing deterioration in the natural history. Br Heart J 1965;27:413–419.
4. **Martin CE, Thomas CS, Bender HW.** Ostium primum atrial septal defect in the adult. South Med J 1976;69:1058–1060.
5. **Goodman DJ, Harrison DC, Schroeder JS.** Ostium primum defect in the adult: Postoperative follow-up studies. Chest 1975;67:185–189.
6. **Roberts WC.** Morphologic features of the normal and abnormal mitral valve. Am J Cardiol 1983;51:1005–1028.

Case 605 "Massive" Calcification of a Right Ventricular Outflow Parietal Pericardial Patch in Tetralogy of Fallot

Elizabeth M. Ross, MD, Charles L. McIntosh, MD, PhD and William C. Roberts, MD

A variety of materials have been used for patches to widen obstructed right ventricular (RV) outflow tracts in patients with tetralogy of Fallot. These materials have included Teflon®, preclotted Dacron®, parietal pericardium and dura mater. Autologous parietal pericardium has the advantage of being readily available, and does not present the problem of suture-line bleeding, which often occurs with the synthetic patches. Both tissue and synthetic patches utilized in the RV outflow tract may become aneurysmal if the RV peak systolic pressure is not returned to normal or near normal levels after operation. Although the intimal lining tissue of the synthetic patch may calcify, the synthetic material itself does not. In contrast, autologous patch material may calcify. Such was the case in the patient described here.

D.H. (#11-37-22), a 16-year-old boy with tetralogy of Fallot, had a Blalock-Taussig anastomosis at age 5 years. He had closure of the ventricular septal defect with insertion of a parietal pericardial RV outflow widening patch at age 9 after catheterization had shown the peak systolic pressure gradient between RV body (105/12 mm Hg) and pulmonary trunk (16/6 mm Hg) to be 89 mm Hg. Another cardiac catheterization was not done until age 16 years, when the peak systolic pressure gradient between RV body (70/2 mm Hg) and pulmonary trunk (15/3 mm Hg) was 55 mm Hg. Chest radiograph showed a large calcific deposit in the RV outflow tract (Figure 1). At reoperation, the RV outflow patch was heavily calcified (Figure 2). It was excised and replaced with a larger patch consisting of Teflon.

Review of several reports[1-6] of patients who underwent insertion of a synthetic or a tissue patch into the RV outflow tract months to years earlier disclosed no mention of grossly visible calcific deposits of the material of the patch itself. Such heavy calcific deposits in our patient may have resulted, in part, from the residual RV outflow gradient which persisted after operation.

From the Pathology and Surgery Branches, National Heart, Lung, and Blood Institute, National institutes of Health, Bethesda, Maryland 20205. Manuscript received and accepted May 30, 1984.

DOI: 10.1201/9781003409342-35

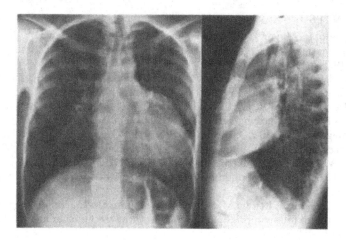

Figure 1 Chest radiograph (**left**, posteroanterior and **right**, lateral) at age 16 years showing calcium in the area of the ventricular outflow tract.

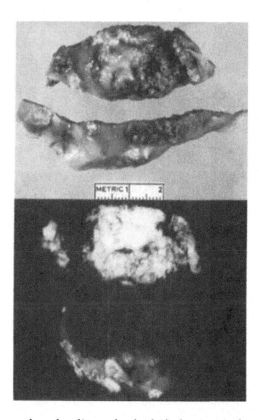

Figure 2 Photograph and radiograph of calcified, operatively excised right ventricular outflow patch.

REFERENCES

1. **Chiariello L, Meyer J, Wukasch DC, Hallman GL, Cooley DA.** Intracardiac repair of tetralogy of Fallot. Five-year review of 403 patients. J Thorac Cardiovasc Surg 1975;70:529–535.
2. **Seybold-Epting W, Chiariello L, Hallman GL, Cooley DA.** Aneurysm of pericardial right ventricular outflow tract patches. Ann Thorac Surg 1977;24:237–240.
3. **Kirklin JW, Bargeron LM, Pacifico AD.** The enlargement of small pulmonary arteries by preliminary palliative operations. Circulation 1977;56:612–617.
4. **Arciniegas E, Farooki ZQ, Hakimi M, Perry BL, Green EW.** Early and late results of total correction of tetralogy of Fallot. J Thorac Cardiovasc Surg 1980;80:770–778.
5. **Fuster V, McGoon DG, Kennedy MA, Ritter DG, Kirklin JW.** Long-term evaluation (12 to 22 years) of open heart surgery for tetralogy of Fallot. Am J Cardiol 1980;46:635–642.
6. **Lane I, Treasure T, Leijala M, Shinebourne E, Lincoln C.** Diminutive pulmonary artery growth following right ventricular outflow tract enlargement. Int J Cardiol 1983;3:175–189.

Case 616 Anomalous Origin of the Left Anterior Descending Coronary Artery from the Pulmonary Trunk with Origin of the Right and Left Circumflex Coronary Arteries from the Aorta

William C. Roberts, MD and Max Robinowitz, MD

Origin of both right and left main (LM) coronary arteries from the pulmonary trunk (PT) rarely allows survival for more than 2 weeks after birth. Origin of the LM from the PT with origin of the right coronary artery from the aorta allows longer survival, but usually (80%) for no more than 1 year after birth. Origin of the right coronary artery from the PT and the LM from the aorta, in contrast, allows survival into adulthood and maybe a normal life span. Because the LM is equivalent to 2 major coronary arteries, whenever the LM arises from the PT, whether in association with the right artery or when isolated, survival is short. However, when 1 major branch of the LM arises from the PT and both the right and the other major LM branch arises from the aorta, the survival rate should be similar to that in patients in whom the right coronary artery arises from the PT and the LM from the aorta. In this report we describe a man in whom the left anterior descending coronary artery (LAD) arose from the PT and the right and left circumflex (LC) coronary arteries from the aorta.

T.J., a 32-year-old man, died suddenly soon after jogging on December 29, 1981. In November 1979 a continuous murmur "similar to that of a patent ductus arteriosus" had been heard during routine physical examination. He was and always had been asymptomatic. The murmur was grade 3/6 in intensity, and loudest in the third left intercostal space. The systemic blood pressure was 120/50 mm Hg. The electrocardiogram was normal. Chest radiograph showed the cardiac silhouette to be at the upper limits of normal. On the M-mode echocardiogram, the left ventricular cavity in end-diastole was 65 mm and the left atrium was 40 mm. Coronary angiography disclosed the origin of the right artery from the right sinus and the origin of only the LC from the left sinus of Valsalva. Both the right coronary artery and LC communicated through collateral vessels with the LAD, which arose from the PT; it was dilated and tortuous. The ejection fraction on the left ventricular angiogram was 48%. The pulmonary to systemic flow ratio was 1.6:1.

On March 9, 1981, thoracotomy was performed for the purpose of ligating the LAD close to its origin from the PT and insertion of saphenous vein graft from aorta to the more distal portion of the LAD. At operation, rather than ligating the LAD, the proximal LC was ligated instead (Figure 1). On the second postoperative day, the continuous precordial murmur was still audible and repeat angiography disclosed that both the LAD and the graft were widely patent. Reoperation was performed on March 12, 1981, and this time the LAD near the PT was ligated (Figure 1).

Reevaluation in May 1981 disclosed mild exertional dyspnea postoperatively, but never chest pain. The patient was working full days as a dentist. The blood pressure was 130/85 mm Hg. No precordial murmurs were present. Electrocardiography disclosed Q waves in leads

---

From the Pathology Branch, National Heart, Lung, and Blood Institute, National Institutes of Health, Bethesda, Maryland, and the Cardiovascular Pathology Department, Armed Forces Institute of Pathology, Washington, DC. Manuscript received and accepted July 24, 1984.

DOI: 10.1201/9781003409342-36

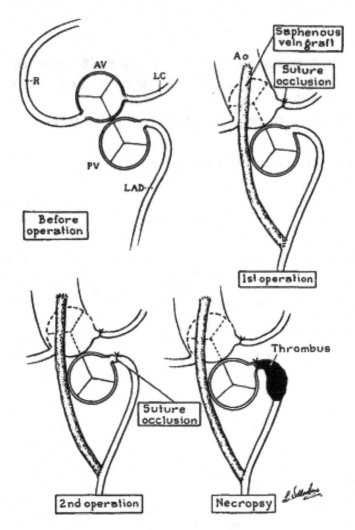

Figure 1 Sequence of development before, during and after operation in the patient described. Ao = aorta; AV = aortic valve; PV = pulmonic valve; LAD, LC and R = left anterior descending, left circumflex and right coronary arteries.

I and aVL and inverted T waves in lead aVL. The Bruce treadmill test to 10 minutes disclosed a heart rate of 175 beats/min, blood pressure 155/75 mm Hg, no symptoms and no ischemic electrocardiographic changes. No symptoms occurred thereafter and he began running 2 miles daily and playing tennis. On December 29, 1981, he complained of dyspnea shortly after a run and died.

Necropsy disclosed the heart weight at 450g. The proximal LAD was occluded by a thrombus and ligature and the graft was patent (Figure 1). A transmural scar involved the lateral wall of the left ventricle and ventricular septum at the base and both papillary muscles were focally scarred (Figure 2).

At least 7 patients (Table 1) have been reported in whom the LAD arose from the PT and both right and LC arteries arose from the aorta.[1–6] At the time of the reports

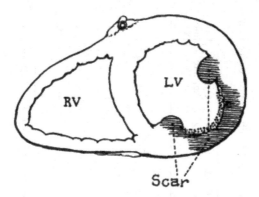

Figure 2 Transverse section of cardiac ventricles at level of left ventricular papillary muscles showing transmural left ventricular scar. LV = left ventricle; RV = right ventricle.

1 patient (patient 1, Table 1), a 7-month old girl, had died of an anterior wall acute myocardial infarct; the other 6 (patients 2 to 7, all women) were aged 18 to 55 years (mean 34). Our patient is the only male thus far described. Of the 6 adults, all were symptomatic: 5 with angina pectoris, 1 of whom also had an anterior wall acute myocardial infarct, and 1 with severe fatigue attributed to severe mitral regurgitation from papillary muscle dysfunction. The angina at some time in all 5 patients was stable, but 3 of the 5 (patients 4, 6 and 7) had unstable angina just before cardiac operation. The age at onset of symptoms of myocardial ischemia in the 6 adults ranged from 18 to 37 years (mean 27). Precordial murmurs were described in 4 of 5 previously reported adults. (No information was provided in the "addendum case" of Donaldson et al.[4]): The murmur apparently was present only in systole in 4 patients, and also in diastole in 1. The intensity of the murmurs was mentioned in 2 patients: "soft" in 1 (patient 4) and grade 2/6 in 1 (patient 6). Findings on the electrocardiogram at rest were described in 4 adults: All had poor R-wave progression in leads V_1 to V_3 and at least 2 (patients 6 and 7) had ST–T-wave changes of ischemia in more than 1 lead. Exercise stress tests in 2 patients (patients 2 and 7) disclosed ST-segment ischemic changes in each. Chest x-rays in 5 of the 6 adults disclosed normal-sized cardiac silhouettes in 2 and cardiac enlargement in 3: mild in 2 (patients 4 and 6) and severe in 1 (patient 3). Right-sided cardiac catheterization, performed in at least 5 patients (patients 2 and 4 to 7) disclosed normal pressures in each and oxygen step-up in the pulmonary trunk in only 1 (patient 6). Coronary angiography with injection of contrast material in the right coronary artery and LC in all 6 adults disclosed that each of these 2 arteries in all 6 patients was large, occasionally also tortuous, and that the LAD was filled with extensive collateral vessels from both the right coronary artery and LC. Injection of contrast material into the PT did not cause filling of the LAD; when the LAD, however, was filled by injections into either the right coronary artery or LC, contrast material did enter the PT through the LAD, which was filled by collateral vessels.

Of the 6 previously reported adults, operative treatment was carried out in 4, all of whom preoperatively had angina: In 2 patients (patients 4 and 5) the PT was opened and the ostium of the LAD was obliterated by sutures, and in 2 (patients 6 and 7) the LAD was ligated just proximal to its entrance into the PT and a reversed saphenous vein was inserted from the ascending aorta to the LAD. Of the 4 patients who had operative treatment, angina disappeared in 3 (patients 4 to 6) and persisted in 1 (patient 7). Patients 6 and 7 had repeat coronary and left ventricular

Table 1: Certain observations in 7 previously reported patients (patients 1 to 7) and in our patient (no. 8) in whom the left anterior descending coronary artery arose from the pulmonary trunk

Pt	First Author	Year	Age (yr) & Sex	Age (yr) Onset Symptoms	First Symptom	AMI	Precordial Murmur		Anterior Wall Ischemia (ECG)	CE by X-Ray	CA A	Ligation LAD	Conduit Aorta to LAD	Alive (mo PO)
							Systole	Diastole						
1	Schwartz[1]	1971	7 moF	—	—	0	0	0	+	+	+	0	0	—
2	Probst[2]	1976	35F	18	AP	0	+	+	+	0	+	0	0	+
3	Baltaxe[3]	1977	18F	18	Fatigue	—	+	0	—	+	+	—	—	—
4	Donaldson[4]	1979	24F	24	AP	0	+	0	+	0	+	+	0	+ (12)
5	Donaldson[4]	1979	26F	—	AP	—	—	—	—	—	+	+	0	
6	Singh[5]	1983	45F	36	AP	0	+	0	+	+	+	+	+	+ (24)
7	Evans[6]	1984	55F	37	AP	+	0	0	+	+	+	+	+	+ (5)
8	Roberts	1984	32M	—	0	0	+	+	0	0	+	+	+	0

A = angiogram; AMI = acute myocardial infarction; AP = angina pectoris; CA = coronary artery; CE = cardiac enlargement; ECG = electrocardiogram; LAD = left anterior descending; PO = postoperatively; + = positive, present or done; 0 = negative or absent; — = no information available or not done or not applicable.

angiography 24 and 36 months, respectively, after operation; in each, the right and LC arteries were much smaller than they had been preoperatively and the collateral vessels between the right coronary artery and LC and the LAD had disappeared; patient 7 had persistent angina postoperatively and the distal portions of both the right coronary artery and LC (36 months postoperatively) were quite narrowed; the cause of narrowing was unclear. Left ventricular angiograms, performed in 4 adults, were normal in 2 (patients 2 and 4), and in the other 2 the apical portion of the left ventricle was akinetic in 1 (patient 6) and aneurysmal in 1 (patient 7). Repeat left ventricular angiography in these latter 2 patients disclosed better overall contractions in 1 and no change in 1 (patient 7).

The presence of both subjective and objective evidence of myocardial ischemia in the 6 previously reported adults and the disappearance of angina and of the collateral vessels between the 2 coronary arteries arising from the aorta and the LAD arising from the PT supports the view that operative treatment is proper for patients with this coronary anomaly. Whether LAD ligation alone is enough or whether ligation plus insertion of a graft between the aorta and LAD is preferable is unclear. Direct connection of the LAD to aorta in this situation appears technically inadvisable. All 4 patients reported in whom operation was performed had angina pectoris. Our patient was asymptomatic preoperatively. Obviously, no data are available on the advisibility of operation in an asymptomatic person in whom the LAD arises from the PT, but it appears reasonable to believe that the operative therapy in this circumstance is proper. If operation is to be performed, however, clear identification of the anomalous artery before ligation is mandatory.

REFERENCES

1. **Schwartz RP, Robicsek F.** An unusual anomaly of the coronary system: Origin of the anterior (descending) interventricular artery from the pulmonary trunk. J Pediatr 1971;78:123–126.
2. **Probst P, Pachinger O, Koller H, Niederberger M, Kaindl F.** Origin of anterior descending branch of left coronary artery from pulmonary trunk. Br Heart J 1976;38:523–525.
3. **Baltaxe HA, Wixson D.** The incidence of congenital anomalies of the coronary arteries in the adult population. Radiology 1977;122:47–52.
4. **Donaldson RM, Thornton A, Raphael MJ, Sturridge MF, Manuel RW.** Anomalous origin of the left anterior descending coronary artery from the pulmonary artery. Eur J Cardiol 1979;10:295–300.
5. **Singh RN, Taylor PC.** Anomalous origin of the left anterior descending coronary artery from the pulmonary artery: Surgical correction in an adult. Cathet Cardiovasc Diagn 1983;9:411–416.
6. **Evans JJ, Phillips JF.** Origin of the left anterior descending coronary artery from the pulmonary artery. Three year angiographic follow-up after saphenous vein bypass graft and proximal ligation. JACC 1984;3:219–224.

Case 617 Asymptomatic Sinus of Valsalva Aneurysm Causing Right Ventricular Outflow Obstruction Before and After Rupture

Carole A. Warnes, MB, BS, MRCP, Barry J. Maron, MD,
Michael Jones, MD and William C. Roberts, MD

Sinus of Valsalva aneurysm (SVA) unassociated with ventricular septal defect does not produce symptoms of cardiac dysfunction until the wall of the SVA ruptures or the aneurysm itself obstructs right ventricular (RV) outflow. If rupture occurs, usually symptoms appear abruptly and congestive heart failure progresses rapidly thereafter. Obstruction to RV outflow by bulging of the SVA into the RV outflow tract has been demonstrated hemodynamically in only 2, or possibly 3, patients.[1–3] The patient described herein is unique because the degree of RV outflow tract obstruction by a SVA was observed to increase with time and symptoms of cardiac dysfunction never occurred despite rupture of the wall of the SVA.

G.P. (#16-40-13-6), a 23-year-old man, had a precordial murmur detected at age 6 weeks. At age 13 years, a grade 4/6 systolic murmur was audible along the left sternal border. At age 16 years, the first cardiac catheterization was performed, and RV outflow obstruction was observed (Figure 1). An aortogram showed aneurysm of the right sinus of Valsalva. The patient remained asymptomatic and worked outdoors in construction. At age 22 years, the presence of the precordial murmur prompted a second cardiac catheterization. RV oxygen content had increased, and the aortogram showed a perforation in the wall of the aneurysm. Five months later, a third catheterization revealed a Qp:Qs ratio of 2.6:1 by Krypton and 3.3:1 by oximetry. Aortogram (Figure 2) confirmed the aortico-RV shunt through the ruptured SVA. Electrocardiogram was compatible with left ventricular hypertrophy. The total QRS voltage in all 12 leads was 376 mm (10 mm = 1 mV). M-mode and 2-D echocardiograms (Figure 2) showed discontinuity between the anterior wall of the aorta and the ventricular septum. In May 1983 the wall of the sinus of Valsalva aneurysm was excised (Figure 1) and aortic valvuloplasty was performed. Six months later, the patient was asymptomatic, and catheterization showed that the RV outflow obstruction had been abolished. He had no left-to-right shunt, but he did have significant regurgitation from the aorta into the left ventricle, a finding not present preoperatively. Total 12-lead QRS voltage 6 months after operation was 379 mm.

Although Sakakibara and Konno[1] described 4 patients and Bulkley et al[2] 3 patients in whom 1 or more sinuses of Valsalva protruded into the RV outflow tract, actual obstruction to RV outflow was unconfirmed because none of the 7 patients had cardiac catheterization, or if performed, the data were not presented. It appears that the 3 patients reported by Bulkley et al had syphilis. Only 2 patients (possibly 3) with hemodynamically documented RV outflow obstruction associated with aneurysm of 1 of the 3 sinuses, as occurred in our patient, have been reported. Gerbode et al[3] described a 47-year-old woman with a 106-mm Hg peak systolic gradient across

From the Pathology, Cardiology and Surgery Branches, National Heart, Lung, and Blood Institute, National Institutes of Health, Bethesda, Maryland 20205. Manuscript received and accepted July 25, 1984.

     DOI: 10.1201/9781003409342-37

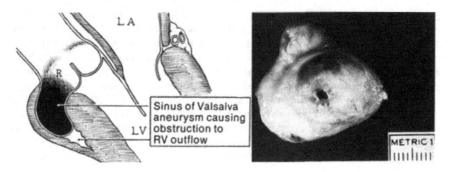

Figure 1 Sinus of Valsalva aneurysm. **Left,** drawing of how the aneurysm obstructs right ventricular (RV) outflow. LA = left atrium; LV = left ventricle; R = right coronary sinus. **Right,** wall of sinus of Valsalva aneurysm excised at operation. A small perforation is visible.

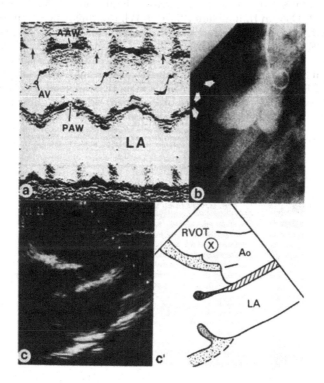

Figure 2 **a,** M-mode echocardiogram showing discontinuity in the anterior aortic wall; **b,** aortogram showing the sinus of Valsalva aneurysm (**arrows**); **c** and **c¹,** 2-dimensional echocardiogram (parasternal long-axis view) showing area of discontinuity between anterior aortic wall and ventricular septum (×). The margins of the aneurysm were not imaged in their entirety in any cross-sectional plane. The discontinuity in **a** almost certainly represents the mouth of the sinus of Valsalva aneurysm. This discontinuity is present in only a portion of the cardiac cycle because movement of the heart allows the intact wall of aorta to pass into the path of the M-mode beam. AAW = anterior aortic wall; Ao = aorta; AV = aortic valve cusp; LA = left atrium; PAW = posterior aortic wall; RVOT = right ventricular outflow tract.

the RV outflow tract associated with an SVA; although the obstruction may have been caused in part by the SVA, an additional "infundibular stenosis" also was present. Taguchi et al[4] described a 35-year-old man in whom the wall of the SVA, which had ruptured, produced a 17-mm Hg peak systolic pressure difference between RV body and pulmonary trunk. Kerber et al[5] described a 62-year-old man with a 60-mm Hg peak systolic pressure gradient caused by an unruptured SVA. Our patient is unique in having hemodynamic documentation of progression of RV outflow obstruction by the SVA in the RV outflow tract, hemodynamic proof of elimination of the gradient after excision of the aneurysm, and no symptoms of cardiac dysfunction despite rupture of the wall of the SVA. The lack of symptoms probably was a result of the small size of the perforation in the aneurysm's wall.

REFERENCES

1. **Sakakibara S, Konno S.** Congenital aneurysms of sinus of Valsalva. Anatomy and classification. Am Heart J 1962;63:405–424.
2. **Bulkley BH, Hutchins GM, Ross RS.** Aortic sinus Valsalva aneurysms simulating primary right-sided valvular heart disease. Circulation 1975;52:696–699.
3. **Gerbode F, Osborn JJ, Johnston JB, Kerth WJ.** Ruptured aneurysms of the aortic sinuses of Valsalva. Am J Surg 1961;102:268–279.
4. **Taguchi K, Sasaki N, Matsuura Y, Uemura R.** Surgical correction of aneurysm of the sinus of Valsalva. A report of forty-five consecutive patients including eight with total replacement of the aortic valve. Am J Cardiol 1969;23:180–191.
5. **Kerber RE, Ridges JD, Kriss JP, Silverman JF, Anderson ET, Harrison DC.** Unruptured aneurysm of the sinus of Valsalva producing right ventricular outflow obstruction. Am J Med 1972;53:775–783.

Case 635 Origin of the Right from the Left Main Coronary Artery (Single Coronary Ostium in Aorta)

Deborah J. Barbour, MD and William C. Roberts, MD

Origin of both the right and left main (LM) coronary arteries from the aortic wall of the *right* sinus of Valsalva frequently is a lethal anomaly.[1] Origin of both the right and LM coronary arteries from the aortic wall of the *left* sinus of Valsalva, in contrast, usually is a benign anomaly.[2] Although many studies have described origin of both LM and right coronary arteries from the aortic wall of the same sinus of Valsalva, few[1, 2] have described origin of the right coronary artery from the LM. Husaini et al[3] described angiographic features of this anomaly in a 52-year-old man who underwent selective coronary angiography after probable acute myocardial infarction. Muus and McManus[4] described this anomaly in a full-term stillborn infant who also had a bicuspid aortic valve. Whether the coronary anomaly played a role in the stillbirth is uncertain. In both of these previously described patients, the anomalously arising right coronary artery coursed between aorta posteriorly and the pulmonary trunk anteriorly.

J.G., a 65-year-old man, never had signs or symptoms of cardiac dysfunction. He did have systemic hypertension and electrocardiographic voltage criteria consistent with left ventricular hypertrophy. He died from carcinoma of the lung. At necropsy, the heart weighed 380 g. The cardiac cavities were of normal size. No foci of myocardial fibrosis or necrosis were present. The origin and courses of the coronary arteries are shown in Figure 1. The anomalous right coronary artery was much smaller than either the left circumflex or left anterior descending branches; it burrowed into the myocardium of the crista supraventricularis for about 2 cm of its length shortly after its origin from the LM. All epicardial coronary arteries were free of atherosclerotic plaque.

This case demonstrates that origin of the right coronary artery from the LM may be a benign anomaly unassociated with either functional or anatomic evidence of myocardial ischemia.

From The Pathology Branch, National Heart, Lung, and Blood Institute, National Institutes of Health, Bethesda, Maryland 20205. Manuscript received and accepted November 7, 1984.

DOI: 10.1201/9781003409342-38

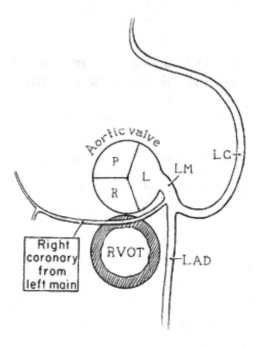

Figure 1   Course of the right coronary artery after its anomalous origin from the left main (LM) coronary artery. It burrowed into the myocardium of the crista supraventricularis for 2 cm shortly after its origin. The entire right coronary artery is small and it virtually disappeared after reaching the right margin of the heart. L = left sinus of Valsalva; LAD = left anterior descending coronary artery; LC = left circumflex coronary artery; P = posterior sinus of Valsalva; R = right sinus of Valsalva; RVOT = right ventricular outflow tract.

REFERENCES

1. **Cheitlin MD, DeCastro CM, McAllister HA.** Sudden death as a complication of anomalous left coronary origin from the anterior sinus of Valsalva. A not-so-minor congenital anomaly. Circulation 1974;50:780–787.
2. **Roberts WC, Siegel RJ, Zipes DP.** Origin of the right coronary artery from the left sinus of Valsalva and its functional consequences: Analysis of 10 necropsy patients. Am J Cardiol 1982;49:863–868.
3. **Husaini SN, Beaver WL, Wilson IJ, Lach RD.** Anomalous right coronary artery arising from left mainstem. Cathet Cardiovasc Diagn 1983;9:407–409.
4. **Muus CJ, McManus BM.** Common origin of right and left coronary arteries from the region of left sinus of Valsalva: Association with unexpected intrauterine fetal death. Am Heart J 1984;107:1285–1286.

Case 642 Mitral Valve Cleft Without Cardiac Septal Defect Causing Severe Mitral Regurgitation but Allowing Long Survival

Charles W. Barth, III, MD, James D. Dibdin, MD, LLB and William C. Roberts, MD

Partial atrioventricular "defect" includes a spectrum of 5 anatomic anomalies. Some patients have all 5 and others have only 1 or 2. The 5 are the following: (1) defect in the lower portion of the atrial septum, so-called primum atrial septal defect; (2) defect in, or absence of, the posterobasal portion of ventricular septum; (3) cleft, anterior mitral leaflet; (4) anomalous chordae tendineae from the anterior mitral leaflet to the crest of the ventricular septum; and (5) partial or complete absence of the septal tricuspid valve leaflet. There are at least 4 potential functional consequences of these 5 anatomic anomalies: (1) shunt at the atrial level, (2) shunt at the ventricular level, (3) mitral regurgitation (MR), and (4) obstruction to left ventricular outflow. Well over 95% of patients with partial atrioventricular defect have a primum type atrial septal defect, and most of those without a primum defect have a shunt at the ventricular level. The occurrence of MR from a cleft in the anterior mitral leaflet unassociated with a defect in either atrial or ventricular septa is extremely rare. Such was the case, however, in the patient to be described herein.

B.P., a 27-year-old man, was found to have a precordial murmur consistent with MR at age 16 years. Atrial fibrillation was also present. Left ventricular angiogram at the time showed 2+/4+ MR. He continued to play recreational basketball and work as a service station attendant without difficulty. At age 27, five months before death, he had a respiratory infection followed by evidence of congestive heart failure. A grade 4/6 holosystolic murmur consistent with MR and a third heart sound were heard. M-mode echocardiogram showed thickened but mobile mitral leaflets; the left atrial dimension was 70 mm, and the left ventricular cavity was 82 mm in diastole and 58 mm in systole. The electrocardiogram showed atrial fibrillation, QRS voltage of left ventricular hypertrophy and inverted T waves in leads II, III and aVF. The pressures in mm Hg were as follows: pulmonary artery wedge mean 15, v wave 16; pulmonary artery 28/14 (mean 18); right ventricle 28/5; right atrial mean 5; left ventricle 120/8; and aorta 120/80 (mean 90). Cardiac index (thermodilution) was 2.3 liters/min/m². Left ventricular angiography now disclosed 4+/4+ MR. After discharge he returned to an active life. He died suddenly from an overdose of cocaine and phencyclidine.

At necropsy the heart weighed 900 g. All 4 cardiac chambers were dilated. A huge cleft was present in the anterior mitral leaflet (Figure 1). The mitral anulus measured 17 cm in circumference and the tricuspid anulus measured 15 cm. The edges of the cleft were thick. The atrial and ventricular septa were intact. The tricuspid, pulmonary and aortic valve leaflets were normal.

We found studies describing 10 patients at necropsy with a cleft in the anterior mitral leaflet unassociated with a defect in either the atrial or ventricular septum.[1-4]

From the Pathology Branch, National Heart, Lung, and Blood Institute, National Institutes of Health, Bethesda, Maryland 20205, and The Medical Examiner's Office, Washington, D.C. Manuscript received December 19, 1984, accepted December 31, 1984.

DOI: 10.1201/9781003409342-39

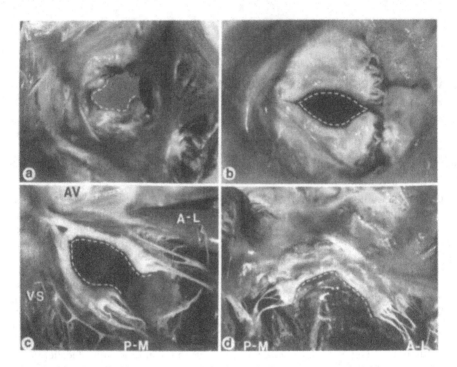

Figure 1 Mitral valve in the patient described. In each of the 4 views the space bordering the cleft in the anterior mitral leaflet is designated by **dashed lines. a**, view from left atrium during simulated ventricular diastole; **b**, close-up view from left atrium during simulated ventricular systole; **c**, view from left ventricle. The apex of the cleft inserts into the crest of the ventricular septum (VS) just caudal to the opened aortic valve (AV). The anterolateral (A-L) papillary muscle actually inserts into the anterior one-half of the cleft anterior mitral leaflet; **d**, opened left atrium, mitral valve and left ventricle. The large amount of anterior mitral leaflet actually missing, i.e., that space bordered by the **dashed lines**, is huge. The circumference of the mitral anulus is about twice normal. P-M = posteromedial papillary muscle. (Photographs by M.M.M. Moore.)

Information on age and gender was available in 6 of the 10 patients: All were males; 5 were younger than age 10 years and 1 was 74 years old. Of the 10 patients, some degree of MR was present in 9; only the 74-year-old man had no MR.[3] Only 2 of the 10 patients were known to have a large cleft—such as occurred in our patient—and both had severe MR and progressive, eventually fatal congestive heart failure.

Our 27-year-old patient appears to be the oldest necropsy patient thus far reported with severe MR from a cleft in the anterior mitral leaflet. Although he had evidence of congestive heart failure for a few months before death, his death was not the result of cardiac disease. What allowed his relatively long survival? Although he had MR during his entire 27 years, the degree of MR worsened through the years. Initially, MR was probably due entirely to the regurgitation through the cleft in the anterior mitral leaflet, but with time the mitral anulus progressively dilated, and this huge anular dilation contributed to the degree of MR, as occurs in patients with mitral valve prolapse.[5]

It is likely that our patient was able to tolerate the MR well because the huge size of the left atrial cavity was able to "absorb" the left ventricular systolic pressure and prevent its reflection into the pulmonary veins and from there into the pulmonary arteries. More than 2 decades ago, Braunwald and Awe[6] demonstrated that patients with pure MR in whom huge left atrial cavities develop do not have pulmonary venous and subsequently pulmonary arterial hypertension; in contrast, those patients with severe MR whose left atrial cavities do not dilate do have severe elevation of their pulmonary venous and pulmonary arterial pressures.[7] The courses in the former group are long and those in the latter group are short. The present patient had a huge left atrial cavity, nearly normal pulmonary wedge pressures and normal pulmonary arterial pressures, and therefore prolonged survival.

REFERENCES

1. **Edwards JE, Dry TJ, Parker RL, Burchell HB, Wood EH, Bulbulian AH.** An Atlas of Congenital Anomalies of the Heart and Great Vessels. Springfield, IL: Charles C Thomas, 1954:41–42.

2. **Berghuis J, Kirklin JW, Edwards JE, Titus JL.** The surgical anatomy of isolated congenital mitral insufficiency. J Thorac Cardiovasc Surg 1964;47:791–798.

3. **Di Segni E, Edwards JE.** Cleft anterior leaflet of the mitral valve with intact septa. A study of 20 cases. Am J Cardiol 1983;51:919–926.

4. **Sellers RD, Lillehei CW, Edwards JE.** Subaortic stenosis caused by anomalies of the atrioventriciular valves. J Thorac Cardiovasc Surg 1964;48:289–302.

5. **Waller BF, Morrow AG, Maron BJ, Del Negro AA, Kent KM, McGrath FJ, Wallace RB, McIntosh CL, Roberts WC.** Etiology of clinically isolated, severe, chronic, pure mitral regurgitation. Analysis of 97 patients over 30 years of age having mitral valve replacement. Am Heart J 1982;104:276–288.

6. **Braunwald E, Awe WC.** The syndrome of severe mitral regurgitation with normal left atrial pressure. Circulation 1963;27:29–35.

7. **Roberts WC, Braunwald E, Morrow Ag.** Acute severe mitral regurgitation secondary to ruptured chordae tendineae. Clinical, hemodynamic, and pathologic considerations. Circulation 1966;33:58–70.

Case 673 Sudden Death in Infancy Associated with Origin of Both Left Main and Right Coronary Arteries from a Common Ostium Above the Left Sinus of Valsalva

*Charles W. Barth III, MD, Michael Bray,
MD and William C. Roberts, MD*

Anomalous origin of the left main coronary artery from the right sinus of Valsalva (SV) with subsequent coursing of the left main artery between the aorta and pulmonary trunk can cause myocardial ischemia, sometimes resulting in sudden unexpected death at a young age.[1] Similarly, anomalous origin of the right coronary artery (RCA) from the left SV with coursing of the RCA between aorta and pulmonary trunk also may cause nonfatal and fatal myocardial ischemia.[2-6] Of 6 reported necropsy patients dying suddenly with 3-cuspid aortic valves and anomalous origin of the RCA from the left SV, 5 were aged 17 to 49 years and 1 was a 9-month-old infant.[2-5] Herein we report an infant who died suddenly with the latter anomaly.

A 4-month-old girl, who previously had been healthy, was found dead in her crib. A nonidentical twin was healthy. At necropsy, both the left main coronary artery and the RCA arose from a common, shallow, oblong ostium situated in the aortic wall just above an imaginary line separating the left SV from the tubular portion of aorta (Figures 1 and 2). The ostium was oriented with its longest dimension in a right-to-left direction. The RCA, which had a round ostium, coursed at an acute angle from the aorta directly to the right between aorta and pulmonary trunk to reach the right side of the heart. The left main coronary artery, which had an oval ostium, arose just to the left of the RCA, and it coursed sharply downward from the ostium to the surface of the heart where it divided into the left circumflex and left anterior descending coronary arteries. The myocardium was normal.

The mechanism by which anomalous origin of the RCA from the left SV with coursing of the RCA between the pulmonary trunk and aorta causes myocardial ischemia is believed to be similar to that when the left main coronary artery arises from the right SV and courses between aorta and pulmonary trunk. The acute angle at which the anomalous RCA arises from the aortic lumen produces a narrowed slit-like orifice at the point it traverses the aortic wall, and it probably is further narrowed by dilatation of the aortic root during exertion, to the extent that impairment of coronary blood flow may result in myocardial ischemia and fatal arrythmia.[1] Benge et al[6] described systolic compression of the origin of the anomalous RCA during coronary angiography in a 25-year-old man with acute myocardial infarction and complete heart block. The course of the anomalous RCA between the great arteries also may result in compression of the anomalous artery and myocardial ischemia.

Our infant differs from the 6 previously reported patients who died unexpectedly in that both the left main artery and RCA arose from the aorta just above the

From the Pathology Branch, National Heart, Lung, and Blood Institute, National Institutes of Health, Bethesda, Maryland 20205, and The Medical Examiner's Office, Washington, D.C. Manuscript received and accepted July 5, 1985.

DOI: 10.1201/9781003409342-40

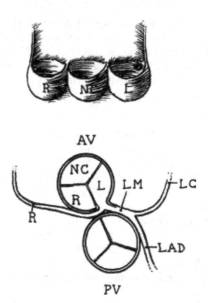

Figure 1 Diagram showing the anomaly in the infant described. AV = aortic valve; L = left aortic valve cusp; LAD = left anterior descending coronary artery; LC = left circumflex artery; LM = left main coronary artery; NC = non-coronary aortic valve cusp; PV = pulmonary valve; R = right aortic valve cusp or right coronary artery.

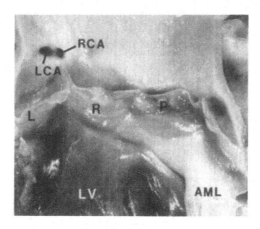

Figure 2 Opened left ventricular outflow tract, aortic valve and ascending aorta in the infant described showing the common ostium of the coronary artery which quickly divides into the left (LCA) and right (RCA) coronary arteries. AML = anterior mitral leaflet; L, R and P = left, right and posterior aortic valve cusps, respectively; LV = left ventricle.

left SV rather than from the aortic wall behind the SV. Although all 6 patients were described as having "slitlike" ostia as a result of the acute angle of takeoff of the RCA from the left SV, the shallow common ostium in our child allowed the acute takeoff of the RCA from the aorta without producing a slit-like orifice. Nevertheless, the RCA could have been compressed between aorta and pulmonary trunk and it could have dilated during a crying spell.

REFERENCES

1. Cheitlin MD, DeCastro CM, McCallister HA. Sudden death as a complication of anomalous left coronary origin from the anterior sinus of Valsalva. A not so minor congenital anomaly. *Circulation* 1974;50:780–787.
2. Roberts WC, Siegel RJ, Zipes DP. Origin of the right coronary artery from the left sinus of Valsalva and its functional consequences. Analysis of 10 necropsy patients. *Am J Cardiol* 1982;48:863–868.
3. Liberthson RR, Gang DL, Custer J. Sudden death in an infant with aberrant origin of the right coronary artery from the left sinus of Valsalva of the aorta: case report and review of the literature. *Pediatr Cardiol* 1983;4:45–48.
4. Isner JM, Shen EM, Martin ET, Fortin RV. Sudden unexpected death as a result of anomalous origin of the right coronary artery from the left sinus of Valsalva. *Am J Med* 1984;76:155–158.
5. Topaz O, Edwards JE. Pathologic features of sudden death in children, adolescents, and young adults. *Chest* 1985;87:476–482.
6. Benge W, Martins JB, Funk DC. Morbidity associated with anomalous origin of the right coronary artery from the left sinus of Valsalva. *Am Heart J* 1980;99:96–100.

Case 725 Aneurysm of the Pulmonary Trunk Unassociated with Intracardiac or Great Vessel Left-to-Right Shunting

Deborah J. Barbour, MD and William C. Roberts, MD

In contrast to aneurysm of the aorta, which is fairly common, aneurysmal dilation of the pulmonary trunk (PT) or of the right or left main pulmonary arteries is rare except in congenital heart disease with an intracardiac or great artery shunt. During the past 27 years we have studied at necropsy 3 patients with aneurysms (diameter more than 4 cm) of the PT and of 1 or both of its 2 major branches unassociated with congenital heart disease. This report describes findings in these 3 patients and summarizes findings in 3 previously reported necropsy patients with PT aneurysms unassociated with congenital heart disease.[1-3]

Certain findings in our 3 patients are summarized in Table 1. All were women aged 40, 58 and 63 years. Patient 1 had hypertrophic cardiomyopathy (Figure 1) and a pulmonary arterial systolic pressure of 54, 51 and 35 mm Hg on 3 occasions in the last 2 years of life. Patient 2 had systemic sarcoidosis and scleroderma with interstitial pulmonary fibrosis (Figure 2) and a pulmonary arterial systolic pressure of 85 mm Hg. In patient 3, the cause of the PT aneurysm, which contained a large intraaneurysmal thrombus, could not be determined (Figure 3). The PT aneurysms were 5, 7 and 7 cm in maximal diameter. Histologic study of the wall of the aneurysm disclosed it to be abnormal in patients 2 and 3 and normal in patient 1. The numbers of elastic fibers in the media in patients 2 and 3 clearly were decreased compared with normal (Figure 3). Histologic study of 34 sections of lung in these 3 patients disclosed the pulmonary arterial intima and media to be thickened in all, but none had plexiform lesions (indicative of irreversible pulmonary hypertension).

Three previously reported patients with PT aneurysms unassociated with shunts included a 57-year-old man and 45- and 64-year-old women. The man had chronic lung disease and was an opium smoker; 1 woman was presumed to have primary pulmonary hypertension with pulmonary plexiform lesions and a pulmonary arterial mean pressure of 66 mm Hg; the other woman had no apparent explanation for the PT aneurysm which, like our patient 3, had an intraaneurysmal thrombus. All 3 had decreased numbers (compared with normal) of elastic fibers in the media of the PT.

Aneurysms of the PT have been reported by other investigators in patients with primary pulmonary hypertension,[2] mitral stenosis,[4] the Marfan syndrome[5-7] and syphilis.[4-8] Since 1959, approximately 8,000 hearts have been examined in our laboratory and only the 3 patients included herein had aneurysms of the PT unassociated with left-to-right shunts. Of our 435 patients studied at necropsy with mitral stenosis, of 25 with primary pulmonary hypertension, and of 26 with the Marfan syndrome, none had an aneurysm of the PT.

The mechanism of development of PT aneurysm unassociated with left-to-right shunting is unclear. Pulmonary hypertension is usually present but it does not have

From the Pathology Branch, National Heart, Lung, Blood Institute, National Institutes of Health, Bethesda, Maryland 20892. Manuscript received and accepted June 18, 1986.

Table 1: Clinical findings in three patients

| Case | Necropsy Number | Age (yr) | Pressures (mm Hg) | | | | | | Diameter (cm) | ↓EF in PT |
			PA (s/d)	RV (s/d)	RA (m)	SA (s/d)	LV (s/d)	PT Aneurysm	
1	A63–77	40	35/17	35/5	4	130/85	125/12	7	0
2	A86–14	58	85/32	85/9	...	140/60	...	7	++
3	A85–29	63	...	...	...	...	...	5	+

EF = elastic fibers; LV = left ventricle; m = mean; PA = pulmonary artery; PT = pulmonary trunk; RA = right atrium; RV = right ventricle; SA = systemic artery; s/d = systolic/diastolic.

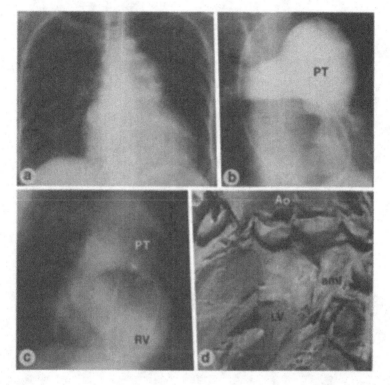

Figure 1 Patient 1 (Table 1). Heart and radiograph. *a*, posteroanterior chest radiogram showing marked dilatation of the pulmonary trunk. *b*, posteroanterior angiogram with injection of contrast material into the huge pulmonary trunk (PT). *c*, lateral view of the same angiogram demonstrating aneurysm. *d*, opened left ventricular (LV) outflow tract showing a mural endocardial plaque in opposition to the anterior mitral leaflet (AMl) and a normal aortic valve. The mural endocardial plaque is typical of hypertrophic cardiomyopathy. Ao = ascending aorta; RV = right ventricle.

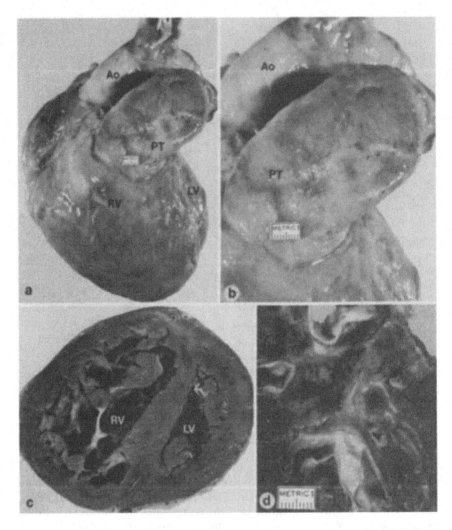

Figure 2 Heart and lung. *a* and *b*, exterior view of the anterior surface of the heart at necropsy showing the severely dilated pulmonary trunk (PT). The right ventricular (RV) cavity is much larger than the left ventricular (LV) cavity. *c*, transverse section through the ventricles at the level of the papillary muscles showing severe right ventricular (RV) wall thickening. *d*, longitudinal section through the lung near the hilum showing atherosclerotic plaques in the pulmonary arteries and enlarged perihilar lymph nodes containing noncaseating granulomas typical of sarcoidosis. Ao = aorta; RA = right atrium.

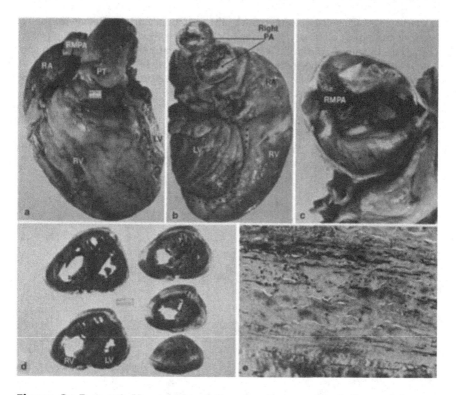

Figure 3 Patient 3. Heart (*a, b and d*) and pulmonary trunk (*b, c and e*). *a*, anterior view of the heart at necropsy. The right ventricle (RV) is massively enlarged and forms the cardiac apex. The pulmonary trunk (PT) and right main pulmonary artery (RMPA) are markedly dilated. *b*, posterior view of heart and right pulmonary artery (PA) at the level of its bifurcation showing extension of the PT aneurysm into the right upper and lower lobe main arterial branches, both of which are filled with organized mural thrombus. *c*, cross section through the right main pulmonary artery (RMPA) showing the aneurysmally dilated lumen to be markedly narrowed by organized thrombus. *d*, transverse sections through right (RV) and left ventricular (LV) chambers extending from base (*top left*) to apex (*bottom right*). The right ventricular cavity is markedly dilated while the left ventricular cavity is of normal dimension. No myocardial necrosis or fibrosis was present. *e*, photomicrograph of portion of wall of PT showing severe depletion of elastic fibers.

to be severe as seen in our patient 1. The wall of the aneurysm may be abnormal as demonstrated by loss of elastic fibers in the media, but the wall may not be abnormal as was observed in our patient 1.

REFERENCES

1. Shilkin KB, Low LP, Chen BTM. Dissecting aneurysm of the pulmonary artery. *J Pathol* 1969;98:25–29.
2. Luchtrath H. Dissecting aneurysm of the pulmonary artery. *Virchows Arch (Pathol Anat)* 1981;391:241–147.
3. Chiu B, Magil A. Idiopathic pulmonary arterial trunk aneurysm presenting as cor pulmonale: Report of a case. *Hum Pathol* 1985;16:947–949.

4. Deterling RA, Clagett OT. Aneurysm of the pulmonary artery: Review of the literature and report of a case. *Am Heart J* 1947;34:471–499.
5. Tung HL, Liebow AA. Marfan's syndrome. Observations at necropsy: With special reference to medionecrosis of the great vessels. *Lab Invest* 1952;1:382–405.
6. Headley RN, Carpenter HM, Sawyer CG. Unusual features of Marfan's syndrome including two postmortem studies. *Am J Cardiol* 1963;11:259–266.
7. Roberts WC, Honig HS. The spectrum of cardiovascular disease in the Marfan syndrome: A clinicomorphologic study of 18 necropsy patients and comparison to 151 previously reported necropsy patients. *Am Heart J* 1982;104:115–135.
8. Boyd LJ, McGavack TH. Aneurysm of the pulmonary artery. A review of the literature and report of two new cases. *Am Heart J* 1939;18:562–578.

Case 848 Retroaortic Epicardial Course of the Left Circumflex Coronary Artery and Anteroaortic Intramyocardial (Ventricular Septum) Course of the Left Anterior Descending Coronary Artery

An Unusual Coronary Anomaly and a Proposed Classification Based on the Number of Coronary Ostia in the Aorta

Allen L. Dollar, MD and William C. Roberts, MD

In recent years a number of articles and books have focused on various coronary anomalies.[1-4] One of the least frequent coronary anomalies is the combination of retroaortic epicardial course of the left circumflex (LC) coronary artery and antero-aortic intramyocardial course of the left anterior descending (LAD) coronary artery. Herein, we describe another such case and provide a classification for such cases based on the present and previously published cases.

A.S., an 87-year-old man, who during life never had evidence of myocardial ischemia or cardiac dysfunction, died from complications of gastrointestinal bleeding. At necropsy, the heart weighed 405 g. None of the 4 chambers was dilated. No grossly visible foci of myocardial fibrosis or necrosis were present. The 4 cardiac valves were normal. The origins and courses of the coronary arteries are shown in Figure 1.

There have been at least 6 previously reported necropsy patients[5-9] with combined retroaortic epicardial course of the LC and anteroaortic intramyocardial course of the LAD coronary arteries (Table 1). None of the 6 previously reported patients had symptoms of cardiac dysfunction or myocardial ischemia. One[9] of the 6 patients, however, was found dead in bed and necropsy disclosed severe atherosclerosis of all 3 major coronary arteries and a left ventricular scar. In these 6 patients, the LC and the LAD arose either from the right coronary artery or from the right aortic sinus.

A useful way to classify this combination of anomalies is according to the number of coronary ostia in the aorta. Three possible variations of this complex exist (Figure 2). If 2 aortic ostia are present, there are 2 further variations based on whether the LC or the LAD arises from the right coronary artery (Figure 2, IIa and IIb).

From the Pathology Branch, National Heart, Lung, and Blood Institute, National Institutes of Health, Bethesda, Maryland 20892. Manuscript received April 18, 1989, and accepted June 26.

DOI: 10.1201/9781003409342-42

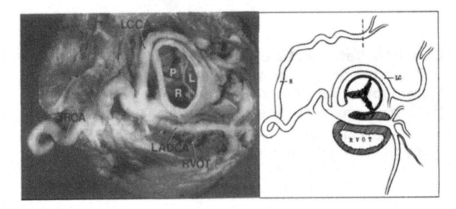

Figure 1 Heart from above in the 87-year-old man. The right coronary artery (RCA) arises from the right (R) sinus of Valsalva and within a centimeter of its origin, it gives rise to the left circumflex coronary artery (LCCA) and the left anterior descending coronary artery (LADCA). The latter artery courses caudally to penetrate into the ventricular septum located posteriorly to the right ventricular outflow tract (RVOT). The LADCA enters epicardium again anterior to the ventricular septum and quickly divides into 3 branches, one of which courses in the usual location of the LADCA. The initial portion of the RCA is very large and after origin of the LCCA and the LADCA, the RCA is very tortuous, so tortuous that R loops around itself. In contrast, neither the retroaortic LCCA nor the intramyocardial portion of the LADCA is tortuous. P = posterior and L = left sinus of Valsalva.

Table 1: Clinical findings and anomaly class of six previously reported necropsy patients with retroaortic epicardial course of the left circumflex and anteroaortic intramyocardial course of the left anterior descending coronary artery

Study (Reference)	Year	Pt Age (yrs), Sex	Cardiac Cause of Death	Anomaly Class[*]
Bachdalek[5]	1867	60, F	—	1
Sanes[6]	1937	4, M	0	1
White[7]	1948	39, M	0	1
Schulte[8]	1985	71, F	0	1
Virmani[†9]	1989	64, M	+	III
Virmani[9]	1989	62, M	0	IIa

[*] See Figure 2. [†] This patient died suddenly in bed at home and at necropsy had extensive coronary atherosclerosis with severe luminal narrowing.
+ = present; 0 = absent; — = no information available.

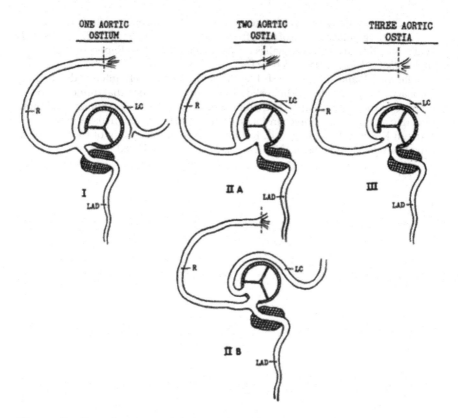

Figure 2 Four drawings of the complex of retroaortic epicardial left circumflex (LC) and anteroaortic intramyocardial left anterior descending (LAD) coronary arteries showing the possible origins of the LC and LAD from either the aorta or from the right (R) coronary artery. In type I (*left*) only a single coronary artery arises from the aorta and both LC and LAD coronary arteries arise from the right. In type II, there are 2 coronary ostia in the right sinus of Valsalva of the aorta, the right coronary artery and either the LAD (Type IIA) or the LC (Type IIB). No reports are available describing the type IIB variety. In type III, there are 3 coronary ostia in the aorta, LC, right and LAD coronary arteries.

REFERENCES

1. Voldaver Z, Neufeld HN, Edwards JE. Coronary Arterial Variations in the Normal Heart and in Congenital Heart Disease. New York: New York Academic Press, 1975:171.
2. Neufeld HN, Schneeweiss A. Coronary Artery Disease in Infants and Children. Philadelphia: Lea and Febiger, 1983:189.
3. Roberts WC. Major anomalies of coronary arterial origin seen in adulthood. *Am Heart J* 1986;111:941–963.
4. Virmani R, Rogan K, Cheitlin MD. Congenital coronary artery anomalies: Pathologic aspects. In: Virmani R, Forman MB, eds. Nonatherosclerotic Ischemic Heart Disease. New York: Raven Press, 1989:153–183.
5. Bachdalek H. Anomaler Verlauf der Kranzarterien des Herzens. *Virchow Arch Pathol Anat* 1867;41:260.

6. Sanes S. Anomalous origin and course of the left coronary artery in a child: So-called congenital absence of the left coronary artery. *Am Heart J* 1937:14:219–229.

7. White NK, Edwards JE. Anomalies of the coronary arteries: Report of four cases. *Arch Pathol Lab Med* 1948:45:766–771.

8. Schulte MA, Waller BF, Hull MT, Pless JE. Origin of the left anterior descending coronary artery from the right aortic sinus with intramyocardial tunneling to the left side of the heart via the ventricular septum: A case against clinical and morphologic significance of myocardial bridging. *Am Heart J* 1985;110:499–501.

9. Virmani R, Chun PKC, Rogan K, Riddick L. Anomalous origin of four coronary ostia from the right sinus of Valsalva. *Am J Cardiol* 1989;63:760–761.

Case 897 Fatal Intrapericardial Rupture of Sinus of Valsalva Aneurysm

Katrina R. Brabham and William C. Roberts, MD
Bethesda, MD

Aneurysmal dilatation of one sinus of Valsalva unassociated with infective endocarditis is rare. Its occurrence generally is attributed to a congenital absence of media in the aortic wall behind the sinus. When a sinus of Valsalva aneurysm ruptures, it does so almost always into an intracardiac chamber. An exception is the case to be described herein, where a sinus of Valsalva aneurysm ruptured outside the heart.

A 32-year-old black woman, who had been well all her life, suddenly collapsed and died while vacuuming the floor of a house. Necropsy disclosed the pericardial sac to be filled with blood. An aneurysm, which had perforated along its right border, was present at the aortic root and it involved the right sinus of Valsalva (Figure 1). The wall of the aneurysm was

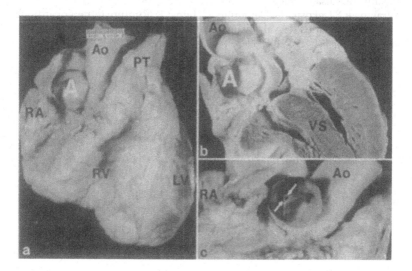

Figure 1 Photographs of the heart in the patient described. **a,** View of heart anteriorly. The sinus of Valsalva aneurysm (*A*) is located between the aorta (*Ao*) and right atrium (*RA*). *LV,* Left ventricle; *PT,* pulmonary trunk; *RV,* right ventricle. **b,** View after excising the anterior portions of both ventricles and of aorta. The thin-walled aneurysm (*A*) is apparent. *VS,* Ventricular septum. **c,** View of the aneurysm from the right side. *Arrows* show the perforation, which led to fatal hemopericardium, in the wall of the aneurysm.

From the Pathology Branch, National Heart, Lung, and Blood Institute, National Institutes of Health.

Reprint requests: William C. Roberts, MD, Bldg. 10, Room 2N258, National Institutes of Health, National Heart, Lung, and Blood Institute, Bethesda, MD 20892.
4/4/24345

DOI: 10.1201/9781003409342-43

much thinner than the wall of either of the other two normal-sized sinuses of Valsalva. The aortic valve cusps were normal, as were each of the other three cardiac valves. None of the four cardiac chambers was dilated. No myocardial foci of fibrosis or necrosis were present. The coronary arteries were normal.

Most congenital sinus of Valsalva aneurysms involve only one or two sinuses. The most common site for an aneurysm is the wall behind the right coronary cusp; next is the wall behind the posterior cusp; the least common is the wall behind the left coronary cusp. Rupture rarely occurs until adulthood. The subject is usually asymptomatic because the nonruptured aneurysm usually causes no cardiac dysfunction. When rupture does occur, a large left-to-right shunt usually develops, along with chest pain, cardiomegaly, plethoric lung fields, a continuous precordial murmur, wide systemic arterial pulse pressures, and collapsing peripheral pulses. Because the rupture of the aneurysm is nearly always intracardiac, death is delayed. If, however, the sinus of Valsalva aneurysm ruptures into the pericardial sac, as in the aforementioned patient, death is instantaneous. We are aware of only two previous reports of rupture of a congenital sinus of Valsalva aneurysm into the pericardial sac.[1, 2]

REFERENCES

1. Killen DA, Wathanacharoen S, Pogson GW Jr. Repair of intrapericardial rupture of left sinus of Valsalva aneurysm. *Ann Thorac Surg* 1987;44:310–311.
2. Defraigne JO, Dekoster G, Demoulin JC, Limet R. Rupture intrapéricardique d'un anévrysme du sinus de Valsalva antéro-droit: Cas clinique et revue de la littérature. *Acta Chir Belg* 1988;88:369–374.

Case 968 Prolonged Survival (74 Years) in Unoperated Tetralogy of Fallot with Associated Mitral Valve Prolapse

Daniel J. Fernicola, MD, Victor R. Boodhoo, MD and William C. Roberts, MD

Prolonged survival in tetralogy of Fallot is rare. About 5% of patients without operative therapy survive >25 years. Recently, we studied at necropsy a man with tetralogy of Fallot who survived 74 years without operation and at necropsy severe mitral valve prolapse also was present. A description of pertinent findings in him are described herein.

S.D., a 74-year-old white man, who worked in a post office as a mail sorter, was cyanotic at birth and had recurrent syncope until the age of 8 years. He was then asymptomatic until age 43 when he developed numbness in his left hand and it recurred. At age 46, the first of 2 cardiac catheterizations was performed and the results are summarized in Table 1. Atrial fibrillation began at age 58, and left ventriculogram at age 68 disclosed moderate mitral regurgitation. From age 46 to 55 he had episodic upper gastrointestinal tract bleeding from a gastric ulcer, and on 1 occasion his blood hematocrit was reduced to 24%. Signs and symptoms of congestive heart failure began at age 73, about 17 months before death. Examination at that time disclosed a grade 4/6 systolic murmur, loudest along the upper left sternal border. His fingers and toes were clubbed and cyanotic. The blood hematocrit was 36% and the systemic oxygen saturation was 80%. An electrocardiogram showed atrial fibrillation,

Table 1: Cardiac catheterization data in the patient described

Site	Age (years) at Study	
	46	68
Right atrium (mean) (mm Hg)	6	10
Right ventricle (s/d) (mm Hg)	95/0 } psg = 70	105/10 } psg = 70
Pulmonary artery (s/d) (mm Hg)	25/0	35/12
Pulmonary artery wedge (mean) (mm Hg)	16	21
Left ventricle (s/d) (mm Hg)	—	105/15
Systemic artery (s/d) (mm Hg)	110/50	105/70
Systemic O$_2$ saturation (%)	89	83
Blood hematocrit (%)	49	40*
Coronary angiogram	—	Single ostium

* Hospitalized for upper gastrointestinal bleed 5 months before catheterization.
O$_2$ = oxygen; psg = peak systolic gradient; s/d = peak systole/end diastole.

From the Pathology Branch, National Heart, Lung, and Blood Institute, National Institutes of Health, Bethesda, Maryland, and the Parrish Medical Center, Titusville, Florida. Manuscript received August 18, 1992; revised manuscript received and accepted September 21, 1992.

DOI: 10.1201/9781003409342-44

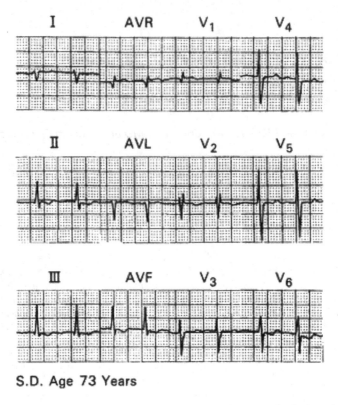

S.D. Age 73 Years

Figure 1 Electrocardiogram of the patient recorded 17 months before death.

incomplete right bundle branch block, right ventricular hypertrophy, and nonspecific ST-T-wave changes (Figure 1). He died of progressive congestive heart failure.

At necropsy, the heart weighed 860 g and the typical features of tetralogy of Fallot, namely ventricular septal defect and right ventricular outflow obstruction were present (Figures 2 and 3). Both mitral leaflets were thickened and both, the posterior more than the anterior, protruded abnormally into the left atrium. Only 1 coronary ostium was present in the aorta and it was located in the left aortic sinus (Figure 4). A radiograph of the heart specimen disclosed heavy calcific deposits in the left circumflex and in its continuation as the right coronary artery, but insignificant luminal narrowing was present (Figure 5). The epicardial coronary arteries were much more dilated than expected (for age 74 years). All 76 five-mm segments of the epicardial coronary arteries were narrowed <50% in cross-sectional area despite heavy calcific deposits within some portions of the walls.

This patient had classic tetralogy of Fallot with a large ventricular septal defect and severe subpulmonic and pulmonic valve obstruction. The pulmonic valve had a unicuspid structure. Additionally, the patient had a single coronary ostium in the aorta, and the very dilated epicardial coronary arteries were devoid of significant narrowing despite heavy calcific deposits. The mitral valve had typical anatomic features of prolapse and the valve was incompetent. Both atria were quite dilated and atrial fibrillation was present.

At least 20 patients >40 years of age with unoperated tetralogy of Fallot and studied at necropsy have been reported (Table 2).[1-18] In contrast to our patient, none

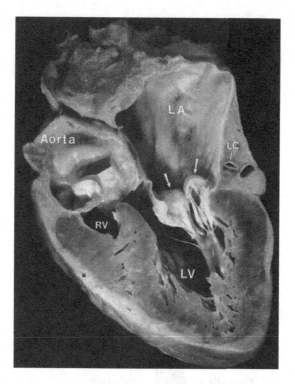

Figure 2 The heart at necropsy after an anteroposterior longitudinal cut. The ventricular septal defect is located just caudal to the overriding aorta. The right ventricular (RV) outflow tract is narrowed. Both mitral leaflets (*arrows*) prolapse into the dilated left atrium (LA). The left ventricular (LV) cavity is moderately dilated. The left circumflex (LC) coronary artery is very dilated.

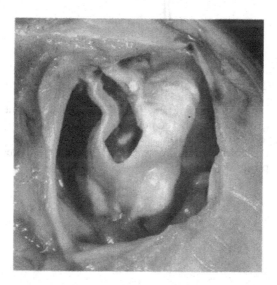

Figure 3 Close-up view of the stenotic pulmonic valve from the arterial side.

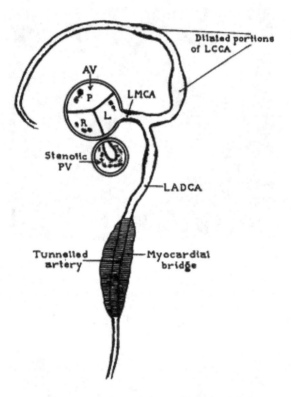

Figure 4 Diagram illustrating the origin and course of the coronary arteries. A single coronary ostium is in the left (L) anterior aortic sinus. The left main coronary artery (LMCA) bifurcates into the left circumflex coronary artery (LCCA) and left anterior decending coronary artery (LADCA). The LCCA continues in the left atrioventricular groove to supply the posterior left ventricular wall and right ventricular wall. A portion of the LADCA was tunnelled. The relative sizes of the aortic valve (AV) and the unicuspid, unicommissural, stenotic pulmonic valve (PV) are also shown. P = posterior; R = right.

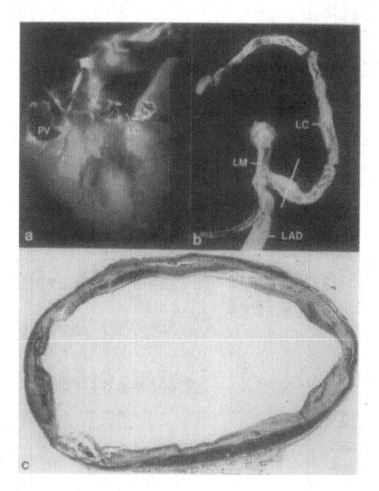

Figure 5 Coronary arteries. *a*, radiograph of the intact heart showing calcific deposits in the epicardial coronary arteries, pulmonic valve (PV) and aortic valve. The left circumflex (LC) coronary artery is heavily calcified. *b*, radiograph of the excised coronary arteries showing extensive calcific deposits in the LC coronary artery. *c*, photomicrograph of a section indicated by the *white line* of the most dilated portion of the LC coronary artery. (Original magnification ×9, reduced by 27%.) Large calcific plaques are present, but the lumen is widely patent. LM = left main; LAD = left anterior descending.

of the 20 patients at necropsy had mitral valve prolapse, and none had a coronary artery anomaly; only 1 survived into the eighth decade, and only 3 had had atrial fibrillation. One (no. 20, Table 2) of the 20 patients was reported to have had mitral valve prolapse with severe mitral regurgitation by M-mode echocardiogram, but the mitral prolapse was not confirmed at necropsy.[18]

Table 2: Clinical and morphologic features of previously published adults > 40 years of age with unoperated tetralogy of fallot and studied at necropsy

Case	First Author	Year of Publication	Ref.	Age (yr) at Death & Sex	Age (yr) at Diagnosis	Age (yr) at Onset of CHF	Duration (yr) of CHF	IE by Hx	NYHA FC (1-4+)	BP (s/d)	C	DC	Highest Hgb (g/dl)	Hct (%)	AF	PR Interval (sec)	VA	Mode of Death CHF	CVA	Other	MVP	HW (g)	Site RV	Site PV
1	White	1929	1	59M	58	58	1	0	4	110/80	+	+	100%[a]	—	0	0.12	0	0	+	0	0	450	+	0
2	Volini	1938	2	41M	41	35	35	0	3	170/100	+	+	100%[a]	—	0	0.28	0	0	0	+[b]	0	750	+	0
3	Strandell	1939	3	56F	56[c]	—	—	0	4	140/70	+	+	18	—	0	0.17	—	0	0	+[d]	0	370[e]	0	+
4	Feigin	1942	4	53M	37	51	2	0	4	140/70	+	+	98%[a]	—	+	0.24[f]	+	+	0	0	0	970	+	0
5				43F	Birth	25	18	0	4	230/160	+	+	98%[a]	—	0	—	0	+	0	0	0	600	+	0
6	Middleton	1947	5	45M	3	44	1	0	4	—	+	+	21	61	0	0.32	0	+	+	0	0	790	0	+
7	Lian	1949	6	55F	Infancy	—	0	0	3	140/85	+	+	—	—	0	—	+	0	+	0	0	—	+	+
8	Civen	1950	7	47M	27	—	0	—	2	140/80	—	—	—	—	0	—	—	0	0	+[g]	0	650	+	0
9	Baguena	1951	8	44M	44[c]	32	12	0	2	125/65	+	+	120%[a]	—	0	—	0	0	0	+[h]	0	—	0	+
10	Miller	1952	9	56M	Childhood	—	0	0	1	120/85	+	+	23	—	+[j]	0.16[f]	+	0	0	+	0	425	+	0
11	Bain	1954	10	69M	1	67	2	0	3	130/75	+	0	13	—	0	—	0	+	0	0	0	450	0	+
12	Bedford	1956	11	53F	32	48	4	—	3	—	0	0	126%[a]	—	0	—	+	0	+	0	—	480	0	+
13	Rosenthal	1956	12	53F	53[c]	—	0	0	1	170/90	0	+	—	—	0	—	0	0	0	+[g]	—	—	+	0
14	Marquis	1956	13	64F	9	—	0	0	3	150/105	+	+	23	—	0	—	—	0	+	0	—	—	+	+
15				47M	4	—	0	0	1	130/100	+	+	23	—	0	0.12	0	0	0	+[j]	0	—	+	0
16	Abraham	1961	14	48F	19	—	—	0	4	140/90	+	+	18	56	0	—	0	0	0	+[k]	0	450	0	+
17	Bowie	1961	15	68F	Childhood	—	—	0	4	140/80	+	+	18	—	0	0.24	+	+	+	0	0	512	0	+
18	Meindok	1964	16	62M	57	62	0[i]	+	4	170/100	+	0	18	—	0	—	+	0	+	+[m]	0	710	0	+
19	Oakley	1966	17	58M	45	53	5	+	4	115/85	+	+	19	62	+	0.08[f]	+	+	0	0	0	660	+	0
20	Thomas	1987	18	77M	77[c]	73	0	+	1	—	+	+	—[l]	—[l]	—	—	0	0	0	0	0	—	+	0

[a] Hemoglobin measurement as a percentage of a standard based on the method used; [b] chronic glomerulonephritis; [c] diagnosis made at necropsy; [d] tuberculosis; [e] patient weighed 48 kg; [f] measured before onset of atrial fibrillation; [g] cancer; [h] sudden death in hospital unassociated with CHF; [i] complication of bowel surgery; [j] CHF developed with acute myocardial infarction; [k] acute myocardial infarction secondary to atherosclerotic coronary artery disease; [m] pneumonia; [n] pulmonary infarct; [l] not polycythemic.

AF = atrial fibrillation; BP = blood pressure; C = cyanosis; CHF = congestive heart failure; CVA = cerebrovascular accident; DC = digital clubbing; F = female; FC = functional class; Hct = hematocrit; Hgb = hemoglobin; HW = heart weight; Hx = history; IE = infective endocarditis; M = male; MVP = mitral valve prolapse; NYHA = New York Heart Association; s/d = peak systole/end diastole; PV = pulmonic valve; Ref. = reference; RV = right ventricle; VA = ventricular arrhythmias.

REFERENCES

1. White PD, Sprague HB. The tetralogy of Fallot. Report of a case in a noted musician who lived to his sixtieth year. *JAMA* 1929;92:787–791.
2. Volini IF, Flaxman B. Tetralogy of Fallot. Report of a case in a man who lived to his forty-first year. *JAMA* 1938;111:2000–2003.
3. Strandell B. Fallot's tetrad—fall av sällsynt duration. *Svenska Läkartidningen* 1939;36:1513–1520.
4. Feigin I, Rosenthal J. The tetralogy of Fallot. *Am Heart J* 1943;26:302–312.
5. Middleton WS, Ritchie G. The tetralogy of Fallot. An account of a patient with this condition surviving over forty-five years. *Am Heart J* 1947;33:250–253.
6. Lian C, Fleury J. Survie jusqú á 55 ans d'une maladie bleue (type Fallot). *Arch Mal Coeur* 1949;42:1209–1210.
7. Civin WH, Edwards JE. Pathology of the pulmonary vascular tree. I. A comparison of the intrapulmonary arteries in Eisenmenger complex and in stenosis of the ostium infundibuli associated with biventricular origin of the aorta. *Circulation* 1950;2:545–551.
8. Báguena R, Tormo V. Coexistencia de tetralogía de Fallot y persistencia del conducto arterioso en una persona de cuarenta y cuatro años. *Med Esp* 1951;26:134–136.
9. Miller SI. Tetralogy of Fallot: Report of a case that survived to his fifty-seventh year and died following surgical relief of gall-stone ileus. *Ann intern Med* 1952;36:901–910.
10. Bain GO. Tetralogy of Fallot: Survival to seventieth year. Report of a case. *Arch Pathol* 1954;58:176–179.
11. Bedford DE. Two cases of Fallot's tetralogy, shown at the section in 1929, exhibiting unusual longevity. *Proc R Soc Med* 1956;46:314–315.
12. Rosenthal L. Longevity and the tetralogy of Fallot. *Br Med J* 1956;1:1107.
13. Marquis RM. Longevity and the early history of the tetralogy of Fallot. *Br Med J* 1956;1:819–822.
14. Abraham AS, Atkinson M, Mitchell WM. Fallot's tetralogy with some features of Marfan's syndrome and survival to 58 years. *Br Heart J* 1961;23:110–112.
15. Bowie EA. Longevity in tetralogy and trilogy of Fallot. Discussion of cases in patients surviving 40 years and presentation of two further cases. *Am Heart J* 1961;62:125–132.
16. Meindok H. Longevity in the tetralogy of Fallot. *Thorax* 1964;19:12–14.
17. Oakley C, Olsen E. A case of long survival with Fallot's tetralogy. *Br Med J* 1966;2:748–753.
18. Thomas SHL, Bass P, Pambakian H, Marigold JH. Cyanotic tetralogy of Fallot in a 77 year old man. *Postgrad Med J* 1987;63:361–362.

Case 983 Coronary Ostial Dimple (In the Posterior Aortic Sinus) in the Absence of Other Coronary Arterial Abnormalities

Jamshid Shirani, MD and William C. Roberts, MD

Normally 2 coronary arteries arise from the aorta, 1 from the aortic wall enclosing the right aortic sinus and the other from the aortic wall enclosing the left aortic sinus; the wall enclosing the posterior, i.e., noncoronary sinus, is smooth and devoid of any "dimples" or "buds" or other suggestions of a residua of a potential coronary ostium. Recently, we examined a heart with 2 normally arising coronary ostia and a dimple of an undeveloped coronary ostium in the third aortic sinus. Such an occurrence has not been seen by us in approximately 10,000 other hearts examined in a similar manner. This report briefly describes the cardiac morphologic finding in this 1 patient.

A 20-year-old man died of gunshot wounds. There was no injury to the heart. At necropsy, the heart weighed 250 g. The left and right ventricular cavities were normal and no grossly visible myocardial scars were seen. The left main and the right coronary arteries arose normally from the left and right aortic sinuses, respectively (Figure 1). The left main coronary artery then divided into the left anterior descending and left circumflex coronary arteries, both of which thereafter coursed normally. In addition to the left main and the right coronary ostia, a coronary ostial dimple was present in the wall of the aorta slightly above the posterior aortic sinus (Figures 1 and 2). It measured 4 mm in diameter and 3 mm in maximum depth.

Coronary artery ostia arise from the wall of the aortopulmonary trunk at the time of embryonic division of the trunk.[1] It is not known why the coronary arteries consistently arise from the left and right aortic sinuses, with only minor variations in their locations in most individuals. It has been suggested that the development of the coronary ostial dimples in the wall of the aortopulmonary trunk require the presence of a developing network of epicardial vessels in the heart.[2] This epicardial vascular network, then, induces the formation of the coronary ostial dimples as it approaches the aortopulmonary trunk. This hypothesis, however, would not explain the presence of coronary ostial dimples in the opposite aortic sinus in patients with "single coronary artery" and in the patient described here.

In addition to the heretofore described patient, at least 6 other cases of coronary ostial dimples or buds have been reported (Table I).[3-8] All 6 cases, however, differed from the present one in that the dimple was at a site where a coronary artery should have arisen but did not. In other words, all 6 previously reported cases of coronary dimple were in actuality examples of single coronary artery.[9] In our patient, on the other hand, a coronary dimple was present at a site where a coronary ostium is not normally present.

From the Pathology Branch, National Heart, Lung, and Blood Institute, National Institutes of Health, Building 10, Room 2N258, Bethesda, Maryland 20892. Dr. Robert's current address is: Baylor Cardiovascular Institute, Baylor University Medical Center, 3701 Junius Street, PO. Box E010, Dallas, Texas 75246. Manuscript received December 7, 1992; revised manuscript received January 29, 1993 and accepted February 1.

DOI: 10.1201/9781003409342-45

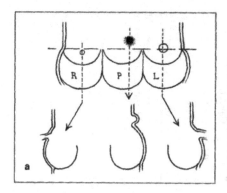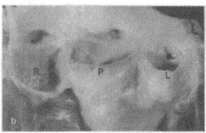

Figure 1 Diagram (*a*) and photograph (*b*) of the longitudinally opened aortic valve showing the positions of the 2 normal coronary ostia in the walls of the left (L) and the right (R) aortic sinuses and the coronary ostial dimple above the posterior (P) aortic sinus. The *horizontal broken line* separates the sinus and the tubular portions of the ascending aorta (sinotubular junction). The right and left coronary ostia are located in the wall of the aorta slightly below and at this sinotubular junction, respectively. The coronary ostial dimple is located slightly above the sinotubular junction.

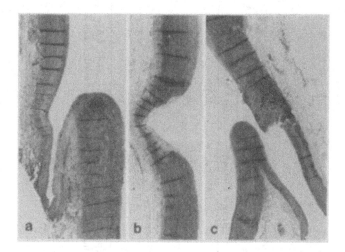

Figure 2 Photomicrograph of longitudinal sections of aorta through the right coronary ostium (*a*), the coronary ostial dimple (*b*) and the left main coronary ostium (*c*). The sections are taken as shown by the *broken vertical lines* through the coronary ostia in Figure la. The aortic media (*darker staining tissue*) continues through the wall of the ostial dimple. Movat stain ×13, reduced by 36%.

Table I: Reported cases of coronary ostial dimple in the presence of "single coronary artery"

Patient	Ref.	Age (yr) & Sex	Location of		AP	AMI	SD	CAD	HW (g)	LV Scar	Cause of Death
			"Single Ostium"	Ostial Dimple							
1	3	37M	LAS	RAS	—	—	—	—	—	—	Infective endocarditis
2	4	68M	LAS	RAS	—	—	—	—	—	—	Cancer
3	5	80F	LAS	RAS	0	0	0	+	340	0	Cancer
4	6	76F	RAS	LAS	0	0	0	0	370	0	Cancer
5	7	84F	RAS	LAS	+	+	+	+	530	+	AMI
6	8	83F	LAS	PAS	0	0	+	+	320	0	Ruptured CA aneurysm

AMI = acute myocardial infarct; AP = angina pectoris; CA = coronary artery; CAD = atherosclerotic coronary artery disease; F = female; HW = heart weight; LAS = left aortic sinus; LV = left ventricular; M = male; PAS = posterior aortic sinus; RAS = right aortic sinus; SD = sudden death; — = information not available; + = present; 0 = absent.

REFERENCES

1. Angelini P. Normal and anomalous coronary arteries: Definitions and classification. *Am Heart J* 1989;117:418–434.
2. Conte G, Pellegrini A. On the development of the coronary arteries in human embryos, stage 14–19. *Anat Embryol* 1984;169:209–218.
3. Plaut A. Versorgung des Herzens durch nur eine Kranzarterie. *Frankf Z Pathol* 1922;27:84–90.
4. Ogden JA, Goodyer AVN. Patterns of distribution of the single coronary artery. *Yale J Biol Med* 1970;43:11–21.
5. Smith JC. Review of single coronary artery with report of 2 cases. *Circulation* 1950;1:1168–1175.
6. Leivo IV, Laurila PK. Atresia of left coronary ostium and left main coronary artery. *Arch Pathol Lab Med* 1987;111:1173–1175.
7. Vlodaver Z, Amplatz K, Burchell HB, Edwards JE. Single coronary ostium in the aorta. In: Coronary Heart Disease: Clinical, Angiographic and Pathologic Profiles. New York: Springer-Verlag, 1976:189–216.
8. Causing WP, Shuster M, Pribor HC, Amboy P. Single coronary artery with ruptured coronary artery aneurysm. *Arch Pathol* 1967;83:419–421.
9. Shirani J, Roberts WC. Solitary coronary ostium in the aorta in the absence of other major congenital cardiovascular anomalies. *J Am Coll Cardiol* 1993;21:137–143.

Case 990 Sudden Death, Right Ventricular Infarction, and Abnormal Right Ventricular Intramural Coronary Arteries in Isolated Congenital Valvular Pulmonic Stenosis

Jamshid Shirani, MD, Abarmard Maziar Zafari, MD and William C. Roberts, MD*

Isolated congenital valvular pulmonic stenosis is a relatively common anomaly of the heart. Fontana and Edwards[1] found pulmonic stenosis in 8 of 357 patients (2%) with congenital cardiac disease studied at necropsy. In unoperated patients with severe forms of this congenital anomaly, death is generally caused by progressive right ventricular failure.[1, 2] In those patients who survive infancy, survival into adulthood is the rule.[2] Sudden death is rare. In a review of 68 previously described fatal cases of isolated congenital valvular pulmonic stenosis, only 2 (aged 19 and 26 years, both men) had died suddenly.[2] Only 1 of 186 sudden deaths in patients with congenital cardiovascular disease (age range 1 to 21 years) was caused by pulmonic stenosis.[3] This report describes a patient with isolated pulmonic stenosis who died suddenly, and at necropsy also was found to have right ventricular infarction and abnormal intramural coronary arteries.

The patient, an 8-year-old black boy, had a precordial murmur since birth. He had normal growth and development, and was asymptomatic until age 5 years when easy fatigability was noted. A diagnosis of "tetralogy of Fallot" was made by physical examination, but the family refused further workup. Although his physical activities apparently were limited, his only symptom was mild exertional dyspnea. He died suddenly at home. At necropsy, the heart weighed 540 g (expected weight approximately 120). The pulmonic trunk was dilated and its diameter was more than twice that of the ascending aorta (2.4 vs 1.1 cm). The major epicardial coronary arteries were normal. The pulmonic valve had a domeshaped structure with a slightly eccentrically located orifice that was 0.4 cm² in area (Figure 1). The right atrial wall was markedly hypertrophied, and the cavity was dilated. The right ventricular wall was markedly hypertrophied; the ventricular septum, which was thicker than the left ventricular wall, was pushed toward the left ventricle, and no defect was present in the ventricular septum. Grossly visible scars were present in the moderator band, right ventricular papillary muscles, and focally throughout the right ventricular free wall (Figures 1 and 2). Histologically, the right ventricular myocytes were larger than those of the ventricular septum and left ventricle, foci of interstitial and replacement fibrosis were present, and many intramural coronary arteries in the right ventricular myocardium had thickened walls, especially in the areas of scarring (Figure 2).

The present findings indicate that sudden death may occur in patients with pulmonic stenosis, despite few symptoms of cardiac dysfunction. Extensive scarring of

From the Pathology Branch, National Heart, Lung, and Blood Institute, National Institutes of Health, Building 10, Room 2N258, Bethesda, Maryland 20892. Manuscript received January 12, 1993; revised manuscript received and accepted March 3, 1993.

* Current address: Baylor Cardiovascular Institute, Baylor University Medical Center, 3500 Gaston Avenue, Dallas, Texas 75246.

   DOI: 10.1201/9781003409342-46

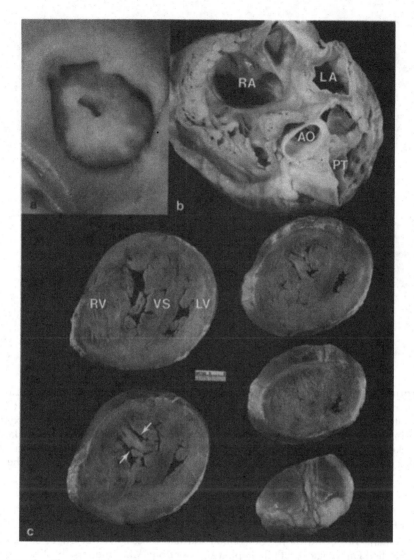

Figure 1 The heart in the patient described. *a,* view of the stenotic pulmonic valve from the pulmonary trunk (PT). *b,* view of the right (RA) and left (LA) atria, and the great arteries after excision of the cephalad portion of both atria showing markedly thickened and dilated right atrium, and the small-sized left atrium. *c, photograph* of the cardiac ventricles after transverse incisions at approximately 1 cm intervals from base (*upper left*) to apex (*lower right*). The right ventricular (RV) wall is enormously thickened, and scars (*arrows*) are visible, particularly in the moderator band. The ventricular septum (VS) is concave toward the left ventricle (LV). AO = aorta.

the right ventricular wall can occur in this congenital cardiac anomaly and may be related to abnormal intramural coronary arteries. Neither right ventricular scarring nor abnormal right ventricular intramural coronary arteries were reported previously in patients with isolated valvular pulmonic stenosis.

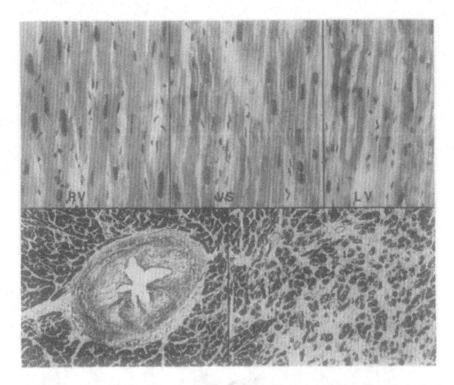

Figure 2 *Photomicrographs* of the ventricular myocardium in the patient described. The nuclei of the right ventricular (RV) myocytes are darker and larger than those of either the ventricular septum (VS) or left ventricular (LV) wall. Hematoxylin-eosin stains each ×400; reduced by 50%. *Bottom left, photomicrograph* showing a large, thickened intramural coronary artery in the RV wall. Movat stain ×100; reduced by 50%. *Bottom right, photomicrograph* showing considerable interstitial fibrosis in the RV wall. Movat stain ×100; reduced by 50%.

REFERENCES

1. Fontana RS, Edwards JE. Congenital Cardiac Disease: A Review of 357 Cases Studied Pathologically. Philadelphia and London: W.B. Saunders, 1962:102–105.
2. Greene DG, Baldwin ED, Baldwin JS, Himmelstein A, Roh CE, Coumand A. Pure congenital pulmonary stenosis and idiopathic congenital dilatation of the pulmonary artery. *Am J Med* 1949;6:24–40.
3. Lambert EC, Menon VA, Wagner HR, Vlad P. Sudden unexpected death from cardiovascular disease in children. *Am J Cardiol* 1974;34:89–96.

Case 1545 "Repaired" Tetralogy of Fallot Mimicking Arrhythmogenic Right Ventricular Cardiomyopathy (Another Phenocopy)

Betsy Ann George, MD[a,d], Jong Mi Ko, BA[d], Forrester Dubus Lensing, MD[b], Johannes Jacob Kuiper, MD[a,d] and William Clifford Roberts, MD[a,c,d], *

Described is a 41-year-old man who at age 6 had partial resection of an obstructed right ventricular outflow tract with insertion of a patch and closure of a ventricular septal defect (tetralogy of Fallot). At age 41, cardiac transplantation was performed because of right ventricular outflow patch aneurysm, numerous episodes of ventricular tachycardia, and chronic heart failure, all features of the familial form of arrhythmogenic right ventricular cardiomyopathy (ARVC). Additionally, the patient had bundle branch block and epsilon waves on electrocardiogram, other features of ARVC. The case is described to introduce the concept of *acquired* ARVC, because the patient had many of the clinically recognized features of familial ARVC.

Arrhythmogenic right ventricular cardiomyopathy (ARVC) is characterized by localized thinning of the right ventricular (RV) wall with the localized portion consisting mainly of fibrofatty tissue.[1-3] The thinning of the RV wall commonly leads to aneurysm formation.[2] ARVC also is characterized by the presence of epsilon waves, bundle branch block, late potentials, and ventricular tachyarrhythmias on the electrocardiogram. ARVC has been recognized exclusively as a familial disease with autosomal dominant inheritance.[1, 2] In this report, we introduce the concept of acquired ARVC in a patient who was operatively treated for tetralogy of Fallot and later developed features of ARVC.

CASE DESCRIPTION

A 41-year-old man, born on October 10, 1969, had a right Blalock-Taussig shunt placed in 1974, at 4 years of age, for tetralogy of Fallot. In 1976, at age 6, he underwent widening of the RV outflow tract using a Dacron patch (4.5 × 3 cm) and closure of a large (2 × 3 cm) subaortic ventricular septal defect. Preoperatively, the peak systolic pressure gradient between the right ventricle and pulmonary trunk had been 85 mm Hg. The patch extended through the nonobstructive pulmonary valve, and 2 of its 3 cusps were excised. The Blalock-Taussig shunt was ligated. Immediately after operation, the peak systolic RV pressure was 70 mm Hg and that in the pulmonary trunk 35 mm Hg. The peak systolic left ventricular pressure was 100 mm Hg.

The patient thereafter was asymptomatic until 26 years of age, when he had his first episode of ventricular tachycardia (VT). Transthoracic echocardiogram performed at age 26 revealed a peak systolic pressure gradient between the right ventricle and pulmonary trunk of 25 mm Hg, marked RV dilatation, a mildly dilated

Departments of [a]Internal Medicine (Division of Cardiology), [b]Radiology, and [c]Pathology and [d]The Baylor Heart and Vascular Institute, Baylor University Medical Center, Dallas, Texas.
Manuscript received January 27, 2011; revised manuscript received and accepted March 7, 2011.
 * Corresponding author: Tel: 214-820-7911; fax: 214-820-7533.
E-mail address: wc.roberts@baylorhealth.edu (W.C. Roberts).

DOI: 10.1201/9781003409342-47

left ventricular cavity, severely depressed right and left ventricular ejection fractions, and severe pulmonary regurgitation. An electrophysiologic study at the time disclosed sustained monomorphic VT with left bundle branch block morphology and superior axis. Mapping disclosed the VT to involve the RV infundibulum (that myocardium between the residual pulmonary valve and tricuspid valve) in a counterclockwise activation pattern. Radiofrequency ablation failed to terminate the VT, and it resulted in acute lengthening of the cycle length from 375 to 420 ms. The VT was then terminated with ventricular burst pacing. Repeat stimulation did not induce further VT. The patient was placed on atenolol and propafenone.

At 27 years of age, 8 months later, the patient had runs of VT again, and a second electrophysiologic study was done. Again, the inducible VT was mapped to involve the RV infundibulum but this time in a bidirectional activation pattern. A total of 23 linear and point radiofrequency ablations were made, and on several occasions the VT was terminated. Nevertheless, the VT was still inducible. Ablation prolonged the cycle length from 380 to 450 ms.

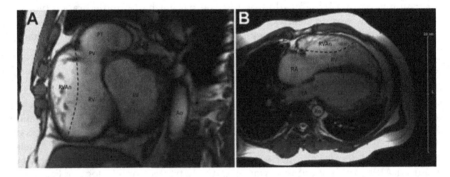

Figure 1 Parasagittal (*A*) and axial (*B*) white blood magnetic resonance imaging scans demonstrating marked right ventricular (RV) dilatation, RV aneurysm (RVAn), left ventricle (LV), left atrium (LA), right atrium (RA), pulmonaric valve (PV), pulmonary trunk (PT), and aorta (Ao).

Table 1: Hemodynamic data late after operative "correction" of tetralogy of Fallot

Variable	Date of Study			
	June 5, 2006	February 3, 2010	August 20, 2010	October 27, 2010
Right atrium (mean) (mm Hg)	10	8	16	11
Right ventricle (mm Hg)	36/15	41/12	45/19	38/5
Pulmonary artery (mm Hg)	34/7	34/5	33/13	35/10
Pulmonary capillary wedge (mean) (mm Hg)	—	9	16	14
Left ventricle (mm Hg)	96/31	—	—	—
Aorta (mm Hg)	91/61	—	—	—
Cardiac index (L/min/m²)	1.69	2.64	2.48	1.59

For several years thereafter, the patient was lost to follow-up. He started using alcohol and marijuana heavily. He quit taking all medications. At 36 years of age, he presented again to the hospital with chest pain, which was preceded by a viral gastroenteritis. His troponin level was 25 ng/ml. An electrocardiogram showed sinus tachycardia, a QRS duration of 200 ms, right bundle branch block, and nonspecific

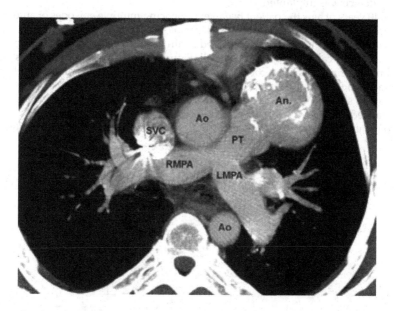

Figure 2 Axial contrast-enhanced computed tomographic scan demonstrating right ventricular (RV) outflow tract aneurysm (An) with heavy calcific deposits in its wall and synthetic graft repair. Ao = aorta; LMPA = left main pulmonary artery; PT = pulmonary trunk; RMPA = right main pulmonary artery; SVC = superior vena cava.

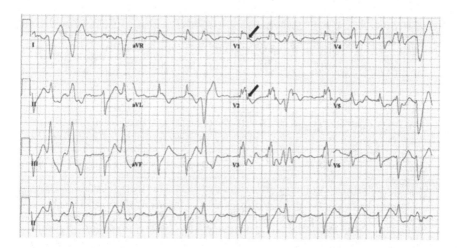

Figure 3 Electrocardiogram depicting epsilon waves (*arrows*) in the right precordial leads and inverted T waves in leads V_1 to V_4 with the presence of a complete right bundle branch block.

ST-T changes. Cardiac catheterization disclosed normal coronary arteries, normal mean pulmonary arterial pressures, no RV outflow obstruction, and no shunts. Transthoracic echocardiogram showed severely depressed RV and left ventricular function. Magnetic resonance imaging disclosed marked dilatation of the RV outflow tract (Figure 1). An automated internal cardiac defibrillator with a biventricular pacing device was implanted.

At 40 years of age, the patient began experiencing multiple episodes of automated internal cardiac defibrillator firings and symptoms of severe heart failure (Table 1). Cardiac computed tomography disclosed again severe dilatation of the RV outflow tract and heavy calcific deposits in its wall (Figure 2). Electrocardiogram now showed epsilon waves in the right precordial leads, T-wave inversions, and complete right bundle branch block (Figure 3). In February 2010, chronic inotropic therapy was initiated. The patient stopped using alcohol and marijuana completely. Six months later, when hospitalized for severe heart failure, runs of monomorphic nonsustained VT were demonstrated (Figure 4). On November 7, 2010, heart transplantation was performed.

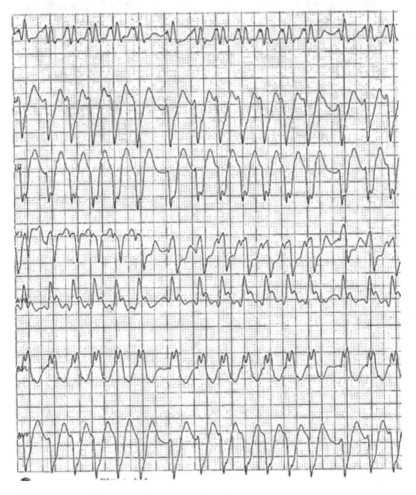

Figure 4 Nonsustained ventricular tachycardia (VT) of left bundle branch morphology with superior axis.

The RV outflow patch was aneurysmal and bulged anteriorly (Figure 5). X-ray revealed a heavily calcified RV outflow tract. The ventricular septal defect was well closed, and a few calcific deposits were present in the closing patch. Both ventricles were dilated. The left ventricular wall had focal scars. The endocardium at the apex of the left ventricle was thickened by white fibrous tissue. The epicardial coronary arteries were wide open and free of plaque.

COMMENTS

The modified International Task Force criteria for the diagnosis of ARVC were published in April 2010.[4] Our patient fulfilled 4 of the 6 major criteria and 1 of the 6 minor criteria: regional RV akinesia and a fractional area change ≤33%, thinning of a large portion of RV wall (by a patch), epsilon waves in the right precordial leads, inducible nonsustained VT of left bundle branch block morphology with superior axis, and inverted T waves in leads V_1 to V_4 in the presence of a complete right bundle branch block. Thus, the patient had criteria of ARVC but in an *acquired* way, after surgical resection of a large portion of the RV outflow tract. One reviewer suggested that the repeated and aggressive ablations in the electrophysiologic studies possibly contributed to the morphologic findings and to the repeated ventricular arrhythmias.

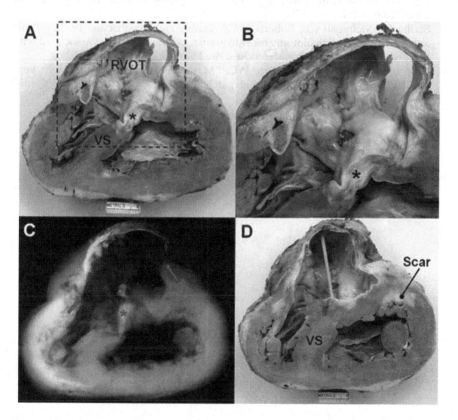

Figure 5 Heart. (*A,B*) View portraying right ventricular (RV) outflow patch aneurysm and marked dilatation of both ventricles. (*C*) X-ray showing a heavily calcified RV outflow tract (RVOT) aneurysm (*arrows*) and a well-closed ventricular septal defect (*asterisk*) with a few calcific deposits in the closing patch. (*D*) The left ventricular wall showing focal scar. VS = ventricular septum.

Aneurysmal development of the RV outflow tract after patch widening for RV outflow obstruction of course has been reported previously.[5] Additionally, the development of calcium deposits within the RV outflow patch also is most unusual but has been reported previously.[6]

REFERENCES

1. Basso C, Thiene G, Corrado D, Angelini A, Nava A, Valente M. Arrhythmogenic right ventricular cardiomyopathy: Dysplasia, dystrophy, or myocarditis? *Circulation* 1996;94:983–991.

2. Basso C, Corrado D, Marcus FI, Nava A, Thiene G. Arrhythmogenic right ventricular cardiomyopathy. *Lancet* 2009;373:1289–1300.

3. Roberts WC, Ko JM, Kuiper JJ, Hall SA, Meyer DM. Some previously neglected examples of arrhythmogenic right ventricular dysplasia/cardiomyopathy and frequency of its various reported manifestations. *Am J Cardiol* 2010;106:268–274.

4. Marcus FI, McKenna WJ, Sherrill D, Basso C, Bauce B, Bluemke DA, Calkins H, Corrado D, Cox MG, Daubert JP, Fontaine G, Gear K, Hauer R, Nava A, Picard MH, Protonotarios N, Saffitz JE, Sanborn DM, Steinberg JS, Tandri H, Thiene G, Towbin JA, Tsatsopoulou A, Wichter T, Zareba W. Diagnosis of arrhythmogenic right ventricular cardiomyopathy/dysplasia: Proposed modification of the Task Force criteria. *Circulation* 2010;121:1533–1541.

5. Saffitz JE, McIntosh CL, Roberts WC. Massive right ventricular outflow tract aneurysm after ventriculotomy for subvalvular pulmonic stenosis associated with peripheral pulmonary arterial stenoses. *Am J Cardiol* 1983;51:1460–1462.

6. Ross EM, McIntosh CL, Roberts WC. "Massive" calcification of a right ventricular outflow parietal pericardial patch in tetralogy of Fallot. *Am J Cardiol* 1984;54:691–692.

Case 1629 Secondary Arrhythmogenic Right Ventricular Cardiomyopathy Decades After Operative Repair of Tetralogy of Fallot

Erin E. Donaldson, DO[a], Jong Mi Ko, BA[b], Gonzalo Gonzalez-Stawinski, MD[c], Shelley A. Hall, MD[d] and William C. Roberts, MD[d,e],*

We describe a 47-year-old man who underwent heart transplantation (HT) for severe right-sided heart failure and periodic episodes of ventricular tachycardia (VT) 43 years after operative repair of tetralogy of Fallot (T of F). The right-ventricular outflow tract, the site where a patch had been placed 4 decades earlier, was aneurysmal. Such development decades after operative repair of T of F of both aneurysm and episodes of VT is probably more common than previously realized.

In July 2011 we reported a 41-year-old man who underwent heart transplantation (HT) because of severe right-sided heart failure and periodic ventricular tachycardia (VT) after operative repair of tetralogy of Fallot (T of F) at age 6.[1] The present report was prompted by studying a similar patient, aged 47, who underwent HT also because of severe right-sided heart failure associated with periodic episodes of VT after operative repair of T of F at age 4. Both patients developed huge right ventricular outflow aneurysms.

CASE DESCRIPTION

A 47-year-old male manual laborer had repair of T of F at 4 years of age. Thereafter, he was asymptomatic until age 33 years, when he had his first symptomatic episode of VT and an intracardiac defibrillator was inserted. Evidence of right-sided failure appeared about the same time and it gradually progressed thereafter. An electrocardiogram before an intracardiac defibrillator was inserted is shown in Figure 1. A computed tomographic image of the heart just before HT is shown in Figure 2. Three months after HT (January 2014) the patient was asymptomatic. Photographs of the explanted heart are shown in Figures 3 and 4.

DISCUSSION

Described herein is a patient who had HT at age 47 for severe right-sided heart failure and episodic VT occurring several decades after repair of T of F at age 4. The patient described is virtually identical to a patient reported 2 years earlier with a

[a]Department of Family Medicine, Methodist Charlton Medical Center, Dallas, Texas and [b]Baylor Heart and Vascular Institute, [c]Department of Cardiothoracic Surgery, [d]Division of Cardiology, Department of Internal Medicine, and [e]Department of Pathology, Baylor University Medical Center, Dallas, Texas. Manuscript received May 7, 2014; revised manuscript received and accepted May 29, 2014.

The study was funded by the Baylor Health Care System Foundation, Dallas, Texas.

See page 806 for disclosure information.

* Corresponding author: Tel: (214) 820–7911; fax: (214) 820–7533.

E-mail address: wc.roberts@baylorhealth.edu (W.C. Roberts).

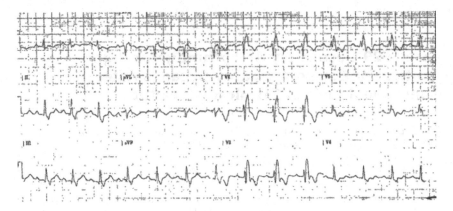

Figure 1 Electrocardiogram in the patient described before an intracardiac defibrillator was inserted. The electrocardiogram discloses a complete left bundle branch block pattern. Shows a complete right bundle branch block pattern. The rhythm is sinus.

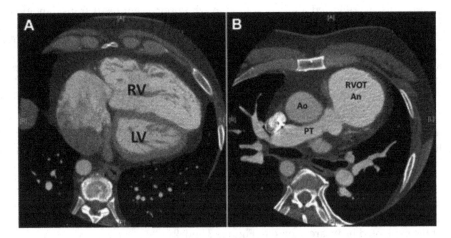

Figure 2 Computed tomographic imaging of the heart in the patient described before cardiac transplantation. (*A*) View showing the right ventricular cavity (inflow portion) and the much smaller left ventricular cavity (LV). The dilated right atrium is also seen as well as the right-sided aortic arch (AO). (*B*) A view showing the marked dilatation of the outflow portion of the right ventricle (RV) just beneath the pulmonic valve (PV). PT = pulmonic trunk; RVOT An = right ventricular outflow tract aneurysm.

similar scenario (Table 1). The earlier report also described a huge right ventricular outflow tract aneurysm involving the widening patch utilized when eliminating the subvalvular right ventricular outflow tract obstruction. To study 2 similar patients in a 2-year period suggests that aneurysmal formation in the right ventricular outflow tract several decades after repair of T of F may not be an uncommon occurrence but indeed potentially a common late occurrence. The development

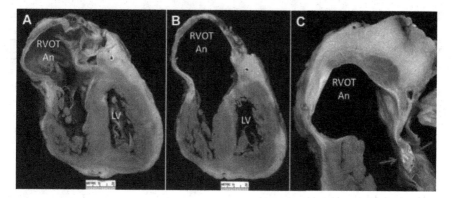

Figure 3 Partial four chamber cuts of the heart in the patient described. (*A*) View of the very dilated right ventricular outflow tract (RVOT), partially destroyed pulmonic valve (PV), left anterior descending coronary artery residing in the excessive subepicardial adipose tissue, right and left ventricular cavities exposing both tricuspid and mitral valves. (*B*) Another view showing the much dilated right ventricular outflow tract and the non-dilated right ventricular inflow tract. The scarring in the cephalad portion of the ventricular septum is the area where the previous ventricular septal defect was closed, approximately 40 years earlier. (*C*) Another view of the right ventricular outflow tract with calcium in the area where a patch (*arrows*) was used to close the ventricular septal defect (CA++). An = aneurysm; LV = left ventricle.

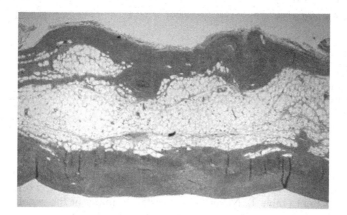

Figure 4 Photomicrograph of a portion of the right ventricular outflow tract showing total absence of myocardial fibers and extensive fibrous deposits in the outer wall and in the inner wall with large deposits of adipose tissue in between. Hematoxylin/eosin stain, ×40.

of episodes of VT with development of the right ventricular outflow aneurysm of course might be described as secondary or acquired arrhythmogenic right ventricular cardiomyopathy/dysplasia.

Table 1: Comparison of certain findings in the 2 men having cardiac transplantation late following repair of tetralogy of Fallot

Variable	Case 1*	Case 2
Age (years)		
At heart transplantation	41 (November 2010)	47 (January 2014)
At repair of tetralogy of Fallot	6	4
When RV outflow tract aneurysm first noted	26	33
At onset of heart failure	26	33
At onset of ventricular tachycardia	26	33
Right-sided aortic arch	0	+
Body mass index (kg/m^2)	25	32
Heart weight (g)	653	505
Calcium in RV outflow tract aneurysm	+	0
RV outflow patch	+ (calcified)	+
Electrophysiology		
Bundle branch block	Left	Right
Intracardiac defibrillator	+ (age 36)	+ (age 33)
Radiofrequency ablation	+	0
Hemodynamics (mm Hg)		
Left ventricle (s/d)	96/31	113/69 (indirect)
Pulmonary artery (s/d)	33/13	44/21
Right ventricle (s/d)	45/19	45/8
Lowest LV ejection fraction (%)	10	50

LV = left ventricle; RV = right ventricular; s/d = peak systole/end diastole.
* From George BA, Jong MK, Lensing FD, Kuiper JJ, Roberts WC. "Repaired" tetralogy of Fallot mimicking arrhythmogenic right ventricular cardiomyopathy. *Am J Cardiol* 2011;108: 326–329.[1]

Shown in Table 2 are selected reports of patients having late follow up after repair of T of F in childhood.[2-9] Of the 1964 patients included none appeared to have a follow up as long as 40 years as did our present patient and our previously described patient (Table 1). Nevertheless, certainly many of the reported patients having pulmonic valve replacement with or without partial excision of the right ventricular outflow tract did have subvalvular aneurysms and some had "arrhythmias" (type not specified).

The other unusual feature here is the use of HT to eliminate both the right-sided severe heart failure and the periodic episodes of ventricular tachycardia. As shown in Table 2, however, HT is infrequently employed for management of late complications after repair of T of F. Only 4 of the previously mentioned 2638 patients (Table 2) underwent HT late after previous "repair" of T of F, and 3 of them previously had homograft replacement of the pulmonic valve.

DISCLOSURES

The authors have no conflicts of interest to disclose.

Table 2: Selected previous publications of patients having repair of tetralogy of Fallot (T of F) early in life with long follow up thereafter

First Author	Publication Year	Age (Years) at Repair of T of F Mean ± SD [Median]	Number of Patients Having Late Survival	Follow Up (Years) Range (Mean ± SD)	Patients Having Cardiac Transplantation
Kirklin[2]	1989	— [5]	791	>2–20 (9 ± 5)	0
Murphy[3]	1997	10 ± 9 [8]	163	0.08–34 (21 ± 13)	0
Nollert[4]	1993	12 ± 9 [-]	490	1.06–35 (25 ± -)	0
Knott-Craig[5]	1998	2 ± 0.2 [-]	193	0.1–26 (11 ± 7)	0
Norgaard[6]	1999	— [13]	109	20–38 (26 ± -)	1
Gatzoulis[7]	2000	8 ± 8 [6]	793	8–41 (21 ± 9)	0
Troost[8]	2007	— [24]	68	1.3–18 (- ± 8)	3*
Munkhammar[9]	2013	— [0.8]	31	2–16 (9 ± 3)	0
Totals			2638		

— = no information available.
* All had homograft replacement of the pulmonic valve.

REFERENCES

1. George BA, Jong MK, Lensing FD, Kuiper JJ, Roberts WC. "Repaired" tetralogy of Fallot mimicking arrhythmogenic right ventricular cardiomyopathy. *Am J Cardiol* 2011;108:326–329.

2. Kirklin JK, Kirklin JW, Blackstone EH, Milano A, Pacifico AD. Effect of transannular patching on outcome after repair of tetralogy of Fallot. *Ann Thorac Surg* 1989;48:783–791.

3. Murphy JG, Gersh MB, Mair DD, Fuster V, McGoon MD, Ilstrup DM, McGoon DC, Kirklin JW, Danielson GK. Long-term outcome in patients undergoing surgical repair of tetralogy of Fallot. *N Engl J Med* 1993;329:593–599.

4. Nollert G, Fischlein T, Bouterwek S, Bohmer C, Klinner W, Reichart B. Long-term survival in patients with repair of tetralogy of Fallot: 36-year follow-up of 490 survivors of the first year after surgical repair. *J Am Coll Cardiol* 1997;30:1374–1383.

5. Knott-Craig CJ, Elkins RC, Lane MM, Holz J, McCue C, Ward KE. A 26-year experience with surgical management of tetralogy of Fallot: Risk analysis for mortality or late reintervention. *Ann Thorac Surg* 1998;66:506–511.

6. Norgaard MA, Lauridsen P, Helvind M, Pettersson G. Twenty-to-thirty-seven year follow-up after repair for tetralogy of Fallot. *Eur J Cardiothorac Surg* 1999;16:125–130.

7. Gatzoulis MA, Balaji S, Webber SA, Siu SC, Hokanson JS, Poile C, Rosenthal M, Nakazawa M, Moller JH, Gillette PC, Webb GD, Redington AN. Risk factors for arrhythmia and sudden cardiac death late after repair of tetralogy of Fallot: A multicentre study. *Lancet* 2000;356:975–981.

8. Troost E, Meyns B, Daenen W, Van de Werf F, Gewillig M, Van Deyk K, Moons P, Budts W. Homograft survival after tetralogy of Fallot repair: Determinants of accelerated homograft degeneration. *Eur Heart J* 2007;28:2503–2509.

9. Munkhammar P, Carlsson M, Arheden H, Pesonen E. Restrictive right ventricular physiology after tetralogy of Fallot repair is associated with fibrosis of the right ventricular outflow tract visualized on cardiac magnetic resonance imaging. *Eur Heart J Cardiovasc Imaging* 2013;14:978–985.

Case 1649 Large Patent Ductus Arteriosus in a 44-Year-Old Woman

Leading to Calcium Deposition in the Left Atrium and Mitral and Aortic Valves

Carey Camille Roberts, BS and William Clifford Roberts, MD

This report describes unusual autopsy findings in a 44-year-old woman who had a large, calcified patent ductus arteriosus that produced substantial left-to-right shunting. The patient died in 1962, 7 days after patch closure of the aortic orifice of the ductus. Numerous calcific deposits were present in the mural left atrial endocardium, the mitral valve leaflets and annulus, and the aortic valve cusps. The cause of the left-sided calcific deposits was perhaps related to the patient's several-decades-old giant aortopulmonary shunt, causing a major increase in the volume of blood passing through the left-sided cardiac chambers in comparison with the volume in the right side. To our knowledge, such findings in a patient with patent ductus arteriosus have not been reported previously. (Tex Heart Inst J 2015;42(3):262–4)

Key words: Adult; calcinosis/pathology; cardiomegaly/etiology/radiography; ductus arteriosus, patent/surgery; heart atria/pathology; heart diseases/physiopathology

A large patent ductus arteriosus (PDA) is now rarely seen in adults in the Western world; however, this was not necessarily the case 50 years ago. We describe noteworthy autopsy findings in a woman who had presented with symptoms after several decades of aortopulmonary shunting through a large PDA.

CASE REPORT

A childless housewife was born in 1917 and died in 1962, at 44 years of age. A precordial murmur had been present since childhood, when she was diagnosed with rheumatic heart disease. She was asymptomatic until 40 years of age, when peripheral edema, abdominal swelling, and exertional dyspnea developed. The patient was seen initially in November 1959 at the National Heart Institute (Bethesda, Md), at

From: Second-year medical student (Ms Roberts), Georgetown University School of Medicine, Washington, DC 20057; Baylor Heart and Vascular Institute (Dr. Roberts and Ms Roberts), Dallas, Texas 75246; Departments of Internal Medicine (Division of Cardiology) and Pathology (Dr. Roberts), Baylor University Medical Center; Dallas, Texas 75246; and Pathology Branch (Dr. Roberts), National Heart, Lung and Blood Institute, Bethesda, Maryland 20205

Address for reprints: William C. Roberts, MD, Baylor Heart and Vascular Institute, Baylor University Medical Center, 3500 Gaston Ave, Dallas, TX 75246

E-mail: wc.roberts@baylorhealth.edu

DOI: 10.1201/9781003409342-49

41 years of age. She was cachectic and in severe right-sided heart failure. Her neck veins were markedly distended. On auscultation, the following were heard: rales in the lung bases, an apical grade 4/6 blowing systolic murmur in association with a thrill that radiated into the left axilla, a diastolic rumble at the apex, a crescendo diastolic grade 3/6 blowing murmur along the left sternal border, and an accentuated P_2. A chest radiograph showed a greatly enlarged cardiac silhouette. An electrocardiogram, measured with normal 10-mm standardization (10 mm=1 mV), showed a total 12-lead QRS voltage of 315 mm (consistent with combined right and left ventricular hypertrophy); the rhythm was atrial fibrillation (Figure 1).[1] Cardiac catheterization via the transbronchial route (involving endotracheal intubation, with the pressure-recording catheter inserted into the left atrium from the trachea) provided only the left-sided cardiac pressures (Table 1). These findings were interpreted as showing "predominant mitral regurgitation." The patient's blood hematocrit was 34%. During her 6-week hospitalization, she was placed on a low-salt diet, chlorothiazide, and acetazolamide, and she lost 40 pounds from her already cachectic frame.

In June 1962, she was readmitted because of similar symptoms and signs. Table I also shows the findings from right-sided and transseptal left-sided cardiac catheterization. The ^{85}Kr and indocyanine green dye curves showed predominant

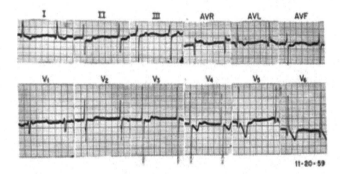

Figure 1 *Electrocardiogram of the patient at 41 years of age shows atrial fibrillation and excessive QRS voltage consistent with both right and left ventricular hypertrophy.*

Table 1: Cardiac hemodynamic values in the patient

Pressure Variable (mmHg)	December 1959	May 1962
Pulmonary artery	—	118/52
Right ventricle	—	118/52
Right atrium		
Mean	—	21
V wave	—	25
Right brachial artery	—	144/60
Femoral artery	150/70	—
Left atrium		
Mean	22	18
V wave	32	27

283

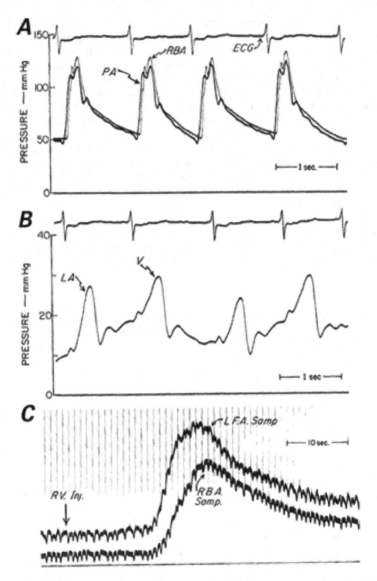

Figure 2 Diagrams show findings in June 1962, approximately one month before closure of the ductus. A) Simultaneous pressure tracings of the pulmonary artery (PA) and right brachial artery (RBA) show similar pressures in each vessel. B) Left atrial (LA) pressure tracing shows tall V waves. C) Drawing shows indocyanine green dye curves upon right ventricular injection (RV. Inj.) and sampling (Samp.) at simultaneous times in the left femoral artery (L.F.A.) and right brachial artery (R.B.A.).

ECG = electrocardiogram

left-to-right shunting (Figure 2). The catheter was passed from the aorta into the major pulmonary arteries through a PDA, which a chest radiograph showed to contain calcific deposits. The patient's right brachial and femoral arterial oxygen saturations were 92% and 89%, respectively. After a course of diuretic therapy, her peripheral edema and ascites completely resolved. In July 1962, the PDA was closed via the surgical placement of a Teflon patch at the aortic entrance of the PDA, with use of extracorporeal circulation during the procedure.[2] Postoperative bleeding necessitated the evacuation of a left hemothorax the next day, at which time the right and left ventricular peak systolic pressures were 105 and 80 mmHg, respectively. Hypotension and renal, hepatic, respiratory, and cerebral failure developed thereafter, and the patient died 7 days after the PDA closure operation. (This patient would not have been a candidate for PDA closure today.)

At necropsy, the heart weighed approximately 520 g. The PDA was 1.5 cm in diameter, and its wall was heavily calcified. All 4 cardiac chambers were dilated and had thicker walls than normal: both the right and left ventricular free walls were approximately 1.3 cm thick. The left atrium was dilated much more than the right atrium. The pulmonary trunk and main right and left pulmonary arteries were very dilated.

Figure 3 shows the locations of calcific deposits in several structures: sprinkled within the mural left atrial endocardium, focal within the mitral and aortic valves (with more in the aortic cusps than in the mitral cusps), and in the mitral annular area behind the posterior mitral leaflet.

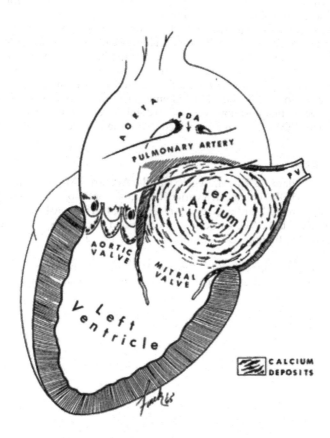

Figure 3 Diagram shows locations of calcific deposits in the patent ductus arteriosus (PDA), mitral valve, aortic valve, and left atrial endocardium.

DISCUSSION

This case is unusual in several aspects. The PDA had been confused with valvular disease for more than 4 decades. The patient's first cardiac catheterization, in 1959, was via the transbronchial route and yielded pressures only in the left side of the heart; these data did not enable a diagnosis of PDA but were consistent with the admitting diagnosis of mitral regurgitation. The right-sided pressures were not determined until 2 years later, and at that time no echocardiography was available for making estimates. The wall of the PDA was heavily calcified at the time of diagnosis, when the patient was 44 years of age. Although the peak systolic pressures were similar in the major pulmonary arteries and in the brachial artery, the shunting through the PDA was overwhelmingly from left to right. Nevertheless, the heart failure was mainly right-sided. The method of closing the calcified PDA was new at the time: inserting a Teflon patch over the aortic entrance into the PDA, with use of extracorporeal circulation.[2] Finally, calcific deposits in the left atrial wall and in the leaflets of the mitral and aortic valves have not to our knowledge been reported previously in patients with PDA.

The reason for the deposits in the left atrial endocardium and in the mitral and aortic valves is unclear. The phenomenon might be explained by the massive volume overload on the left side of the heart—caused by the left-to-right shunting through the PDA—while much smaller volumes of blood passed through the right side of the heart. The increased volume and therefore increased work of the left side of the heart might have caused rapid aging, such that the condition of that side more resembled typical findings in an 85-year-old patient than those expected in a 44-year-old. The calcific deposits in the left atrial endocardium might have resulted in part from the considerable stretching of that chamber due to increased volume and pressure, and from the superimposed mitral regurgitation. In patients with mitral stenosis, calcific deposits have been seen in the left atrial endocardium when a thrombus has organized into calcific plaques; however, this patient never had evidence of left atrial thrombus.[3] Her PDA was heavily calcified, a finding in older patients with a large PDA.

REFERENCES

1. Roberts WC, Filardo G, Ko JM, Siegel RJ, Dollar AL, Ross EM, Shirani J. Comparison of total 12-lead QRS voltage in a variety of cardiac conditions and its usefulness in predicting increased cardiac mass. *Am J Cardiol* 2013;112(6):904–909.
2. Morrow AG, Clark WD. Closure of the calcified patent ductus. A new operative method utilizing cardiopulmonary bypass. *J Thorac Cardiovasc Surg* 1966;51(4):534–538.
3. Roberts WC, Humphries JO, Morrow AG. Giant right atrium in rheumatic mitral stenosis. Atrial enlargement restricted by mural calcification. *Am Heart J* 1970;79(1):28–35.

Case 1686 Full Development of Consequences of Congenital Pulmonic Stenosis in Eighty-Four Years

William C. Roberts, MD*, Paul A. Grayburn, MD, Joseph
M. Guileyardo, MD and Robert C. Stoler, MD

Described herein is an 84-year-old woman, the oldest reported, with severe pulmonic stenosis who underwent a highly successful pulmonic valvotomy at age 77 and highly unsuccessfully attempted percutaneous pulmonic valve implantation at age 84. During the 84 years she developed nearly all clinical and morphologic consequences of pulmonic stenosis, including heavy calcification of the pulmonic valve, heavy calcification of the tricuspid valve annulus, severe right ventricular wall thickening without ventricular cavity dilation, aneurysm of the pulmonary truck, multiple focal ventricular wall scars without narrowing of the epicardial coronary arteries, wall thickening and luminal narrowing of the intramural coronary arteries, and extremely low 12-lead QRS electrocardiographic voltage.

In the January 2010 issue of the *Baylor University Medical Center Proceeding*, Ayad et al[1] reported a 77-year-old woman with severe congenital pulmonic stenosis (PS) successfully treated with percutaneous balloon valvotomy.[1] The peak systolic transpulmonic gradient was reduced from 114 to 25 mm Hg. The authors indicated that their patient was the oldest at that time to undergo percutaneous balloon pulmonic valvuloplasty. The present report was prompted to provide a 7-year follow-up on their patient, and to describe several full-blown morphologic consequences of this congenital valvular anomaly.

CASE DESCRIPTION

An 84-year-old white woman had been asymptomatic until about age 70 when she initially noted exertional dyspnea and fatigue and they progressively worsened. In her 20s she had had 3 sons without difficulties. At age 77, cardiac catheterization (June 2009) disclosed the following pressures in mm Hg: pulmonic artery, 23/5; right ventricle, 133/16; left ventricle, 150/12; and pulmonary artery wedge mean, 4. Selective angiography disclosed normal epicardial coronary arteries. The left ventricular ejection fraction was 60%. Both ventricular cavities were of normal size. Pulmonic valvuloplasty reduced the peak transvalvular pulmonic gradient by 78%. Her symptoms improved considerably by the procedure until age 83 when exertional dyspnea with minimal exertion and leg edema reappeared. Electrocardiogram (Figure 1) showed right bundle branch block (QRS width 0.146 mm), sinus rhythm

From the Baylor Heart and Vascular Institute, the Departments of Internal Medicine (Division of Cardiology) and Pathology, Baylor University Medical Center, Dallas, Texas. Manuscript received November 29, 2016; revised manuscript received and accepted November 29, 2016.

See page 1287 for disclosure information.

* Corresponding author: Tel: (214) 820–7911; fax: (214) 820–7533.

E-mail address: william.roberts1@bswhealth.org (W.C. Roberts).

DOI: 10.1201/9781003409342-50

(63 beats/min), and a total 12-lead QRS voltage of 78 mm (standard 10-mm voltage). Echocardiogram (August 2016) disclosed a 50 mm Hg peak and a 25 mm Hg mean transpulmonic valve gradient. Moderate pulmonic value regurgitation was also present (Figure 2). Computed tomographic angiogram disclosed a heavily calcified pulmonic valve and aneurysmal dilatation of the pulmonic trunk.

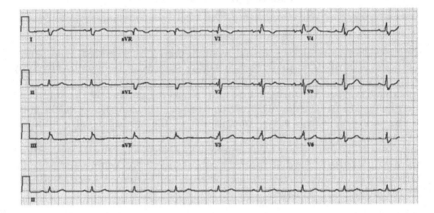

Figure 1 Electrocardiogram recorded 2 weeks before the attempted percutaneous pulmonic valve implantation. It shows sinus bradycardia (53 beats/min) and right bundle branch block (QRS duration 156 ms). An earlier electrocardiogram showed occasional ventricular premature complexes.

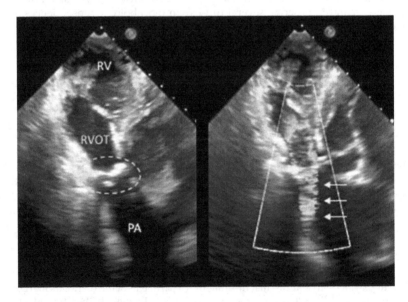

Figure 2 Deep transgastric right ventricular outflow views showing the heavily calcified pulmonic valves at end-systole (*left panel, yellow oval*) and the color Doppler jet of pulmonic stenosis (*right panel, with arrows*). PA = pulmonary artery; RV = right ventricular cavity; RVOT = right ventricular outflow track.

In August 2016, she underwent pulmonic valve balloon angioplasty using a 22 mm × 4 cm Z-Med balloon. An attempt was made to place a #23 Sapien S3 valve across the pulmonic valve but the procedure was unsuccessful because the substitute valve could not be moved from the right ventricular inflow to the pulmonic valve position. The patient became progressively more hypoxic from sudden development of right-to-left shunting at the atrial level, probably because of severe tricuspid valve regurgitation due to the bulk of the valve implantation equipment in the tricuspid valve orifice. An Amplatzer 24-mm balloon was successfully inflated across a patent foramen ovale and the right-to-left shunting was eliminated. Nevertheless, hypoxia persisted and electrical activity ceased. The Sapien S3 valve was then successfully implanted into the nonbeating heart in the pulmonic valve position. Resuscitation efforts, however, were unsuccessful.

Necropsy disclosed the heart to weigh 385 g (Figures 3 and 4). Both ventricular cavities were extremely small and their walls quite thick. Multiple focal scars were present in the right ventricular free wall and were fewer in the ventricular septum and left ventricular free wall (Figure 4). The pulmonic valve was heavily calcified as was a large portion of the tricuspid valve annulus (Figure 4). The epicardial coronary arteries were widely patent. Histologic examination of the walls of the ventricles disclosed many intramural coronary arteries with thick walls and narrowed lumens. A valvular-competent patent foramen was present. Focal calcified deposits were present in the descending thoracic and abdominal aorta.

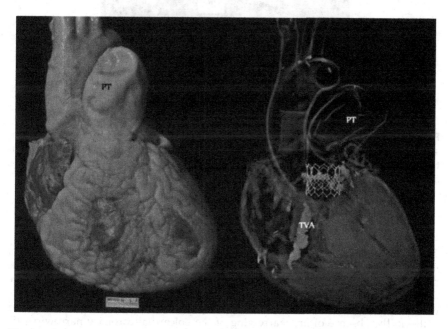

Figure 3 Anterior view of the heart (*left*) and radiograph of the heart at autopsy (*right*). The PT is aneurysmal. The quantity of subepicardial tissue is excessive. The x-ray shows the bioprosthesis in the pulmonic valve position and heavy calcific deposits in the pulmonic valve. The TVA is heavily calcified. Focal calcific deposits are present in the epicardial coronary arteries but their lumens are wide open. PT = pulmonary trunk; TVA = tricuspid valve annulus.

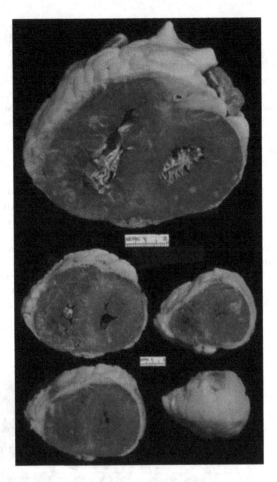

Figure 4 Photographs of the heart. (*Upper*) Basal portion showing numerous (non-subendocardial) scars in their right ventricular free wall and fewer scars in the ventricular septum and left ventricular free wall. (*Bottom*) Cross section of the ventricles caudal to the more basal portion. Note the minute sizes of the ventricular cavities.

DISCUSSION

The hitherto described patient illustrates the full development of complications of severe PS associated with intact ventricular septum: (1) heavy calcification of the pulmonic valve; (2) heavy calcification of the tricuspid valve annulus; (3) severe right ventricular wall thickening and the absence of ventricular cavity dilatation; (4) multiple focal ventricular wall scars—mainly involving the right ventricular wall—in the absence of any narrowing of the epicardial coronary narrowing; (5) the presence of wall thickening and luminal narrowing of many intramural coronary arteries in the ventricular walls; (6) aneurysmal dilatation of the pulmonary trunk; (7) the incredibly low 12-lead QRS voltage on the electrocardiogram; (8) the difficulty in implanting a bioprosthesis via the percutaneous route in the face of severe thickening of the right ventricular free wall and the extremely small right ventricular cavity; and (9) the lack of a right-to-left atrial shunt despite the presence of a valvular-competent patent foramen ovale until the attempted insertion of a bio-prosthesis into the pulmonic valve position.

Heavy calcific deposits in stenotic pulmonic valves have been recognized to occur for over 50 years.[2, 3] The deposits are never present at birth and occur only in adults with a considerable degree of PS. The older the patient with PS, the greater the likelihood of calcific deposits in the valve.

Although it is well appreciated that calcified deposits are common in the mitral annulus in patients with aortic stenosis, their presence in the tricuspid valve annulus in patients with severe PS, as occurred in the present patient, is unappreciated.[4]

The degree of right ventricular and ventricular septal thickening and its effects on the right ventricular cavity size is probably inadequately appreciated in these patients. The right ventricular wall may become thicker than the left ventricular free wall and the contribution of the right ventricular portion of the ventricular septum may result in the septum's being thicker than the left ventricular free wall and that situation occurred in the present patient. The present patient, however, not only had right ventricular pressure elevation but also left ventricular systolic pressure elevation, the latter consequence of systemic hypertension.

Focal scars in the right ventricular free wall in the absence of narrowing of the epicardial coronary arteries was described initially by Shirani et al[5] in 1993. Their luminal narrowing may well be responsible for the focal right ventricular scars in these patients. Thus, congenital PS joins the list of causes of abnormalities of the intramural coronary arteries: amyloidosis, hypertrophic cardiomyopathy, and the neurogenic heart diseases (Friedreich's ataxia, myotonia congenita, and Duchenne muscular dystrophy).

Aneurysmal dilatation of the pulmonary trunk in patients with PS is uncommon. Tami and McElderry[6] described a single patient and summarized findings in 3 previously reported patients. The 4 patients ranged in age from 24 to 57 years, the pulmonary trunk had a diameter of 5.5 to 6.8 cm, and the 3 patients had high (52 to 150 mm Hg) transvalvular peak systolic pressure gradients. The media in the pulmonary trunk was not described. In the present case, histologic study of the pulmonary trunk disclosed marked disorganization of the medial elastic fibers and thinning of the media.

Electrocardiographic abnormalities are present in all adults with moderate to severe PS: some evidence of right ventricular hypertrophy, atrial and/or ventricular arrhythmias, and, right bundle branch block. Examination of total 12-lead QRS voltage has proved to be the best electrocardiographic evidence of left ventricular hypertrophy.[7] Its usefulness in patients with right ventricular hypertrophy unassociated with left ventricular hypertrophy is unclear. In the present patient, total 12-lead QRS voltage was only 78 mm, an astoundingly low voltage in a patient with both right and left ventricular hypertrophy. Its explanation is unclear.

Pulmonic valve replacement for isolated PS by either the surgical or percutaneous routes has proved in general to be quite beneficial.[8, 9] Such procedures, to our knowledge, have not been attempted previously in a patient as old as ours, namely 84 years. The attempt to put the bioprosthesis in the pulmonic valve position in our patient was unsuccessful and led to acute tricuspid valve regurgitation and sudden development of arterial oxygen desaturation because of a right-to-left shunt through the valvular-competent patent foramen ovale. With sudden onset of tricuspid regurgitation, cardiac arrest occurred. The bioprosthesis was then successfully placed in the pulmonic valve position but the heart was not beating at the time of its manipulation through the small right ventricular cavity. In retrospect, a repeat pulmonic valvuloplasty alone would probably have been satisfactory.

Shunting at the atrial level is fairly common, of course, in patients with isolated PS. Roberts et al[10] in 1980 reported 127 patients with PS with intact ventricular septum treated by valvotomy: 95 (75%) had no shunt at the atrial level and 30 (14%) had an interatrial shunt detected preoperationally by dye-dilution curves. In 19 of the 30 patients, the atrial shunt was right-to-left and the defect was simply a patent foramen ovale; in the other 11 patients, the shunt was left-to-right and these patients had a true fossa ovalis atrial septal defect. The peak pressure gradient across the pulmonic valve was much higher in the group with a patent foramen ovale than in the group with a true atrial septal defect (120 ± 11 vs 60 ± 5 mm Hg). Shunning at the atrial level in the present patient never occurred until acute tricuspid regurgitation from the valve replacement equipment in the tricuspid valve orifice led to the sudden appearance of a right-to-left shunt through the previous valvular-competent patent foramen ovale.

DISCLOSURE

The authors have no conflicts of interest to disclose.

REFERENCES

1. Ayad RF, Johnston SB, Grayburn PA, Schmidt TT, Choi JW. Congenital pulmonic stenosis in a 77-year-old woman successfully treated with percutaneous balloon valvuloplasty. *Proc (Bayl Univ Med Cent)* 2010;23:21–23.
2. Roberts WC, Mason DT, Morrow AC, Braunwald E. Calcific pulmonic stenosis. *Circulation* 1968;37:973–978.
3. Covarrubias EA, Sheikh MU, Isner JM, Gomes M, Hufnagel CA, Roberts WC. Calcific pulmonic stenosis in adulthood. Treatment by valve replacement (porcine xenograft) with postoperative hemodynamic evaluation. *Chest* 1979;75:399–402.
4. Roberts WC, Vowels TJ, Filardo G, Ko JM, Mathur RP, Shirani J. Natural history of unoperated aortic stenosis during a 50-year period of cardiac valve replacement. *Am J Cardiol* 2013;112:541–553.
5. Shirani J, Zafari AM, Roberts WC. Sudden death, right ventricle infarction, and abnormal right ventricular intramural coronary arteries in isolated congenital valvular pulmonic stenosis. *Am J Cardiol* 1993;72:367–370.
6. Tami LF, McElderry MW. Pulmonary artery aneurysm due to severe congenital pulmonic stenosis: Case report and literature review. *Angiology* 1994;45:383–390.
7. Roberts WC, Filardo G, Ko JM, Siegel RJ, Dollar AL, Ross EM, Shirani J. Comparison of total 12-lead QRS voltage in a variety of cardiac conditions and its usefulness in predicting increased cardiac mass. *Am J Cardiol* 2013;112:904–909.
8. Blalock A. The surgical treatment of congenital pulmonic stenosis. *Ann Surg* 1946;124:879–888.
9. Coberly L, Harrison JK, Bashore TM. Percutaneous balloon pulmonic valvuloplasty following treated endocarditis in a patient with congenital pulmonary valve stenosis. *Cathet Cardiovasc Diagn* 1990;21:245–247.
10. Roberts WC, Shemin RJ, Kent KM. Frequency and direction of interatrial shunting in valvular pulmonic stenosis with intact ventricular septum and without left ventricular inflow or outflow obstruction. An analysis of 127 patients treated by valvotomy. *Am Heart J* 1980;99:142–148.

Case 1697 Combined Atresia of One Left-Sided and One Right-Sided Cardiac Valve in a Premature Newborn

William C. Roberts, MD, Alan C. Sing, MD and Joseph M. Guileyardo, MD

Described herein is the heart of a 2-day-old newborn, the product of a 25-week gestation, with atresia of two cardiac valves, one on the right side and one on the left side, apparently a previously undescribed entity.

The worst heart disease—the one allowing the shortest survival—is aortic valve atresia, the most common cause of death in the first month of life.[1,2] About 25% of these newborns with aortic valve atresia also have mitral valve atresia. The second most common condition associated with an atretic cardiac valve is pulmonic valve atresia. The occurrence of one right-sided atretic valve and one left-sided atretic valve in the same heart must be incredibly rare, but such was the case in the newborn described herein.

CASE DESCRIPTION

A 2-day-old female newborn after a 25-week gestation weighed 550 g. An electrocardiogram shortly after birth disclosed a prolonged P-R interval and sinus bradycardia. A technically difficult echocardiogram disclosed a dilated right ventricle, a normal-sized left ventricle, a large atrial septal defect with bidirectional flow, a large ventricular septal defect with bidirectional flow, a small (1 mm) patent ductus arteriosus with left-to-right flow, severe "pulmonic stenosis," and an unobstructed aortic valve and aortic arch. The echocardiographic findings were interpreted as being consistent with tetralogy of Fallot.

The newborn died in the intensive care unit on the second day of life. At necropsy, the heart weighed 4.15 g. The cardiac findings are illustrated in the *Figure*. Both the mitral and pulmonic valves were atretic, the atrial septum was absent, and a ventricular septal defect was located caudal to the aortic valve, which arose from the dilated right ventricle. A narrowed patent ductus was present, and it was the only source of blood to the lungs.

In addition to the cardiac anomalies, a cleft lip was present, and it extended to involve the entire hard and soft palate. Cytogenetic SNP microarray analysis performed on an ante-mortem blood sample disclosed a normal female chromosome pattern with no deletions or duplications of known or potential clinical significance. Postmortem chromosome analysis also showed a normal female 46 XX karyotype.

From the Baylor Heart and Vascular Institute (Roberts) and the Departments of Pathology (Roberts, Guileyardo) and Internal Medicine (Division of Cardiology) (Roberts), Baylor University Medical Center at Dallas; and the Department of Pediatric Cardiology, Texas Health Presbyterian Hospital, Dallas, Texas (Sing).

Corresponding author: William C. Roberts, MD, Baylor Heart and Vascular Institute, 621 N. Hall Street, Suite H-030, Dallas, TX 75226 (e-mail: William.Roberts1@bswhealth.org).

DOI: 10.1201/9781003409342-51

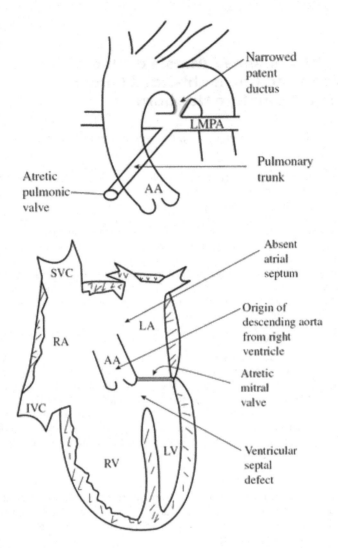

Figure Cardiac findings of a premature newborn with combined pulmonic and mitral valve atresia. AA indicates ascending aorta; IVC, inferior vena cava; LA, left atrium; LMPA, left main pulmonary artery; LV, left ventricle; RA, right atrium; RV, right ventricle; SVC, superior vena cava.

No numerical or structural aberrations were seen at the 500 G-band resolution. Examination of the placenta disclosed a three-vessel cord, premature villous architecture, severe acute chorioamnionitis, and mild acute funisitis.

DISCUSSION

Our patient had combined pulmonic and mitral valve atresia. Such a combination, to our knowledge, has not been reported previously. Death was probably the consequence of progressive narrowing of the ductus arteriosus.

REFERENCES

1. Roberts WC, Perry LW, Chandra RS, Myers GE, Shapiro SR, Scott LP. Aortic valve atresia: A new classification based on necropsy study of 73 cases. *Am J Cardiol* 1976;37(5):753–756.
2. Perry LW, Scott LP III, Shapiro SR, Chandra RS, Roberts WC. Atresia of the aortic valve with ventricular septal defect: A clinicopathologic study of four newborns. *Chest* 1977;72(6):757–761.

Case 1766 Huge Right Ventricular Outflow Tract Aneurysm Late Following Total Repair of Tetralogy of Fallot Leading to Orthotopic Heart Transplantation

William C. Roberts[1,2,3,] and Shaffin Siddiqui[1,#]*

1. INTRODUCTION

Operative correction of patients with tetralogy of Fallot (T of F) has been one of the seminal developments in medicine in the last century. Many such patients as a consequence have had entirely normal life spans compared to patients without operative intervention whose mean span is 5 years.[1] Despite these phenomenal operative results, some of the operative survivors develop debilitating right-sided heart failure, arrhythmias, right-ventricular outflow tract (RVOT) patch aneurysms, and other forms of cardiac dysfunction. We describe herein 3 men who developed huge RVOT aneurysms, a relatively infrequently described consequence of the corrective operation for patients with T of F, and right-sided heart failure; simultaneously, 2 of them developed refractory ventricular tachycardia (VT). All 3 patients subsequently underwent orthotopic heart transplantation (OHT).

1.1. Patients Studied

Findings in the 3 men are summarized in Table 1. Each had successful OHT 35, 43, and 59 years, respectively, after the corrective operation at ages 6, 4, and 6 years, respectively. Two developed recurring episodes of VT, one of whom had multiple ventricular ablations without preventing the VT. All 3 had evidence of right-sided heart failure, worse in the patient without VT. The RVOT patch in all 3 patients was parietal pericardium. Follow-up after OHT (11 years in case #1; 7 years in case #2;

[1] *Baylor Scott & White Heart and Vascular Institute, Baylor Scott & White Health, Dallas, Texas, USA*

[2] *Department of Internal Medicine (Cardiology), Baylor Scott & White Health, Dallas, Texas, USA*

[3] *Department of Pathology, Baylor University Medical Center, Baylor Scott & White Health, Dallas, Texas, USA*

Article history:

Received 2 February 2021, Revised 24 February 2021, Accepted 25 February 2021, © 2021 Elsevier Inc. All rights reserved.

Declaration of competing interest: The authors declare that they have no known competing financial interests or personal relationships that could have appeared to influence the work reported in this paper.

* Corresponding author.

E-mail address: william.roberts1@bswhealth.org (W.C. Roberts).

Shaffin Siddiqui, Junior, Princeton University, Princeton, New Jersey.

DOI: 10.1201/9781003409342-52

and 5 months in case #3) disclosed that all 3 patients were asymptomatic and quite active.

Table 1: Comparison of findings in the 3 men having cardiac transplantation decades after total repair of tetralogy of Fallot.

Variable	Case 1*	Case 2**	Case 3
Age (years)			
At repair of tetralogy of Fallot	6	4	6
When RV outflow tract aneurysm first noted	26	33	60
At onset of heart failure	26	33	60
At onset of ventricular tachycardia	26	33	No VT
At orthotopic heart transplantation	41	47	65
At January 2021) ****	51	54	65
Patch = Parietal pericardium	+	+	+
RV outflow patch calcified	+++	+	+++
Body mass index (kg/m²)	29 →25(OHT) →33	32	29
Bundle branch block	+(Left)	+(Right)	+(Right)
Total 12-lead QRS voltage (mm)	156	71	84
Intracardiac defibrillator (age)	+(36)	+(33)	+(61)
Radiofrequency ablation	+	0	0
Pre-OHT Hemodynamics			
Left ventricle (s/d) (mm Hg)	95/30	—	—
Pulmonary artery (s/d) (mm Hg)	35/15	45/20	45/5
Right ventricle (s/d) (mm Hg)	45/20	45/10	45/5
Lowest LV ejection fraction (%)	10	50	20
Heart weight (g)	655	505	590
Cardiac adiposity (floating heart)	+	+	+
Coronary artery disease	0	0	0

LV= left ventricular; RV = right ventricular; s/d = peak systolic/end diastolic; OHT = orthotropic heart transplant.

* From George BA, Jong MK, Lensing FD, Kuiper JJ, Roberts WC. "Repaired" tetralogy of Fallot mimicking arrhythmogenic right ventricular cardiomyopathy. *Am J Cardiol* 2011;108:326–329.

** From Donaldson EE, Jong MK, Gonzales-Stawinski G, Hall SA, Roberts WC. Secondary arrhythmogenic right ventricular cardiomyopathy decades after operative repair of tetralogy of Fallot. *Am J Cardiol* 2014;114;806–809.

2. DISCUSSION

Each of the 3 patients described developed huge RVOT aneurysms involving the transannular patches decades after the operative correction of T of F. Calcific deposits developed in the parietal pericardial patches of all 3 patients, minimal in one and massive in 2. Confirmation of the presence of calcific deposits in the patches has been infrequent.[2-7] Calcific deposits in the patch can develop relatively early after its insertion. Seybold-Epting et al.[3] reported 10 patients among 252 patients with corrected T of F who had a parietal pericardium RVOT patch inserted, and 4 of them were confirmed to have developed microscopic-sized patch calcific deposits 6 to 36 months after the operation. This time span is too short to recognize patch calcific deposits by imaging studies or grossly. In contrast, the patients of this study accumulated the calcific deposits over the course of 35, 43, and 59 years. Ross et al.[8] reported a 16-year-old boy who developed massive calcific deposits in a parietal pericardial RVOT patch within 7 years after its insertion.

Two of the 3 patients described had recurring VT, uncontrolled by either multiple antiarrhythmic agents or repeated ablation procedures. One of the 2 patients with VT had classic epsilon waves on the electrocardiogram, characteristic of arrhythmogenic right ventricular cardiomyopathy.

The occurrence of OHT after repair of T of F is an uncommon event (Table 2). Each of the 3 patients described herein returned to normal activities after their OHT. All 3 are asymptomatic as of January 2021.

A previously unreported finding in patients with repaired T of F is excessive cardiac adipose tissue. The hearts in all 3 patients described herein floated in a container of formaldehyde indicating excessive cardiac adipose tissue (adipose tissue is lighter than myocardium). The fat surrounding the left ventricle was especially extensive, an unusual feature. All 3 patients were overweight.

This manuscript, of course, has limitations: 1) Only 3 cases are described but OHT is, as Table 2 demonstrates, uncommon after total "correction" of T of F. Few other studies, however, have had such long intervals between the corrective operation and the OHT. 2) Although all 3 patients had huge RVOT aneurysms and right-sided heart failure, 2 patients had recurring VT prior to OHT (Figures 1–3).

Table 2: Previous publications of patients having repair for tetralogy of Fallot (T of F) with insertion of right ventricular outflow tract (RVOT) patch with follow-up thereafter.

First author (reference)	Publication year	Patients with T of F	Patients receiving RVOT patch	Material of patch	Age (years) at total repair of T of F range (mean ± SD) [median]	Duration of follow-up (years) range (mean ± SD) [median]	Patients developing patch aneurysm	Patients developing VT	Patients having OHT
Payne[9]	1961	58	26	Ivalon	—	0.75-4 (1.9)	3	—	—
			6	Ivalon-Teflon	—	0.66-2 (1.3)	0	—	—
			26	Teflon	—	0.5-1.5 (0.6)	0	—	—
Rosenthal[10]	1972	—	135	Pericardial	—	—(0.5)	8	—	—
Kaplan[11]	1973	150	54	Pericardial	0-26	0.5-14	16	—	—
			13	Homograft	0-26	0.5-14	1	—	—
Rieker[12]	1975	60		Teflon	4-20	—	0	—	—
Chiariello[2]	1975	403	144	Pericardial	0.25-41	—(1.25)	7	—	0
Seybold-Epting[3]	1977	252	252	Pericardial	—	0.5-3	10	—	—
Fuster[6]	1980	396	—	Ivalon or Teflon	0-54	12-22	3	1	0
Kirklin[13]	1989	791	255	Dacron	—[5]	>2-20 (9 ± 5)	2	—	0
Nollert[14]	1993	490	—	—	—(12 ± 9)	1.06-35 (25 ± 13)	—	0	0
Knot-Craig[15]	1997	193	—	—	—(2 ± 0.2)	0.1-26 (11 ± 7)	—	—	—
Nørgaard[16]	1999	109	60	Dacron or Pericardial	—[13]	20-28 (26)	—	—	1
Gatzoulis[17]	2000	793	274	274	—(8 ± 8) [6]	8-41 (21 ± 9)	—	33	0

Troost[18]	2007	68	—	—	—[24]	1.3–18 (— ± 8)	—	3
Munkhammar[19]	2013	31	—	—	—[0.8]	2–16 (9 ± 3)	—	0	0
Kotani[20]	2013	41	11	Dacron	0.5–3.5 (0.9)	—[5.9]	—	0	0
Cuypers[21]	2014	80	48	—	1.7–6.6 (4.3)	31–43	—	26	0
Galicia-Tornell[22]	2015	52	52	Dacron	—(4 ± 2)	—(6 ± 2)	0	0	0
Dłuzniewska[23]	2018	83	54	—	0–30 [3]	—(30)	—	13	0
Simon[24]	2019	38	27	—	—(3.3 ± 1)	19.5–35.8 (30.9)	—	15	—
Castilhos[25]	2019	206	65	—	2–4 [3]	—(21 ± 8.2)	—	15	0
Padalino[26]	2019	720	435	Pericardial or homograft	3.7–11.7 (5.7)	1–21	—	—	0
TOTALS		5014	1937 (2.58%)				50 (0.03%)*	103 (0.06%)*	4 (0.002%)*

OHT = orthotopic heart transplant; VT = ventricular tachycardia; — = no information available.
* These percentages are out of the number of patients with RVOT patch (1,937 patients).

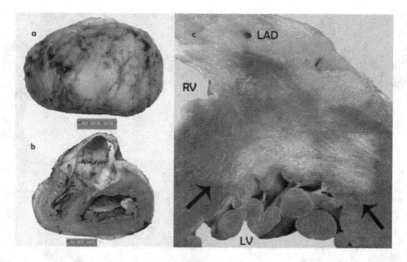

Figure 1 Case #1. The heart. (a) Outside of the heart showing a huge quantity of adipose tissue covering both ventricles. (b) Opened right ventricle showing the huge aneurysm in the outflow tract. (c) Anterior wall of the left ventricle showing a healed ablation site, consisting of fibrous tissue and adipose tissue. The coronary arteries are free of plaque. The ablation had been performed 20 years earlier. LAD = left anterior descending; LV = left ventricular cavity; RV = right ventricular cavity.

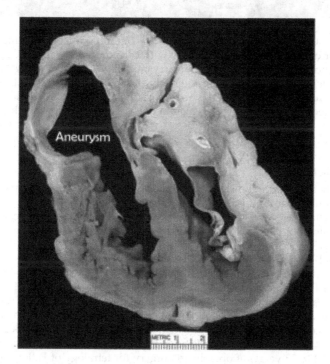

Figure 2 Case #2. Opened right ventricle showing the huge aneurysm in the outflow tract. Both ventricles are nearly covered by adipose tissue. The coronary arteries are wide open.

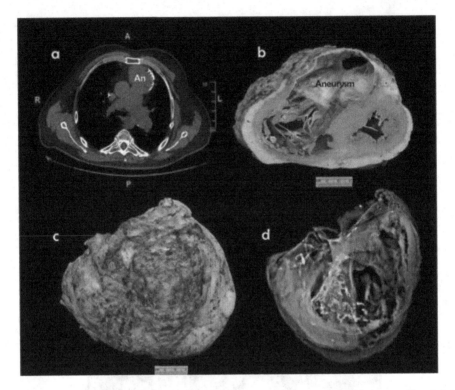

Figure 3 Case #3. Heart. (*a*) Computed tomographic image showing the right ventricular outflow tract aneurysm (An) with calcium in its wall. (*b*) Opened right ventricle showing the outflow tract aneurysm. Adipose tissue nearly covers both ventricles. (*c*) Outside of the heart anteriorly showing the portion of the right ventricle that had been attached to the undersurface of the sternum. (*d*) Radiograph of the explanted heart displaying the calcium present in the outflow patch.

REFERENCES

1. Campbell M. Natural history of cyanotic malformations and comparison of all common cardiac malformations. *Br Heart J* 1972;34:3–8.
2. Chiariello L, Meyer J, Wukasch DC, Hallman GL, Cooley DA. Intracardiac repair of tetralogy of Fallot. Five-year review of 403 patients. *J Thorac Cardiovasc Surg* 1975;70:529–535.
3. Seybold-Epting W, Chiariello L, Hallman GL, Cooley DA. Aneurysm of pericardial right ventricular outflow tract patches. *Ann Thorac Surg* 1977;24:237–240.
4. Kirklin JW, Bargeron LM, Pacifico AD. The enlargement of small pulmonary arteries by preliminary palliative operations. *Circ* 1977;56:612–617.
5. Arciniegas E, Farooki ZQ, Hakimi M, Perry BL, Green EW. Early and late results of total correction of tetralogy of Fallot. *J Thorac Cardiovasc Surg* 1980;80:770–778.
6. Fuster V, McGoon DC, Kennedy MA, Ritter DG, Kirklin JW. Long-term evaluation (12 to 22 years) of open heart surgery for tetralogy of Fallot. *Am J Cardiol* 1980;46:635–642.

7. Lane I, Treasure T, Leijala M, Shinebourne E, Lincoln C. Diminutive pulmonary artery growth following right ventricular outflow tract enlargement. *Int J Cardiol* 1983;3:175–185.

8. Ross EM, McIntosh CL, Roberts WC, Massive calcification of a right ventricular outflow parietal pericardial patch in tetralogy of Fallot. *Am J Cardiol* 1984;54:691–692.

9. Payne WS, Kirklin JW. Late complications after plastic reconstruction of outflow tract in tetralogy of Fallot. *Ann Surg* 1961;154:53–57.

10. Rosenthal A, Gross RE, Pasternac A. Aneurysms of right ventricular outflow patches. *J Thorac Cardiovasc Surg* 1972;63:735–740.

11. Kaplan S, Helmsworth JA, McKinivan CE, Benzing G, Schwartz DC, Schreiber JT. The fate of reconstruction of the right ventricular outflow tract. *J Thorac Cardiovasc Surg* 1973;66:361–374.

12. Rieker R, Berman M, Stansel HC. Postoperative studies in patients with tetralogy of Fallot. *Ann Thorac Surg* 1975;19:17–26.

13. Kirklin JK, Kirklin JW, Blackstone EH, Milano A, Pacifico AD. Effect of transannular patching on outcome after repair of tetralogy of Fallot. *Ann Thorac Surg* 1989;48:783–791.

14. Nollert G, Fischlein T, Bouterwek S, Böhmer C, Klinner W, Reichart B. Long-term survival in patients with repair of tetralogy of Fallot: 36-year follow-up of 490 survivors of the first year after surgical repair. *JACC* 1997;30:1374–1383.

15. Knott-Craig CJ, Elkins RC, Lane MM, Holz J, McCue C, Ward KE. A 26-year experience with surgical management of tetralogy of Fallot: Risk analysis for mortality or late reintervention. *Ann Thorac Surg* 1998;66:506–511.

16. Nørgaard MA, Lauridsen P, Helvind M, Pettersson G. Twenty-to-thirty-seven-year follow-up after repair for tetralogy of Fallot. *Eur J Cardiothorac Surg* 1999;16:125–130.

17. Gatzoulis MA, Balaji S, Webber SA, Siu SC, Hokanson JS, Poile C, et al. Risk factors for arrhythmia and sudden cardiac death late after repair of tetralogy of Fallot: A multicentre study. *Lancet* 20;356:975–981.

18. Troost E, Meyns B, Daenen W, Van de Werf F, Gewillig M, Van Deyk K, et al. Homograft survival after tetralogy of Fallot repair: Determinants of accelerated homograft degeneration. *Eur Heart J* 2007;28:2503–2509.

19. Munkhammar P, Carlsson M, Arheden H, Pesonen E. Restrictive right ventricular physiology after tetralogy of Fallot repair is associated with fibrosis of the right ventricular outflow tract visualized on cardiac magnetic resonance imaging. *Eur Heart Jl—Cardio Imag* 2013;14:978–985.

20. Kotani Y, Chetan D, Ono N, Mertens LL, Caldarone CA, Van Arsdell GS, et al. Late functional outcomes after repair of tetralogy of Fallot with atrioventricular septal defect: A double case-match control study. *J Thorac Cardiovasc Surg* 2013;145:1477–1484.

21. Cuypers JA, Menting ME, Konings EE, Opic P, Utens EM, Helbing WA, et al. Unnatural history of tetralogy of Fallot: Prospective follow-up of 40 years after surgical correction. *Circ* 2014;130:1944–1953.

22. Galicia-Tornell M, Reyes-López A, Ruíz-González S, Bolio-Cerdán A, González-Ojeda A, Fuentes-Orozco C. Treatment of Fallot tetralogy with a transannular patch. Six years follow-up. *Cir* 2015;83:478–484.

23. Dłuzniewska N, Podolec P, Skubera M, Smas-Suska M, Pajak J, Urbanczyk-Zawadzka M, et al. Long-term follow-up in adults after tetralogy of Fallot repair. *Cardiovasc Ultrasound* 2018;16:28.

24. Simon BV, Subramanian S, Swartz MF, Wang H, Atallah-Yunes N, Alfieris GM. Serial follow-up of two surgical strategies for the repair of tetralogy of Fallot. *Semin Thorac Cardiovasc Surg* 2019;31:515–523.

25. de Castilhos GM, Ley ALG, Daudt NS, Horowitz ESK, Leiria TLL. Routine detection of atrial fibrillation/flutter predicts a worse outcome in a cohort of tetralogy of Fallot patients during 23 years of follow-up. *Pediatr Cardiol* 2019;40:1009–1016.

26. Padalino MA, Pradegan N, Azzolina D, Galletti L, Pace Napoleone C, Agati S, et al. The role of primary surgical repair technique on late outcomes of tetralogy of Fallot: A multicentre study. *Eur J Cardiothorac Surg* 2020;57:565–573.

Index

Note: Page numbers in *italics* indicate a figure and page numbers in **bold** indicate a table on the corresponding page.

Printed in the United States
by Baker & Taylor Publisher Services